MW00835265

Groupthink in Science

David M. Allen • James W. Howell
Editors

Groupthink in Science

Greed, Pathological Altruism, Ideology, Competition, and Culture

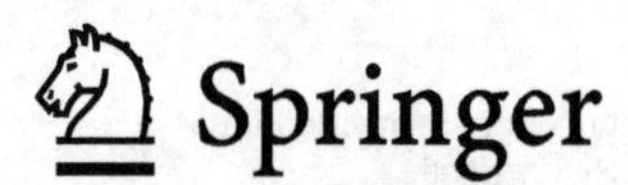

Editors
David M. Allen
Department of Psychiatry
University of Tennessee Health
Science Center
Memphis, TN, USA

James W. Howell
Department of Psychiatry
University of Tennessee Health
Science Center
Memphis, TN, USA

ISBN 978-3-030-36821-0 ISBN 978-3-030-36822-7 (eBook)
https://doi.org/10.1007/978-3-030-36822-7

This Springer imprint is published by the registered company Springer Nature Switzerland AG
The registered company address is: Gewerbestrasse 11, 6330 Cham, Switzerland

This book is dedicated to
S. Hossein Fatemi, MD, PHD,
a true scientist, physician, and friend.
Professor, Department of Psychiatry
Medical School
University of Minnesota

Acknowledgments

We, the editors, owe a debt of gratitude to E.O. Wilson, Gregg Henriques, and Jonathan Haidt for their pioneering work on groupthink and the evolution of logic in human beings.

We would like to thank the production team at Springer, including Lilith Dorko and Arun Pandian.

We would like to thank our wives, Harriet Allen and Marcia Coesta Chia, for their unwavering support and understanding.

We would like to thank Barbara Oakley for initiating this project as a follow-up to her book, *Pathological Altruism*, and for suggesting several of our chapter authors.

Additionally, we would like to thank the following for their assistance and support:

Harrison Ambrose, III
Sonny Anand
James R. Barr
Meegan Barrett-Adair
Kathy Brooks
George Casaday
Maggie Debon
Harry and Dee Rinehart
S. Hossein Fatemi
Carol Hardy
Casonja Harris
Detlef Heck
Linda Heffner
Golden Leon Howell
Hank Herrod
Charles Hicks
David Howard
Carol Jacks

Jannae Jacks
Kathie Kirkpatrick
Wayne Kuenzel
Sagman Kayatekin
Queen Titilé A. Keskessa
Sam Leonard
John Lienhard
Scott O. Lilienfeld
Robert and Ellen McGowan
Mark Muesse
Dick Nesbitt
Walter Pagel
John Richardson
Linda Hefner Richardson
Dee Rinehart
Bob Sasser
Minè Teague
Barbara Tharp
Ari van Tienhoven
Fran Tylavsky
Henning Willeke
Robert W. Williams
Don Young
Yueuing (Angela) Zhang

Contents

Contributors

David M. Allen Department of Psychiatry, University of Tennessee Health Science Center, Memphis, TN, USA

Augustine Brannigan University of Calgary, Calgary, AB, Canada

Loretta Breuning Inner Mammal Institute, California State University, East Bay, Hayward, CA, USA

Curt Dudley-Marling Lynch School of Education, Boston College, Chestnut Hill, MA, USA

David C. Geary Department of Psychological Sciences, Interdisciplinary Neuroscience Program, University of Missouri, Columbia, MO, USA

Bradley Harris Rhodes College, Memphis, TN, USA

Paul Harris Southern College of Optometry, Memphis, TN, USA

Gregg Henriques Department of Graduate Psychology, James Madison University, Harrisonburg, VA, USA

James W. Howell Department of Psychiatry, University of Tennessee Health Science Center, Memphis, TN, USA

Jay F. Kirkpatrick The Sience and Conservation Center, Billings, MT, USA

Joel Lexchin School of Health Policy and Management, Faculty of Health, York University, Toronto, ON, Canada

Brian Martin Humanities and Social Inquiry, University of Wollongong, Wollongong, NSW, Australia

Florencia Peña Saint Martin Graduate Program of Physical Antrhopology, National School of Anthropology and History, Mexico City, Mexico

John M. Norwood Medicine-Infectious Disease, University of Tennessee College of Medicine, Memphis, TN, USA

Cailin O'Connor Logic and Philosophy of Science, University of California Irvine, Irvine, CA, USA

Andrew C. Papanicolaou The University of Tennessee, College of Medicine, Knoxville, TN, USA

David R. Penberthy Virginia Radiation Oncology Associates, Richmond, VA, USA

J. Kim Penberthy University of Virginia School of Medicine, Charlottesville, VA, USA

Nicole Prause Liberos LLC, Los Angeles, CA, USA

Elizabeth A. Reedy Penn State University, College of Nursing, University Park, Abington, PA, USA

David B. Resnik National Institute for Environmental Health Sciences, National Institutes of Health, Bethesda, MD, USA

Nestar Russell University of Calgary, Calgary, AB, Canada

Elizabeth Schriner Division of Quality of Life (QoLA), St. Jude Children's Research Hospital, Memphis, TN, USA

Elise M. Smith National Institute of Environmental Health Sciences, Durham, NC, USA

Gijsbert Stoet Department of Psychology, University of Essex, Colchester, Essex, UK

John W. Turner Jr. Department of Physiology & Pharmacology, University of Toledo College of Medicine, Toledo, OH, USA

Ah Young Wah Regional One Health – East Campus, Memphis, TN, USA

James Owen Weatherall Logic and Philosophy of Science, University of California, Irvine, Irvine, CA, USA

D. J. Williams Social Work, & Criminology, Idaho State University, Pocatello, ID, USA

Center for Positive Sexuality (Los Angeles), Los Angeles, CA, USA

Abbreviations

AAVE	African-American Vernacular English
AML	Appropriate Management Level
BIT	Behavioral Investment Theory
BLM	Bureau of Land Management
CMS	Centers for Medicare & Medicaid Services
DNC	Maryland Department of Natural Resources
DOI	Digital Object Identifier
EPA	Environmental Protection Agency
FIIS	Fire Island National Seashore
HEI	Higher Education Institutions
HMA	Herd Management Areas
JH	Justification Hypothesis
KOL	Key Opinion Leader
NIST	National Institute of Standards and Technology
NPS	National Park Service
RSVI	Relational Value/Social Influence
USDA	United States Department of Agriculture

Groupthink in Science: An Introduction

One of the hottest topics in science today is concern over certain problematic practices within the scientific enterprise. Richard Horton (2015), editor of the respected medical journal *The Lancet*, recently summarized some of the issues involved: studies with small sample sizes, tiny effects, invalid exploratory analyses, and flagrant conflicts of interest, together with an obsession for pursuing fashionable trends of dubious importance. *Groupthink in Science* will elucidate in depth a widespread phenomenon that is often at the heart of this—problematic aspects of the psychology and behavior of people in groups.

Now of course, the fact that this book acknowledges that science can be done in problematic ways is not in any way an indictment of science per se. When it works well, science is by far the best way to discover accurate information about how the universe works and to gain objective knowledge. We are huge proponents of the scientific method. However, we do not buy in to the proposition that scientists are beyond reproach. In fact, this book is meant to *advance* the cause of science, not to attack science.

Groupthink is when a group of people, in an effort to demonstrate harmony and unity, fail to consider alternative perspectives and ultimately engage in deeply problematic decision-making. Haidt (2012) points out that if we focus on behavior in groups of people who know each other and share goals and values, "our ability to work together, divide labor, help each other, and function as a team is so all-pervasive that we don't even notice it" (p.198). He adds that "Words are inadequate to describe the emotion aroused by prolonged movement in unison that drilling involved" (p.221). "It doesn't mean that we are mindless or unconditional team players; it means [we] are selective" (p.223). However, groupthink may lead to a great deal of bias when the psychological drive for consensus is so strong that any divergence from that consensus is ignored or rejected.

In scientific research, groupthink may lead researchers to reject innovative or controversial ideas, hypotheses, or methodologies that challenge the status quo. Philosophers, historians, and sociologists have observed that scientists often resist new ideas, despite their reputation for open-mindedness (Barber, 1961; Kuhn, 1962). The great quantum physicist Max Planck has been quoted as saying: "A new scientific truth does not triumph by convincing its opponents and making them see the light, but rather because its opponents eventually die, and a new generation grows up that is familiar with it" (Planck, 1962:33–34).

In his seminal work on the history of science, *The Structure of Scientific Revolutions*, Kuhn described the role of conformity and close-mindedness in scientific advancement. According to Kuhn (1962), science progresses through different stages. In the first stage, known as normal science, scientists conduct their research within a paradigm that defines the field. A paradigm is a way of doing science that includes basic assumptions, beliefs, principles, theories, methods, and epistemic values that establish how one solves problems within the normal science tradition; normal science involves consensus within a scientific community. For example, Newtonian physics was a normal science tradition that established ways of solving problems related to motion and electromagnetic radiation (Kuhn, 1962).

During the normal science stage, scientists attempt to apply the paradigm to problems they can solve and resist certain theories, methods, and ideas that challenge the paradigm. At this stage, scientists tend to think within the theoretical limits of the paradigm, limiting novel ideas. However, as problems emerge that cannot be solved within the paradigm, scientists start to consider new ideas, theories, and methods that form the basis of a new and emerging paradigm. A scientific revolution occurs when the new paradigm replaces the old. For example, during the early twentieth century, Newtonian physics succumbed to quantum mechanics and relativity theory (Kuhn, 1962). However, a paradigm shift is not a purely rational process driven by logical argumentation and empirical evidence; rather, it involves a change in perception or a willingness to see the world in a different way (Kuhn, 1962). After the revolution, a new paradigm takes hold and the process once again starts to repeat itself.

Some philosophers have argued that a certain amount of closed-mindedness, known as epistemological conservatism, is justified in scientific research. The rationale for this epistemological stance is that change in a network of beliefs should be based on substantial empirical evidence. Since changes in beliefs can consume a considerable amount of time and effort and our cognitive resources are limited, we should not change our beliefs, especially ones that play a central role in our worldview, without compelling evidence (Lycan, 1988; Quine, 1961; Resnik, 1994; Sklar, 1975). For example, because Einstein's general theory of relativity contradicted the fundamental principle of Newtonian physics that space and time are immutable, it took an extraordinary proof—i.e., that observation of the sun's gravity bending light from a star during a solar eclipse in 1919—to confirm the theory (Buchen, 2009). While it seems clear that a certain amount of conservatism makes sense in research, scientists should be careful to avoid dogmatism. Although scientists should practice a degree a skepticism pertaining to hypotheses and theories that challenge the status quo, they should be open to new ideas (Resnik, 1994).

So, despite idealization by some students and practitioners, scientists are of course human beings and as such are subject to anything that can adversely affect the thinking of all human beings. In particular, scientists are not immune from acting in the interests of the groups to which they belong, be they financial, bureaucratic, political, or ideological. They can lie to others and even to themselves, engage in fraudulent practices, design studies in ways that lead to predetermined and preordained outcomes, draw conclusions based on false a priori assumptions that are never acknowledged, act together as a mob, or shun other scientists who have evidence for viewpoints which are at odds with their own. They can be bought off by profiteering industries.

Human beings also are highly prone to forming hierarchies, as well as cults of personality, in which leaders can then be lionized and followed like sheep unthinkingly. This is particularly true in universities and organizations which fund research, where the funding of projects and the publication of data can be subject to the arbitrary whims of the department heads or of well-thought-of, fully tenured professors at the expense of those lower down on the academic totem pole. Academic politics is widely known to be a cutthroat competition in which members of a department jockey and maneuver for influence with the powers that be.

The tendency of human beings to form hierarchies has an evolutionary advantage as described by Loretta Breuning in Chap. 1. Unfortunately in some instances, it has an impactful downside. People at the top of the hierarchy may let the power of the position go to their heads in a sense, especially if they have narcissistic tendencies to begin with due to their own individual upbringing. David Robson, in his book *The Intelligence Trap: Why Smart People Make Dumb Mistakes* (2019), looks at the problem from the perspective of people with relatively high intelligence do stupid things. Two processes stand out:

Earned dogmatism: Our self-perception of expertise can lead to a feeling that we have gained the right to be closed-minded and to ignore other points of view. We see this too often among established professionals who think that their accepted success level gives a deserved weight to their words, ideas, and opinions. This is especially true if the person has made a lot of money (in any field) or is the recipient of accolades and awards.

Entrenchment: A high-ranking expert's ideas often become rigid and fixed. When accepted by others lower in status, as is often the case, such ideas can become the foundation of the group's ideology and, effectively, become a "fashion" in a particular field of science. This usually includes a belief held by many simply because they have reached a certain "level of expertise" within a community and the benefits of following the leader's beliefs become entrenched.

Robson also points out how the most effective leaders in science benefit from being at least somewhat humble. One needs this in order to best interact with and consider the opinions of other people. Considering alternative views helps us all to avoid dogmatic thinking. Too often, outside arguments against ideas held by groupthink and defended by blind bias can be stifling to anyone who has the effrontery to challenge those ideas. In fields like medicine, this can sometimes have a literally fatal effect.

One of the most deadly examples of this was the experience of Dr. Sunny Anand when he was in his last year in medical school at Oxford University (Paul, 2008). Dr. Anand's ambition was to work with premature babies. He worked with these preemies in the nursery at the hospital in his spare time. After a while, he noticed that when babies were taken away for surgery, some of them came back to the nursery blue and some did not come back at all.

Of course, he became concerned about this, but at the time, he was a mere senior medical student and he did not know if he could find out what caused this problem. Finally, he went to the head of the nursery and asked if he could go to the operating room with one or two of these babies to see what was happening. He found that the babies were being operated upon without the benefit of anesthesia.

The reason given was that there was a consensus, not only at this hospital but pretty much around the world, that newborns did not feel pain and thus they were not exposed to the possible negative effects of anesthesia. The babies were going into shock and many did not survive.

Another reason that academics can also reject important truths is due to political correctness concerns. This is easiest to see in the social sciences and humanities, where professors are thought to be far more progressive than the general public. Their conclusions are often labeled as "left-leaning." Their approach to "free speech" on university campuses is ironically associated with repressive actions that actually suppress free speech (Beinhart, 2017). This process seems to have become more extreme in recent years on college campuses, where groups sometimes turn even on their own members for not exhibiting the proper orthodoxy (Lukianoff & Haidt, 2018).

The problem is not, however, limited to the social sciences and the humanities. In the hard sciences, scientific education may operate as a kind of indoctrination that privileges certain theories or methods and leads to selective perception and validation of evidence. A symposium at the Wellcome Trust in London in association with the Academy of Medical Sciences in 2015 reviewed a growing failure in the reliability and reproducibility of biomedical research suggestive of this sort of bias. The situation was attributed variously to "data dredging" to impose expectations on the data; the non-publication of negative results; the use of small, unreliable samples; underspecified methods; and weak research designs—all of which make it difficult to reject the null hypothesis (which means that there is no significant difference between two specific populations and that any observed difference is due to sampling or experimental error).

Another symposium—"Is Science Broken?"—was held at University College London by experimental psychologists and came to similar conclusions (Woolston, 2015). It acknowledged widespread "p-hacking" to arbitrarily rerun quantitative models in search of the statistical significance of pet theories and the cherry picking of conclusions favorable to the proponents' perspective.

These problems can sometimes create setbacks for entire fields for significant periods of time. In psychology, for example, one of the biggest deceptions perpetrated on the American public has been the idea that "self-esteem" is the key to success and self-improvement (Lilienfeld, Lynn, Ruscio, & Beyerstein, 2010). We were told that if we just improved the self-esteem of students and other individuals in this country, everyone would be happier and more successful. This idea has been carried on to this day in many sectors of mental health and is still supported by a large number of professionals despite a multitude of studies exposing the concept as useless. There is a major difference between self-esteem and self-confidence. Psychology has also become increasingly aware of failures by independent experimentalists to replicate allegedly robust discoveries (Baker, 2015).

The reliability of much of the neuroscience literature is also questionable, usually because of the small sample sizes used. With some of her colleagues, Dr. Katherine S. Button, now of Bath University, reviewed the statistical power of a large spectrum of the neuroscience literature (Button et al., 2013). They found the statistical power to be quite low at approximately 20 %. This makes it almost impossible to make a statement about any effects being studied.

In 2010, Ivan Oransky and Adam Marcus created a web site, *retractionwatch.com*, to record the public repudiation and retraction of refereed publications, not only in social sciences but in every sort of refereed scientific publication. In both the London venues, the chief supposition of participants was that the crisis in contemporary science in these diverse areas is more the failure of unconscious biases and regrettable (but not deliberate) sloppy methods and procedures—the sorts of things predicted by Kuhn's normal science. This does not rule out cases of scientific misconduct based on outright fabrication of data for career advancement. This does occur and is more likely to be unearthed through whistle-blowers than through failures to replicate or the peer-review process (Stroebe, Postmes & Spears, 2012). However, this is not usually created by groupthink.

When researchers and academic administrators sacrifice any modicum of scientific objectivity, and perhaps even their own ethical standards, in their behavior in order to support a particular group's interests, or that of group's leaders, doing so not only impedes scientific progress for the rest of us but can backfire and adversely affect the interests of the group to which a scientist belongs. Problems with the science that are never addressed often begin to show up and become very intense, negatively affecting group processes. In addition, other scientists from competing groups who are pushing more accurate ideas tend to eventually prevail, and the first group can suffer a precipitous fall from grace.

Oakley (2012) deemed this aspect of the behavior of systems—the process in which individuals who sacrifice themselves for the good of a group eventually cause harm to their group—*pathological altruism*. Of course, such behavior is altruistic only toward their in-group, not toward outsiders. We are particularly interested in how established leaders in a field often block the work of challengers for real or proffered reasons of "doing the right thing" or "helping others."

Many of the problems in science created by processes that often occur during groupthink have been highly exacerbated in recent decades due to several developments:

1. The increasing industrialization of all academic endeavors.
2. Research quality has been slowly giving way to excessive quantity, as several peer-reviewed publications per year are required for promotion and tenure—and even continued employment—at universities and professional schools.
3. The increasing emphasis on production and on attracting funding that gives universities more and more the appearance of businesses and scientists more and more that of merchants.

4. The proliferation of professional journals that must attract research papers or perish.
5. The increasingly loud siren calls of travel around the world's resorts for the presentation of "new" scientific facts and theories by the same conferees two to five times in a single year.

Group allegiances can cause adverse effects on science at every stage of the scientific process. As mentioned, researchers pick statistical tests based on how they want their research to come out and in their journal articles do not write about the assumptions that they are making which, if clarified, might lead readers to be highly skeptical of their conclusions. Certain journals are ranked higher than others, often on the basis of a past history which may no longer be valid, and findings published in "lesser" journals can be ignored. Peer reviewers for both journal editorial panels and grant review panels may subconsciously favor papers and proposals which are in line with their theoretical and professional group prejudices. Editors of journals can reject articles even when well-reviewed. Newspapers and television news show may highlight findings that are sensational without balancing the implications of their headlines with important caveats.

An understanding of this process is a major contribution by those who advocate for *systems thinking* (Senge, 1990). Systems thinking is a holistic approach to analyzing how events and processes that are often distant in time and space interrelate with each other in ways that are not often obvious but lead to various outcomes. The constituent parts within any one "system" also function within the context of larger systems.

The objective of the book is to educate scientists, health professionals, political advocacy groups, and interested members of the general public about these issues and to suggest solutions to help minimize the propagation of questionable science.

The book starts with a discussion of the evolutionary and cultural origins of group processes and then looks in detail at a wide variety of manifestations in science today of "going along with the crowd" that are adopted at the expense of the truth. It describes the many techniques scientists can employ to bias their research in order to further the interests of an "in-group" and through which others are unwittingly induced to go along. In order for ourselves to avoid maladaptive groupthink, we include in this volume chapter authors who have a wide variety of differing and sometimes opposing political viewpoints.

University of Tennessee Health Science Center David M. Allen
Memphis, TN, USA

The University of Tennessee Health Science Center James W. Howell
Memphis, TN, USA

References

Baker, M. (2015, August 27). Over half of psychology studies fail reproducibility test. *Nature*. https://doi.org/10.1038/nature.2015.18248.

Barber, B. (1961). Resistance by scientists to scientific discovery. *Science, 134*(3479), 596–602.

Beinhart, P. (2017). A violent attack on free speech at Middlebury. *The Atlantic*, March 6 online. https://www.theatlantic.com/politics/archive/2017/03/middlebury-freespeech-violence/518667/. Retrieved 3 November 2017.

Buchen, L. (2009, May 29). May 29, 1919: A major eclipse, relatively speaking. *Wired*. Available at: https://www.wired.com/2009/05/dayintech_0529/. Accessed: 17 April 2017.

Button, K. S., Ioannidis, J. P. A., Mokrysz, C., Nosek, B. A., Flint, J., Robinson, E. S. J., et al. (2013). Power failure: Why small sample size undermines the reliability of neuroscience. *Nature Reviews Neuroscience, 14*(5), 365–376. https://doi.org/10.1038/nrn3475.

Haidt, J. (2012). *The Righteous Mind: Why Good People Are Divided by Politics and Religion*. New York: Pantheon.

Horton, R. (2015, April 11). *Offline: What is medicine's 5 sigma?* www.thelancet.com Vol 385.

Kuhn, T. S. (1962). *The Structure of Scientific Revolutions*. Chicago: University of Chicago Press.

Lilienfeld, S. O., Lynn, S. J., Ruscio, J., & Beyerstein, B. L. (2010). *50 Great Myths of Popular Psychology: Shattering Widespread Misconceptions about Human Behavior*. Hoboken, NJ: Wiley Blackwell.

Lukianoff, G., & Haidt, J. (2018). *The Coddling of the American Mind: How Good Intentions and Bad Ideas Are Setting Up a Generation for Failure*. New York: Penguin Press.

Lycan, W. G. (1988). *Judgment and Justification*. Cambridge, UK: Cambridge University Press.

Oakley, B., Knafo, A., Madhavan, G., & Wilson, D. S. (Eds.). (2012). *Pathological Altruism*. Cambridge: Oxford University Press.

Paul, A.M. (2008, February 10). The first ache. *New York Times Magazine*. https://www.nytimes.com/2008/02/10/magazine/10Fetal-t.html

Planck, M. (1962). *Quoted in Kuhn TS. 1962. The Structure of Scientific Revolutions* (pp. 33–34). Chicago, IL: University of Chicago Press.

Quine, W. V. (1961). *From a Logical Point of View*. New York: Harper and Rowe.

Resnik, D. B. (1994). Methodological conservatism and social epistemology. *International Studies in the Philosophy of Science, 8*(3), 247–264. New York: W.W. Norton.

Robson, D. (2019). *The Intelligence Trap: Why Smart People Make Dumb Mistakes*. New York: W.W. Norton.

Senge, P. (1990). *The Fifth Discipline: The Art & Practice of the Learning Organization*. New York: Doubleday Business.

Sklar, L. (1975). Methodological conservatism. *Philosophical Review, 84*(3), 374–400.

Stroebe, W., Postmes, T., & Spears, R. (2012). Scientific Misconduct and the Myth of Self-Correction in Science. *Perspectives on Psychological Science, 7*(6), 670–688.

Woolston, C. (2015). *Is Science Broken?* Symposium held at University College London.

Part I
Introduction: Definition, Manifestations, and Theoretical Issues

Chapter 1
The Neurochemistry of Science Bias

Loretta Breuning

Dr. Ignaz Semmelweis was shunned by the nineteenth-century medical establishment for telling doctors to wash their hands. His belief in invisible disease-causing agents was ridiculed by his peers. We hope this could not happen today because the scientific method keeps us focused on replicable data. But Semmelweis's critics likewise perceived themselves as defenders of evidence-based science (Nuland, 2003). They invoked the greater good in their dismissal of his findings. How is it possible for people intent on objectivity to dismiss essential information?

Two familiar answers are *confirmation bias* and *paradigm shift,* but neither explains it entirely. Confirmation bias is incomplete because it typically omits the investigator's own bias. For example, Semmelweis's critics could accuse him of confirmation bias without acknowledging their own biases. Paradigm shift is incomplete because it does not explain how a brain actively rejects information without conscious awareness.

Brain chemistry offers a new way to understand information-processing biases. Brain chemicals cause positive feelings about one chunk of information and negative feelings about another (Damasio, 1994). Feelings are presumed irrelevant to empirical analysis, but they are highly relevant to the brain's constant extraction of meaning from an overload of inputs. The neurochemicals of emotion are easily overlooked because they do not report themselves to the verbal brain in words. Their absence from our verbal inner dialog leads to the presumption that we are not influenced by them. The impact of emotion on empirical inferences is often more observable in others. The ability to recognize our own neurochemical responses to information is a valuable scientific tool. This paper explains these responses in animals, which illuminate their nonverbal motivating power in humans. Some examples of this motivating power are drawn from modern social science.

L. Breuning (✉)
Inner Mammal Institute, California State University, East Bay, Hayward, CA, USA
e-mail: Loretta@InnerMammalInstitute.org

D. M. Allen, J. W. Howell (eds.), *Groupthink in Science*,
https://doi.org/10.1007/978-3-030-36822-7_1

Nature's Operating System

The reward chemicals and threat chemicals in humans are inherited from earlier mammals. These chemicals evolved to promote survival, not to make a person feel good all the time. Each chemical has a specific survival job that is observable in animals. Here is a simple introduction to the natural function of three reward chemicals (dopamine, oxytocin, and serotonin) and the threat chemical, cortisol. (This discussion will be somewhat oversimplified for heuristic purposes, because the various neurotransmitters often regulate one another in various complex feedback loops, making the overall picture somewhat more complicated.)

The operating system we share with animals motivates survival behavior by releasing a chemical that feels good when it sees something good for its survival, and a chemical that feels bad when it sees something bad for its survival. The human brain differs from other animals of course. The differences get a lot of attention, particularly our large cortex, so it is useful to review the similarities. Our neurochemicals are controlled by brain structures common to all mammals, including the amygdala, hippocampus, hypothalamus, and pituitary. This core operating system does not process language, yet it has allowed mammals to make complex survival decisions for 200 million years. It works by tagging inputs as reward or pain, which motivates approach or avoidance. A pleasant-feeling chemical motivates an organism to go toward a reward, while an unpleasant-feeling chemical motivates withdrawal from potential threats (Ledoux, 1998).

Humans define survival with the aid of a large cortical capacity to store, retrieve, and match patterns in information inputs. But we make these patterns meaningful by responding to them with a chemical that says, "this is good for me" or "this is bad for me" (Gigerenzer, 2008).

Natural selection built a brain that defines survival in a quirky way. It cares about the survival of its genes, and it relies on neural pathways built in youth. Anything relevant to the survival of your genes triggers a big neurochemical response. Neurons connect when the chemicals flow, so old rewards and threats build the neural pathways that alert us to new potential rewards and threats. This happens throughout life, but the pathways connected in youth become myelinated, which allows electricity to flow through them almost effortlessly. This is why old responses feel reliable, even when they conflict with new knowledge. And it is why our positive and negative neurochemistry is so poorly explained by our conscious verbal thoughts about survival (Kahneman, 2013).

The electricity in the brain flows like water in a storm, finding the paths of least resistance. The cortex can define rewards and pain in complex ways with its huge reserve of neurons, but it can only process a limited amount of new information at a time. Thus, we are heavily influenced by the pathways we already have. We are not consciously aware of these pathways, so we tend to overlook their influence over our thought process and presume that our declarative reasoning is the whole story (Ledoux, 2002).

No one consciously sifts new inputs through an old filter, but this is how the brain is equipped to make sense of its information environment. We have 10 times more neurons going from the visual cortex to the eyes than we have in the other direction (Pinker, 1997). This means we are 10 times more prepared to tell our eyes what to look for than we are to process whatever happens to come along. Our ancestors survived because they could prompt their senses to find information relevant to their survival. Neurochemicals are central to the prompting mechanism. The mammalian brain evolved to honor its neurochemical signals as if its life depended on it, not to casually disregard them. Here is a closer look at some chemicals of reward (dopamine, oxytocin, and serotonin) and pain (cortisol) and their role in our inferences about the empirical world.

Dopamine

The brain releases dopamine when a reward is at hand. A person may think they are indifferent to rewards because they do not respond to rewards that others value. But each brain scans the world with pathways built from its own past dopamine experiences. When it sees an opportunity to meet a need, dopamine produces a great feeling. This motivates us to do things that trigger it, and to lose interest in things that do not trigger it (Schultz, 1998).

Dopamine releases the energy that propels a body toward rewards. We humans experience this as excitement, but the physical sensation makes more sense when viewed from an animal perspective. A lion cannot get excited about every gazelle that crosses its path because its energy would be used up before it found something it could actually catch. A lion survives by scanning the world for a reward it realistically expects based on past experience. When a lion sees a gazelle within its reach, dopamine! That releases the energy needed for the hunt. Most chases fail, so a lion's brain constantly reevaluates its course of action. If it succeeds at closing in on the gazelle, dopamine surges, which tells the body to release the reserve tank of energy.

We are designed to survive by reserving our energy for good prospects, and dopamine guides these decisions. Our hunter-gatherer ancestors scanned for evidence of food before investing energy in one path or another. A modern scientist meets needs in different ways, but the same operating system is at work.The good feeling of dopamine motivates us to approach rewards, as defined by the neural pathways we have.

Dopamine is metabolized in a few minutes, alas, and you have to do more to get more. This is why we keep scanning the world for new opportunities to meet our needs. The brain habituates quickly to old rewards, so it takes new reward cues to turn on the dopamine (Schultz, 2015). When berries are in season, they stop triggering dopamine in a short time because they no longer meet a need. Then, protein opportunities turn on the good feeling, until nuts are in season. Dopamine focuses our attention on unmet needs by making it feel good. Today's scientists seek new discoveries because they stimulate dopamine.

Social rewards are as relevant to a mammal's survival as material rewards. Once physical needs are met, social needs get the brain's attention. The brain makes predictions about which behaviors will bring social rewards in the same way that it predicts which path is likely to lead to a berry tree: by relying on the neural pathways built by past experience (Cheney & Seyfarth, 2008). One may believe they are indifferent to social rewards, but anything that brought social rewards in your past sends electricity to your dopamine, which motivates an approach.

The brain defines social rewards in ways that are not obvious to one's verbal inner dialog. Mammals are born helpless and vulnerable, and thus need reliable attachments to survive. They evolved a survival strategy based on safety in numbers. To the mammal brain, isolation is a survival threat and social alliances are a valuable reward. Alliances with kin are especially rewarding to the brain built by natural selection (Wilson, 1975). (More on this in the "Oxytocin" section below.)

Our mirror neurons activate when we see others get rewards (Iacoboni, 2009). This wires us to turn on the dopamine in ways we see work for others. Our brain promotes survival by observing the patterns of rewards and pain around us, which helps us create a better hunting tool or a better grant proposal.

Oxytocin

Social alliances promote survival, so natural selection built a brain that rewards you with a good feeling when you build social alliances. Oxytocin causes the feeling that humans call "trust" (Zak, 2013). Oxytocin is not meant to flow all the time because trusting every critter around you does not promote survival. The mammal brain evolved to make careful decisions about when to trust and when to withhold trust. It releases the good feeling of oxytocin when there is evidence of social support.

Safety in numbers is a mammalian innovation. Reptiles avoid their colleagues except during the act of mating, when they release an oxytocin-equivalent. Reptiles produce thousands of offspring and lose most of them to predators. Mammals can only produce a small number of offspring, so they must guard each one constantly in order to keep their genes alive. Oxytocin makes it feel good. It causes attachment in mother and child, and over time it builds pathways that transfer this attachment to a larger group.

A mammalian herd or pack or troop is an extended warning system. It allows each individual to relax a bit as the burden of vigilance is spread across many eyes and ears. This only works if you run when your herd mates run. Mammals who insisted on seeing a predator for themselves would have poor survival prospects. We are descended from individuals who trusted their herd mates. We humans are alert to the risks of herd behavior, of course. But when we distance ourselves from our social alliances, our oxytocin dips and we start to feel unsafe. Even predators feel unsafe without a pack: a lone lion's meal gets stolen by hyenas and a lone wolf cannot feed its children. We have inherited a brain that constantly monitors its social support.

But life with a pack is not all warm and fuzzy. Trust is hard to sustain in proximity to other brains focused on their own survival. And the social alliance that protects you today can embroil you in conflict tomorrow. Yet, mammals tend to stick to the group because the potential pain of external threats exceeds the potential pain of internal threats. Common enemies cement social bonds, and oxytocin makes it feel good. Each brain turns it on with the pathways of its unique individual oxytocin past. Each scientist recognizes the rewards of social alliances and potential threats to those alliances, whether they put it into words or not.

Serotonin

An uncomfortable fact of life is that stronger mammals tend to dominate weaker group-mates when food and mating opportunity are at stake. Violence is avoided because the brain anticipates pain and retreats when it sees itself in the weaker position. Yet, an organism must assert itself some of the time for its genes to survive. Serotonin makes it feel good. Serotonin is not aggression but the nice calm sense that you can meet your needs. When you see an opportunity to take the one-up position, your mammal brain rewards you with the good feeling of serotonin (Raleigh, McGuire, Brammer, Pollack, & Yuwiler, 1991). We can easily see this in others, even though we reframe it in ourselves.

The mammalian brain evolved to compare itself to others, and hold back if it is in the weaker position. Avoiding conflict with stronger individuals is more critical to survival than any one meal or mate. When a mammal sees itself in the stronger position, the safe feeling of serotonin is released. But it is metabolized in a few minutes, which is why the mammal brain keeps scanning for more opportunities to be in the one-up position (Palmer & Palmer, 2001). You may insist you do not compare yourself to others or enjoy a position of social importance. But if you filled a room with people who said that, they would soon form a hierarchy based on how much disinterest each person asserts. That is what mammals do, because each brain feels good when it advances its unique individual essence.

Cooperation is one way to gain a position of strength, and larger-brained mammals will cooperate when it meets their needs. They work together to advance their position in relation to common rivals, and serotonin is stimulated when they succeed (Breuning, 2015). The pursuit of social importance may threaten social alliances at times, but it strengthens social alliances at other times. Each brain is constantly weighing complex trade-offs in its path to survival.

Each serotonin spurt connects neurons that tell you how to get more in the future. The serotonin of your early years builds myelinated pathways that play a big role in your social navigation through life. These pathways generate expectations about which behaviors are likely to enhance social power and which behaviors might threaten it. Every researcher has expectations about which actions might bring respect or lose respect. One research outcome might trigger the expectation of social reward while another set of data might trigger social pain. It is easy to see why people go toward one slice of information and avoid another without conscious intent. And it is easy to ignore one's own efforts to compare favorably, even as we lament such efforts in others.

Cortisol

The mammalian brain releases the bad feeling of cortisol when it encounters a potential threat (Selye, 1956). Bad feelings promote survival by commanding attention. For example, a gazelle stops grazing when it smells a lion, even if it is still hungry. Cortisol motivates an organism to do what it takes to make the bad feeling stop (Sapolsky, 1994).

Cortisol is the brain's pain signal, but waiting until one is in pain is not a good survival strategy. That is why the brain is so good at learning from pain. Each cortisol surge connects neurons that prepare a body to respond quickly to any input similar to those experienced in a moment of pain. The brain evolved to anticipate pain because your prospects fall quickly once a lion's jaws are on your neck.

Social pain triggers cortisol. In the state of nature, social isolation is an urgent survival threat. Cortisol makes a gazelle feel bad when it wanders away from the herd, even when it is enjoying greener pastures. Cortisol creates alarm in a monkey who experiences a loss of social status because that is a threat to the monkey's genetic survival prospects. Conscious concern for one's genes or one's status is not needed to get the cortisol flowing. Natural selection built a brain that warns you with a bad feeling when your prospects encounter a setback. You may try to ignore it, but if you do not act to relieve the perceived threat, the alarm is likely to escalate.

A big brain brings more horsepower to the task of identifying potential warning signals. Cortisol turns on when we see anything similar to neurons activated by past cortisol moments. It is not surprising that people are so good at finding potential threats, and so eager to relieve them. And it is easy to see how social threats can get our attention as much as we presume to disregard them.

The Survival Urge in Science

Scientists are presumed to be indifferent to social rewards and threats as they comb the world for empirical truths. But like all mammals, scientists can easily see the potential for rewards and threats in their information environment; and like other mammals, they respond neurochemically to this information.

For example, dopamine is released when a scientist sees an opportunity to step toward a reward. Oxytocin is released when scientists cooperate with peers. Serotonin is released when an investigator gets respect. Cortisol is released when a scientist sees an obstacle to rewards, cooperation, or respect. These responses are shaped by neural pathways built from unique individual life experience, but the urge to do things that relieve cortisol and stimulate happy chemicals is common to all brains.

While our responses depend on our individual pathways, those pathways overlap to the extent that the experiences creating them overlap. Science training is a common set of experiences that help to wire individuals with common responses. For example, professional training prepares an individual to invest enormous effort in a long series of tasks in anticipation of distant rewards (social and/or material). It prepares an individual to collaborate within a particular theoretical framework. And it builds circuits that confer respect in specific ways and expect to receive respect accordingly. In short, science training builds specific expectations about how to gain rewards, social trust, and respect, and thus stimulate dopamine, oxytocin, and serotonin.

Expectations about threat and cortisol relief are likewise shaped by professional training. The credentialing process of each discipline prepares the mind to recognize potential threats to the discipline and respond in a way that promotes the well-being of the discipline. This need not be said in words because expectations are real physical pathways in the brain. Scientists surge with cortisol when they see a potential threat to their discipline and their place within it, and like any mammal, they are motivated to do what it takes to relieve that cortisol.

Fortunately for the state of knowledge, a scientist can gain rewards, cooperation, respect, and threat relief through objective empirical analysis. But even if this works in the long run, it does not always work in the short run. Thus, every scientist can recognize opportunities to stimulate immediate positive neurochemistry in ways that violate the scientific method.

It would be easy to point accusing fingers here, given the universality of these responses. But our brains are already skilled at seeing bias in others. The challenge is to recognize these mammalian motivations in one's self. In that spirit, I present two empirical biases I discovered in my own life. Before that, let us return to the Semmelweis story, where short-run motivations prevailed and in the long run we're all dead.

The Survival Brain's Potential for Bias

The hand-washing Dr. Semmelweis was of course interested in his own survival. The colleagues who disdained him were too. Each brain defined survival with networks of associations built from past experience. Those networks make it easy to process inputs that fit, and thus to respond in ways that worked before.

In the state of nature, objectivity promotes survival. To find food and procreate, an animal must interpret cues realistically. However, an animal that looked at the world with fresh eyes each morning instead of relying on old pathways would starve, and be socially ostracized. Old neural pathways equip us to scan the overload of detail that surrounds us and zero in on cues relevant to meeting our needs.

In the natural world, rewards fit old patterns so often that old neural networks are an efficient way to find new rewards. Scientists learn the value of relying on old pathways through lived experience and formal training. Yet, we expect scientists to reject old interpretations instantly when they bias interpretations of new data. Alas the brain did not evolve to instantly discard old circuits. They are real physical changes in neurons that speed electricity to the on switch of reward chemicals and pain chemicals. Hence, it is not too surprising that Semmelweis's peers filtered the new message through their old lenses.

It would be easy to accuse them of greedy preoccupation with their own survival needs at the expense of others. But the germ theory of disease had not been established yet, so Semmelweis's allusion to invisible disease carriers was superstitious nonsense in the science paradigm of his day. Leading doctors claimed that the public needed protection from such dangerous misinformation (Nuland, 2003).

Curing a major killer of the day, "childbed fever" (septicemia), may seem like a huge reward, but without a perceived link between hand-washing and health, there is no expectation of that reward. Doctors could easily anticipate a threat to their respect and social alliances as a result of Semmelweis's findings. The consequent bad feeling would not be offset by the expected good feeling of rewards, leaving doctors with antipathy that they could explain with verbiage unrelated to their own neurochemistry.

One may wonder why Semmelweis persisted in isolation. His biography is full of clues. First, his closest associate died from "childbed fever" after cutting his finger during surgery. This rewired Semmelweis's view of the disease. People often fail to rewire their views in response to new information, but the bigger neurochemical surge, the more the rewiring. Losing a best friend so quickly with such a clear chain of evidence would easily do that.

Second, Semmelweis was not wired to trust the safety of the herd in the way that his peers were. Some people attain professional credentials by cooperating with mentors in their discipline, while others satisfy credentialing requirements by going their own way. Semmelweis had been rejected numerous times by the community of science in his formative years, so he was already wired to rely on his own perceptions by the time the natural experiment with septicemia occurred in his hospital. When he observed that mothers attended to by midwives did not die of the disease the way postoperative doctors did, he was ready to rely on his own survival responses instead of trusting the survival responses of the herd.

If we are angered by his colleagues' indifference to the facts, we must hold ourselves to the same standards. We must be willing to invest our own energy in new information that conflicts with shared expectations, even when it threatens our social support. Often we do not. Often I did not. Here are two examples.

I was trained in International Management at a time when Japanese methods were celebrated and American methods were disparaged. I was wired to effortlessly process information about the glories of Japanese management and the misguidedness of American management. Then one day in 1995, while lecturing to 150 students, I suddenly realized that Japan had been in a deep depression for 5 years. US productivity was booming, and I had not adjusted my rhetoric one bit. Why? It is easy to see the rewards and threat contingent on the new data. My survival was not really at stake because I was a tenured full professor. As hard as it is to admit, I was influenced by the threat that the new facts posed to my whole constellation of expected rewards. To state it more boldly, I feared social sanction. I might have continued to ignore the unwelcome truth if the terror of perceiving my bias midsentence on the stage of a large auditorium had not triggered enough cortisol to connect neurons to sear in the facts.

I was also trained to believe that children are better off in daycare. I put my children in daycare with the belief that "studies show" a neutral or even positive impact. Despite my pretensions to objectivity, I know that I cheered any data that fit my beliefs and disdained any data that did not. Now that the daycare generation is grown and there are causes for concern, I can see the many obstacles to new information. Anyone trained in the social sciences could easily see the potential rewards for findings consistent with the prevailing mindset and the potential threat of contradicting it. A researcher who stumbled on negative effects of daycare might fear reporting them. They could easily repeat the study with adjustments until they got results consistent with expected rewards. And if they did report anomalous findings, that information might get ignored by mass communication channels. They might also get ignored by the science community, leading to a lack of replication and a consensus that the findings are an aberration.

We can never have data on studies not performed, so we can never know the full extent of bias. But we can explore the extent of our own biases. I only noticed my bias on daycare because the survival stakes for my DNA triggered large cortisol surges. Yet, my accumulation of discrepant data over the years has fostered a willingness to notice biases in my own mindset – a paradigm shift on an individual level.

Science Bias Today

Though we aspire to objectivity, we end up seeing the world through the lens of old neural pathways. This lens is hard to notice because it is built from shared experience and thus overlaps with the lens of those around us. Consider, for example, the Rousseauian lens embedded in today's social science. Rousseau asserted that nature is good, and "our society" is the cause of that which is bad. A social scientist who finds evidence to support this presumption can expect rewards. The result is an accumulation of evidence that:

1. Animals are good (they cooperate and nurture each other)
2. Children are good (they grow to perfection automatically, unless miseducated by society)
3. Preindustrial people are/were good (in harmony with nature and each other)

A reader may think these assertions are indisputable facts because the effortless flow of electricity through well-developed pathways gives us a sense of truth. No one notices the neural network they built from repeated experience. No one accounts for their natural anticipation of rewards and pain as they process each new input. We can only have realistic information if researchers feel safe reporting what they find and we feel safe receiving it. Here are some simple examples of data being shaped to fit the Rousseauian framework, despite the shared presumption of objectivity.

1. Animals are naturally good Mountain lions are endangered in the hills around my hometown, and measures to protect them are in effect. Every effort is made to rehabilitate an injured mountain lion; but the animal cannot be returned to the wild when it recovers because it would be killed instantly by the lion that dominates the territory it is released into. This raises an uncomfortable problem. No one wants to admit that animals routinely kill intruders (Lorenz, 1966). "Only humans kill" is a widely shared belief, and a person is likely to get ostracized from a social alliance if they violate such a core belief. Just thinking of that risk is enough to trigger a neurochemical alarm that discourages a person from stating obvious facts. So animal rescuers struggle to do the necessary without acknowledging the reasons.

For most of human history, animal conflict was observed first hand. It is true that animals rarely kill their own kind, but that is because the weaker individual withdraws to save itself (Ardrey, 1966). Animals are at the edge of conflict a lot because asserting promotes their genes. Today's researchers "prove" that animals share and empathize by crafting "studies" that ignore all behaviors except that which supports the message of animal altruism (de Waal, 2010). Every researcher understands the reward structure, and no researcher wants to invalidate his or her prior investments of effort. Researchers believe they are motivated by the greater good rather than the urge to seek rewards and avoid pain because those words are part of the learned framework and people tend to believe their verbal explanations of their motives. If no one will risk reporting animal conflict, then we can say there is "no evidence" of animal conflict, and it will be true.

2. Children are naturally good Children flourish if left to their own impulses according to widely held beliefs in social science (Montessori, 1949). Any developmental problems that occur are quickly explained as a failure of "our society," and letting a child do what feels good is the widely embraced solution (Rousseau, 1762). Credentialed professionals point toward "proof" that fun is the core of learning, and they know they will be rebuked if they expect a child to do something unfun (Gatto, 2008). If the student has not learned, the teacher has not made it fun.

For most of human history, survival depended on children pulling their weight. Each child carried water, firewood, or a younger sibling, as parents deemed necessary, whether it felt good or not. Children looked for ways to make it fun, but adults did not substitute children's fun-meter for their own judgment. A young brain learned survival skills not by following its bliss but by being held accountable for essential tasks – often harshly. Experiencing the repetitive, backbreaking labor of one's parents (a challenging concept explained in Sect. 3 below) built core self-management skills such as focusing attention on steps that meet needs.

We have been trained to believe that children frolicked happily in the past. If you violate this shared presumption, it is hard to survive as a member in good standing of a social-science profession. Just taking a step toward information that violates a shared framework is difficult because one's neurochemical alarm signals the risk. It is not surprising that people step where rewards are expected, without consciously telling themselves that in words. The result may be more research on how to make things "fun," and more children who do not learn basic survival skills.

3. Preindustrial societies were/are good Traditional people only worked a few hours a day, according to social scientists, and spent the rest of their time making art, making love, and making their group-mates feel valued and understood (Pink, 2011). Research that enhances this paradigm gets recognition. Research that conflicts with it gets ignored, ridiculed, or attacked. This reward structure surrounds a researcher's choices about where to invest their energy.

The higher form of this paradigm offers higher rewards: the concept that traditional people never worked at all, because work is what you have to do, and early humans could survive by doing only what felt good (Diamond, 1987). Researchers can support this assertion with inferences about the time period before recorded history but after the separation between humans and apes – the time when no data are available except that produced by social science itself. Evidence is also easy to generate by defining the labor of prehistory as "creativity" or "fun." Of course, foraging feels good when you are hungry, so the premise is true as long as you ignore all the facts that do not fit.

A researcher has no reason to investigate the pain and suffering of the past if there is no expected reward. They have reason to fear social pain if they step toward evidence that our ancestors did mind-numbing labor in service to tyrants in hopes of getting protection from endless attackers. The result is the prevailing belief that life is sheer hell today, compared to past times. One wonders how those aggrieved by modern society would feel about vermin-infested open-pit toilets and neighboring tribes stealing their food stocks and their daughters.

The Greater Good Tautology No one likes to imagine themselves sifting data for opportunities to meet their own survival needs. It feels better to imagine one's self serving the greater good. The verbal brain can always define the greater good in ways that rationalize the mammal brain's quest to meet its needs. Semmelweis's critics invoked the greater good without acknowledging their own survival motives. Today's science community focuses on verbal abstractions about the greater good and overlooks the role of neurochemical survival responses in their thinking. This makes it hard for individuals to recognize biases that may occur. The brain is designed to go toward things that feel good, and believing in the superiority of one's ethics feels good. But no brain is indifferent to rewards and pain because that information drives our operating system. If we want good data, we are better off understanding our brain than masking our biases with abstractions about the greater good.

References

Ardrey, R. (1966). *Territorial imperative*. New York: Dell.

Breuning, L. (2015). *Habits of a happy brain: Retrain your brain to boost your serotonin, dopamine, oxytocin and endorphin levels*. New York: Simon & Schuster.

Cheney, D., & Seyfarth, R. (2008). *Baboon metaphysics: The evolution of a social mind*. Chicago: University of Chicago Press.

Damasio, A. (1994). *Descarte's error: Emotion, reason, and the human brain*. New York: Penguin.

de Waal, F. (2010). *The age of empathy: Nature's lessons for a kinder society*. New York: Broadway Books.

Diamond, J. (1987). The worst mistake in the history of the human race. *Discover Magazine, 5*, 64–66.

Gatto, J. (2008). *Weapons of mass instruction: A schoolteacher's journey through the dark world of compulsory schooling*. Gabriola Island, BC: New Society.

Gigerenzer, G. (2008). *Gut feelings: The intelligence of the unconscious*. New York: Penguin.

Iacoboni, M. (2009). *Mirroring people: The new science of how we connect with others*. New York: Farrar, Straus and Giroux.

Kahneman, D. (2013). *Thinking fast and slow*. New York: Farrar, Straus and Giroux.

Ledoux, J. (1998). *The emotional brain: The mysterious underpinnings of emotional life*. New York: Simon & Schuster.

Ledoux, J. (2002). *Synaptic self: How our brains become who we are*. New York: Viking Adult.

Lorenz, K. (1966). *On aggression*. London: Methuen Publishing.

Montessori, M. (1949). *The absorbent mind*. New York: Holt, Rinehart and Winston.

Nuland, S. (2003). *The Doctors' plague: Germs, childbed fever, and the strange story of Ignac Semmelweis*. New York: Norton.

Palmer, J., & Palmer, L. (2001). The biochemistry of status and the function of mood states. In *Evolutionary psychology: The ultimate origins of human behavior* (pp. 173–177). Boston: Allyn and Bacon.

Pink, D. (2011). *Drive: The surprising truth about what motivates us*. New York: Riverhead Books.

Pinker, S. (1997). *How the mind works*. New York: Norton.

Raleigh, M., McGuire, M. T., Brammer, G. L., Pollack, D. B., & Yuwiler, A. (1991). Serotonergic mechanisms promote dominance acquisition in adult male vervet monkeys. *Brain Research, 559*(2), 181–190.

Rousseau, J. J. (1762). *Emile, or on education*. Public domain, Penguin Classics, London UK.

Sapolsky, R. (1994). *Why zebras don't get ulcers*. London: WH Freeman.

Schultz, W. (1998). Predictive reward signal of dopamine neurons. *Journal of Neurophysiology, 80*(1), 1–27.

Schultz, W. (2015). Neuronal reward and decision signals: From theories to data. *Physiological Reviews, 95*, 853–951.

Selye, H. (1956). *The stress of life*. New York: McGraw-Hill.

Wilson, E. (1975). *Sociobiology: The new synthesis*. Cambridge, MA: Belknap Press.

Zak, P. (2013). *The moral molecule: How trust works*. New York: Plume.

Chapter 2
Groupthink and the Evolution of Reason Giving

Gregg Henriques

A short while ago I witnessed what I considered to be an excellent example of "political groupthink" at my university. Because the "truth" of political opinions is inevitably tied to one's own position and political values, I should be clear that my political views are left of center, are consistent with a more classic liberal view than a modern progressive identity political view (see, e.g., Lilla, 2017), and I am concerned that the university academy is too dominated by left leaning political perspectives such that I am a member of the heterodox academy, which is explicitly concerned about the lack of political "view point diversity" in university settings.

The context was a faculty discussion following the disturbing events in Charlottesville, VA, which included a large number of white supremacists marching on the city, carrying Nazi flags, and ultimately committing a horrendous act of violence such that an innocent protester perished. It received national attention, and I had offered a commentary on my *Psychology Today* blog about why I believed President Trump's response that "both sides were to blame" was disheartening (Henriques, 2017). I argued that if we were guided by a clear moral compass, this would not have been the response of our government leader. It was because of the blog that I was asked to be a participant leader in an open faculty discussion about the implications of the incident for college campuses.

What happened, at least from my "center left" political perspective, was that a group of liberal professors engaged in a discussion that proceeded to move from a heavily "left leaning" to ultimately considering an activist stance that, if actually carried forth, I believe would have been an excellent example of the horrible dangers of groupthink. The progression of the discussion was as follows: After a few opening remarks, one professor commented that the conservative commentaries and critiques in the media seemed mean-spirited and off-base, such that the picture being painted about the university academy was "unrecognizable." Then an African

G. Henriques (✉)
Department of Graduate Psychology, James Madison University, Harrisonburg, VA, USA
e-mail: henriqgx@jmu.edu

D. M. Allen, J. W. Howell (eds.), *Groupthink in Science*,
https://doi.org/10.1007/978-3-030-36822-7_2

American professor, one of the two in the group, asked if we wanted to have a "real" conversation about race. She talked about her experiences at James Madison University (JMU), especially since the election of President Trump, and claimed that there were really two cultures at JMU, one for whites another for blacks, and that the JMU culture was racist in many ways. Then a number of historians offered perspectives on the emergence of confederate statues and why they were constructed largely at the time of Jim Crow laws and many were explicitly placed near or around black communities to send a clear message about intimidation and racist attitudes.

Then a professor commented that it is our duty as professors to help students recognize just how racist and sexist our society truly was and is, and how much more needs to be done to level the playing field. Then a self-described "activist" stated that professors were good at talking, but what was really required was action. He argued we needed to march or to demand change. Finally, another activist-professor claimed that what was needed was to send a real statement. He suggested we start a petition to change the name of our university from James Madison to that of a slave who had worked toward freedom. No one objected directly. The meeting was near the end and adjourned shortly thereafter.

One of the main characteristics of groupthink is that, in an effort to demonstrate harmony and unity, people fail to consider alternative perspectives and ultimately engage in deeply problematic decision-making. From my position on the political spectrum, this is exactly what happened in this case. First, there was a general comment that "we" do not recognize the negative ways in which conservatives characterize "us." This created a groupthink element of us versus them and justified the notion that "they" do not know what we are about so we do not need to listen to them. Then claims were made, such as those regarding the institutionally racist culture of the university that almost could not have been challenged, given the context and immediate social dynamics. Then evidence was offered about the racist nature of the culture in general. Then there were proposals about our roles both to educate others about this and to take active steps to dismantle the institutions that emerged historically from our racist past, including cleansing the university of association with the slaveholder, James Madison.

While there certainly are elements of truth and logic to this kind of thinking, the chain of logic was clearly blind to many realities. First, the conversation, its content, process, and evolution of proposals were an exemplar of exactly the kinds of thinking that or about which conservative political theorists object and critique the liberal academy for engaging in. In other words, it was notably ironic that the discussion began with a comment about how a professor claimed the conservative press painted an "unrecognizable" picture of the academy, and then the group proceeded to engage in precisely the kinds of arguments and rhetoric that political conservatives complain about. Second, the progression of stronger and stronger claims, ending with a claim that we should disavow the primary organizing symbol of the university and the father of the United States Constitution. What are the implications if James Madison is deemed to be no longer worthy of admiration?

Third, there were virtually no reflections about the consequences of this proposal. Consider that it was the proposal that we needed to remove the statue of

Robert E. Lee that sparked the initial confrontation in Charlottesville and provided justification for white supremacists and the alt-right for an organized march. Could one imagine the response to changing the name of the university of the Father of the Constitution? In fact, President Trump was roundly criticized for asking, in the context of removing confederate statues, "Who is next, George Washington?" Removing James Madison and replacing it with a former slave would say that we need to completely cleanse ourselves of any association. with our "founding fathers." No one in the group, including myself, pointed these things out. All I could muster was the following comment, "I think we would need much more discussion about these issues to determine if there is a consensus in the group about actions that might make sense to take." Why did I not stand up and strenuously object and say that the discussion had clearly gone off the rails? The power of social influence in group contexts is enormously strong.

There were many elements in this situation that made it ripe for a groupthink dynamic. Specifically, we are living in a hyperpolarized political environment and a highly emotional and polarizing event had occurred. The academy is quite liberal in general and this particular event and open discussion would have been appealing to individuals who were particularly liberal. There was a need to "do something" in response and it was important that "we" were united in that response. Indeed, if one was not with the group, then questions would be raised about whether one supported Trump or white supremacy in general.

Social psychologists have long documented the empirical reality of groupthink (Turner & Pratkanis, 1998). However, what is generally not present in such analysis is a deeper understanding regarding the nature of human consciousness and social motivation, such that the reasons why humans are so prone to groupthink are laid clear. Indeed, a general critique I have long made regarding the field of psychology is that it lacks a unified conceptual framework that grounds and ties together the various lines of empirical work that currently defines the field. My scholarly efforts have been devoted to the development of a new, unified theory of psychology (Henriques, 2003, 2011) that pulls together many different threads within the field and related social science perspectives and offers a way to see the whole in a way that is more coherent than the current fragmented arrangement of theories and findings.

The remainder of this chapter focuses briefly on two key ideas that are part of the unified theory of psychology that maps human consciousness and the evolution of human culture. The first idea we will cover is called the *Justification Hypothesis*, which provides an evolutionary account of human consciousness and culture and provides a clear framework for understanding why humans do not come equipped as abstract, analytic reasoners, but in fact operate primarily as socially motivated "reason givers." The second frame is the *Influence Matrix*, which is a map of the human relationship system, specifically the social motivations and emotions that intuitively guide people in relationships and social exchanges. Together, these two ideas capture the complex interplay between the social context and how humans justify their actions to themselves and to others, and provide us with a general lens from which to understand groupthink and related phenomena.

The Justification Hypothesis

The Justification Hypothesis (JH) is really several interlocking ideas bundled in one, and we will highlight two of its main features here. First, it is a theory of the origins of human self-consciousness, filling in the crucial missing link regarding the evolutionary forces that transformed the human mind into its modern form and gave rise to the explosion of human culture. The idea about the origins of human self-consciousness is what the "hypothesis" actually references. Second, the JH specifies the key domains of human consciousness and maps how they are interrelated via an updated "Tripartite Model."

The Justification Hypothesis on the Origins of Human Self-Consciousness

Human consciousness has always been the source of much fascination and mystery. Whether and how it emerged via evolution and natural selection has been controversial since the beginning of evolutionary models. Over the past several decades, a number of pieces of the evolutionary puzzle have come into view. Many scholars have highlighted how complex social interactions drive the evolution of higher intelligence in social mammals. The JH complements and adds to these perspectives via making an explicit connection between the modern design features of the human consciousness system and a novel evolved selection pressure that gave rise to it. Specifically, the JH points to how language changed the social environment, in particular by giving rise to a fundamentally new adaptive problem. The adaptive problem that emerged with a linguistic environment was the problem of social justification. The adaptive solution was an interpreter (see Gazzaniga, 1998) that provided justifications for actions that took social influence into account. Stated differently, as human language and cognitive capacities emerged, such that individuals began to ask questions that forced reason-giving accounts, the social psychological environment changed rapidly. This in turn shaped evolution of the human self-consciousness system into the "mental organ of justification" (Henriques, 2003).

Anyone who has raised a child knows that kids first learn simple commands and descriptions for objects (e.g., no, mommy, juice). After they obtain some mastery with descriptive language, a transformation happens, usually around the age of two; they start asking questions. The JH posits that the emergence of the "Q&A" capacity that tipped human evolution into a completely different phase. Why? Because, although asking questions is relatively easy, answering questions raises a completely new series of problems. To see what I mean, hang out with an intelligent, curious four-year-old who has discovered "why questions": "Why don't we eat cookies before we eat dinner?"; "Why are you going bald?"; "Why is the sky blue?" As such children readily demonstrate, asking questions is much easier than answering them. That is why exasperated parents eventually say, "That is just the way it is!"

Once language had tipped from descriptions and commands to a Q&A format, individuals could be held to account for why they did believe and act the way that they did. Although a chimpanzee can clearly send the message she is angry or scared, without a symbolic language it is almost impossible for her to communicate the reasons why she feels that way. In contrast, a "Q&A" language environment means humans can ask and be asked about the thought processes associated with their behaviors. Questions such as "Why did you do that?"; "What gives you the right to behave that way?" and "Why should I trust you?" force the issue. Obtaining information about what others think, what they have done, and what they plan to do is obviously important for navigating the social environment in modern times and, given that humans have always been an intensely social species, there is every reason to believe that it was equally essential in the ancestral past. The first basic claim of the JH is that once people developed the capacity to use language to access the thought patterns of others, they likely did so with vigor.

Now consider why the answers to those questions would have been so important. If you strike a comrade with a stick, it matters whether you tell him it was done by accident or on purpose. If you take more than your proportional share of meat, it matters how you explain that action. If you are bargaining with a stranger, you can get more resources if you emphasize why the resources you are trading are valuable, and so on. A second basic claim is that the kinds of explanations people offer for their behavior have real-world consequences.

A third claim is that human interests diverge and this complicates the interpretation process significantly. If one's interests always fully coincided with the interests of others, communicating the reasons for one's behavior would primarily be a technical problem of translating one's nonverbal thoughts into a symbolic form that could be understood. But because interests always diverge to some extent and the explanations given for one's behavior have real-world consequences, the communication task becomes one of justification rather than simple translation. These claims about the problem of social justification point directly to the design features we would expect the human self-consciousness system to exhibit. That is, to the extent that the adaptive problem of justification can be thought of as a "lock," the human self-consciousness system should look like a "key" that fits it.

So according to the Justification Hypothesis, what is the self-consciousness system? It is the language-based portion of your mind that is narrating what is happening, why it is happening, and why you are doing what you are doing in that context. This formulation clearly predicts that the self-consciousness system should be designed in such a way that it allows humans to effectively justify their actions to others in a manner that, all things being equal, tends to maximize social influence. An examination of some of the characteristics of human self-consciousness, as elucidated by neuropsychology, social, cognitive, and developmental psychology, demonstrates that there is a large body of general human psychological research that is highly consistent with this proposition. Specifically, Henriques (2011) reviews how the JH accounts for the "interpreter" function of the left hemisphere, cognitive dissonance, self-serving biases, motivational reasoning biases, findings on the differences between implicit and explicit attitudes, and research on reason-giving and social accounts. In sum, the JH allows us to get the correct frame on the evolution of the self-consciousness system, and in so doing allows us to map the key domains of human consciousness and their interrelationship. This sets the stage for us to tackle a closely related concept, that of the human self.

The Updated Tripartite Model of Human Consciousness

The value of the Justification Hypothesis is not simply in that it provides a plausible story for why the human self-consciousness system might have evolved, but rather it sheds new light on understanding human consciousness. For example, the JH gives rise to an "updated" Tripartite Model of human consciousness (Fig. 2.1). It is referred to as an updated Tripartite Model because it divides human consciousness into three domains (the experiential system, the private self-consciousness system, and the public self-consciousness system) that parallels Freud's famous structural model in some regards (Henriques, 2003), although there are also crucial differences.

The experiential portion of human consciousness is quite different from the id that Freud envisioned. It is not an unconscious caldron of sex and aggression. Instead, it is a primary process, experiential system (see Epstein, 1994). This means

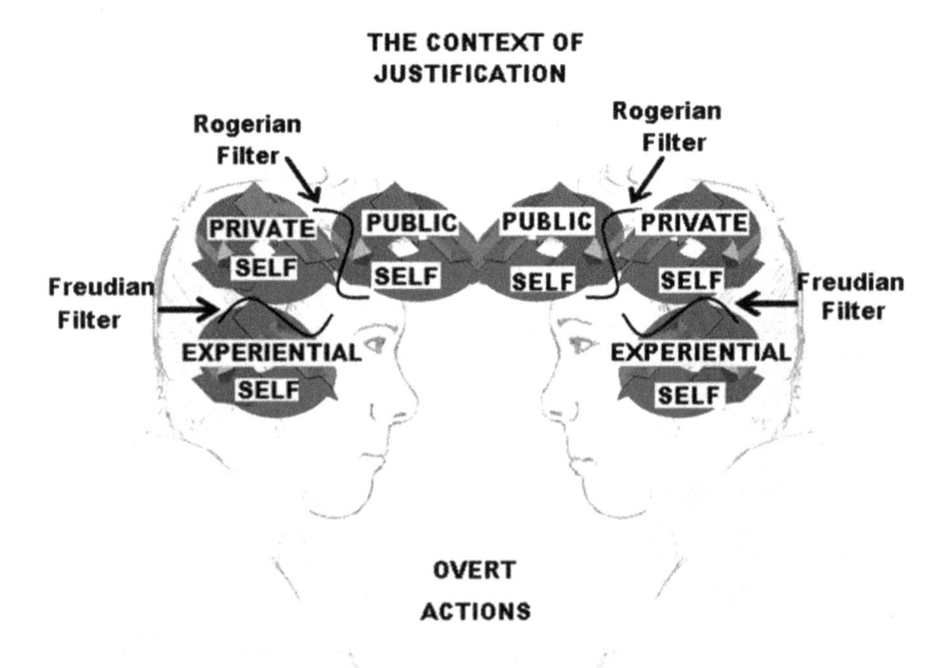

Fig. 2.1 The Updated Tripartite Model of Human Consciousness

that it is fast and relatively automatic. Everyday perception does not require conscious effort. Rather, you simply open your eyes and are presented with the world around you. The structure of the experiential system is framed in part by the Influence Matrix described in the subsequent section. As such, we can note here that the experiential system is part of the larger mind that is guided by positive and negative feeling states that function to orient an individual toward valued goals and away from dangers.

The private narrator portion shares some overlap with Freud's concept of an ego. However, Freud's conception of the ego was fuzzy. The JH achieves clarity because it comes with an explicit evolutionary account of the origin of the private self-consciousness system that helps us understand its design features, as described previously. The private narrator is a reflective reason-giving system that helps to navigate the relational world. It is clearly not fully formed at birth, but instead develops with experience. It requires the cognitive capacity to become the object of one's own attention. It also requires the capacity for symbolic language because it is fundamentally a reason-giving structure. In young children, the system operates to learn the rules of conduct. In adolescence, it emerges as a potentially separable identity, such that the teenager can reflect on the distinction between how they are actually and how they wished they might be. Finally, in adults it becomes a full narrator, an active self-concept that is weaving together one's life story (see McAdams, 2013).

With its central focus on justification and reason giving in a social context, the JH highlights a crucial distinction between private and public domains of justification. Anyone who has accidently shared a thought or action publicly that was meant to be private will quickly and powerfully experience the distinction. For example, on an e-mail listserv, I once accidently sent a message that was meant to be back channel to a single individual and not to the entire group. As soon as I hit send and saw the message appear on the board for everyone to see, a jolt of fear and anxiety rippled through me, and I literally let out a yelp. The distinction of private and public becomes very salient when barriers that are supposed to function to separate the two fail.

One of the most powerful pieces of evidence for the JH is the way it characterizes the relationship between the three domains of consciousness. Specifically, it highlights the presence of filters between the experiential and the private, and the private and the public. These are the "Freudian" and "Rogerian" filters, respectively, and they are clearly framed by the logic of the JH, which is why they are explicitly labeled in the diagram.The Freudian filter (or experiential-to-private filter) works via the process of inhibiting disruptive or problematic feelings, images, or thoughts, and shifting attention away from them. Why are certain impulses filtered? According to the Justification Hypothesis, the reason is to maintain a consistent, relatively stable justification narrative of the self and to maintain a justifiable image in the eyes of others. In his book *Ego Defenses and the Legitimization of Behavior*, Swanson (1988) made exactly this point, explicitly arguing that we should think of all ego defenses as "justifications that people make to themselves and others—justifications so designed that the defender, not just other people, can accept them" (p. 159). Part of the filter also involves a shift in attention, which can be called repression or, in behavioral terms, "experiential avoidance." Such experiential avoidance is often supported by justifications, such as "There is no point in my feeling sad about that, it only brings up pain."

The Rogerian (or private-to-public filter) refers to the extent to which we share or do not share our narrative with others. It also refers to the way we share such information. Any time that you are thinking about whether or not to share a piece of information with another person or group of people, this is an example of the private-to-public filter. The JH posits that we all have significant experience filtering our thoughts, depending on who the audience is and what we want them to see in us. The example I referenced regarding the e-mail accidently going out to the whole group demonstrates that this filtering process is not just one on one, but refers to how we navigate our identities to different audiences across the levels of human interaction, from self to dyad to small group to full public identity. When diaries are sealed or doors are closed or memos are marked "confidential," we can see clearly the private-to-public filter at work.

The three domains of consciousness are not the only aspects in Fig. 2.1. Above the two figures is labeled "The Context of Justification," which refers to the network of symbolically based beliefs and values that provide the interacting members a shared frame of reference for their interaction. The context can be considered on the dimensions of time and scope. Scope refers to the size and scale of the context one is considering. Urie Bronfenbrenner's (1979) Ecological Systems Theory provides a useful framework for considering the scope of the system, although I should note that he was concerned with the whole societal context, which would include the biophysical ecology and technology, in addition to the systems of justification. There is also the concept of action, which refers to the overt activities of each individual.

The Influence Matrix

The above description offers some details on the domains of justification (i.e., the private and the public) and argues that humans create and live in contexts of justification, but the model does not clearly articulate what exactly drives the system. That is, where does the energy come from to justify one's actions in a certain way? The unified theory of psychology answers this question in the form of *Behavioral Investment Theory* (BIT). The BIT posits that the "mind/brain system" is evolved as a computational control center that computes the animal's actions on an energy investment value system built via natural and behavioral selection (or evolution and learning), such that animals are inclined to move toward "the good" (which they seek and approach) and away from "the bad" (which they avoid and withdraw from). The Influence Matrix is an extension of BIT, applied to human social motivation and emotion.

Based on much research in *personality* and social psychology, *the Influence Matrix* (Fig. 2.2) offers a map of our foundational relational strivings. The Matrix identifies one core relational motive and then highlights several other key relational

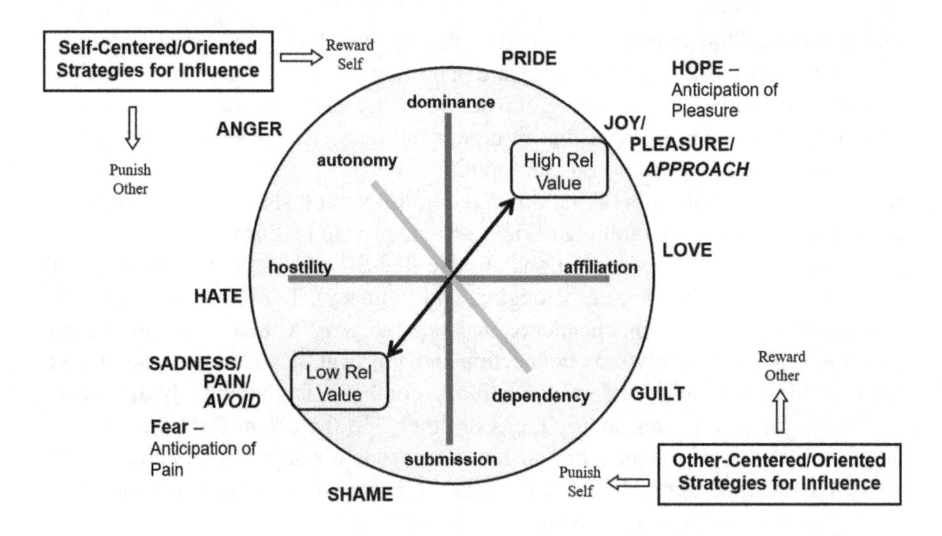

Fig. 2.2 The Influence Matrix

motives that are connected in various ways to the core motive. The core motive is called the Relational Value/Social Influence (RV-SI) motive, and is represented on the center diagonal line in the diagram, with high relational value on one end and low relational value on the other. This line refers primarily to the degree to which you feel known and valued by important others (i.e., family, friends, lovers, groups one belongs to). Behaviorally, it refers to the extent to which important others will share and invest in your interests, which is the degree of social influence one has – you put them together to get the RV-SI line. From this perspective, people are energized to be respected, valued, appreciated, cared for, or admired. And they are also energized to avoid the opposites (i.e., being rejected or held in contempt or ignored by important others) and we can see these are things folks generally fear and try to avoid. The vast majority of people can see that these are major themes in their relational world.

Although RV-SI is the core motive, we can go further and assert there are various ways folks try to gratify their RV-SI needs. There are two "competitive" (or vertical) ways folks try to obtain RV-SI. One common and directly competitive way is via power. *Power* in the form of direct dominance, *leadership*, and control over others is a way to insure social influence. Another competitive relational process, but one that is more indirect, is *achievement*. Achievement refers to accomplishing markers of skill and status which are valued in a society or group. These two motives (i.e., direct and indirect competitive influence) are represented by the vertical line.

There are also two forms of positive "horizontal" or cooperative relating to acquiring social influence and relational value. These motivational forces and kinds of relating involve affiliating and joining one's interests with the interests of others.

One form of affiliative motive is called belonging, which refers to being a part of a group or *identity*. So, if you take pleasure in rooting for a sports *team* or feel a close identification with your *religious* group or nationality, then you are experiencing the motive to belong. The other affiliative urge is intimacy. This involves letting others know more about "the real you" and joining with them at a much more personal level. Intimacy involves breaking down public filters and sharing authentically to allow for a more genuine joining of interests and private feelings.

We have identified a core relational motive (RV-SI) and four common relational strivings (achievement, power, belonging, and intimacy). Two other common relational strivings include independence and *self-reliance*. Although we are clearly social animals and deeply seek connection and approval, it is also the case that we are in need of separation and individuation to combat being completely dependent on the whims and desires and opinions of others. To the extent that an individual advertises one's self-reliance, diminishes their needs for approval and connection, or tries to buck the trend, defy social norms, and carve their own unique path, they are engaged in autonomous strivings.

Finally, there are relational "avoidance strategies," where individuals strive to avoid the negative consequences of trying to achieve the approach strivings. Submitting or surrendering in *competition* is one such avoidance strategy. Many individuals are plagued by self-conscious, shameful thoughts about how inferior they are. The root of this behavior is that these folks are striving to avoid competition or conflict which would then cause them to lose respect or be embarrassed. Whereas *shame* and submission are about avoiding relational conflict and competition, hostility and contempt are about avoiding affiliation or connection (and often then justifying power). These are "othering" strategies designed to avoid betrayal and others' control and to remove any sense of obligation to them (i.e., make them unimportant). In existing affiliative relations, we use *anger* and hostility to remind those close to us of their obligations to us and to remove or diminish their tendency to betray us (or we use it to move away from them after we feel they have betrayed us and we can no longer have an intimate relation with them). Notice that a difference between avoidance strategies and approach strategies is that folks do not engage in avoidance strategies just for the sake of doing so. Very few people strive to be hostile or ridden with shame. But they are activated in the service of avoiding some even worse outcome.

Implications for Understanding Groupthink and Other Related Phenomena

Why do people believe what they do? How do social dynamics influence how people reason? Why would a group of people, who say averaged a left leaning "8" on a political scale ranging from 1 to 10, come up with a political "solution" that would be rated an "11" by individuals external to the group? The empirical elements that contribute to groupthink are well documented. When there is pressure on a group to believe a certain way, when there is a strong need for unity, often spurred by the identification of an "other" group that is seen as a polar opposite, when emotions are stoked, and when there is a charismatic leader who wants to see certain things done, the stage is set for groupthink. What these empirical findings do not answer are ultimate questions about why humans believe, feel, and act in this way. They do not provide models regarding the architecture of the human mind or its motivational systems that clearly delineate why these processes unfold.

It is this latter gap that the combination of the Influence Matrix and Justification Hypothesis fills. When taken together, these models state very clearly that human reasoning is not a cold analytic process, designed to take in information and calculate pros and cons via some "rational actor." Rather, human consciousness is guided by the need for social influence and relational value, and more specific needs for power and achievement or belonging and intimacy or the avoidance of the loss of such things. And human consciousness functions, first and foremost, as a social reason-giving system, one that seeks a personally and publicly socially justifiable path to legitimize action. If we understand this as the fundamental model by which humans operate, then the phenomena of groupthink, along with many other social psychological processes, become readily understandable.

References

Bronfenbrenner, U. (1979). *The ecology of human development: Experiments by nature and design*. Cambridge, MA: Harvard University Press.

Epstein, S. (1994). Integration of the cognitive and the psychodynamic unconscious. *American Psychologist, 49*, 709–724.

Gazzaniga, M. S. (1998). *The mind's past*. Berkeley, CA: University of California Press.

Henriques, G. R. (2003). The tree of knowledge system and the theoretical unification of psychology. *Review of General Psychology, 7*, 150–182.

Henriques, G. R. (2011). *A new unified theory of psychology*. New York: Springer.

Henriques, G. R. (2017, August). A moral compass for troubling times. *Theory of Knowledge on Psychology today*. Retrieved February 14, 2019, from https://www.psychologytoday.com/us/blog/theory-knowledge/201708/moral-compass-troubling-times.

Lilla, M. (2017). *The once and future liberal: After identity politics*. New York: Harper Collins.

McAdams, D. P. (2013). The psychological self as actor, agent, and author. *Perspectives on Psychological Science, 8*, 272–295.

Swanson, G. E. (1988). *Ego defenses and the legitimation of behavior*. New York: Cambridge University Press.

Turner, M. E., & Pratkanis, A. R. (1998). Twenty-five years of groupthink theory and research: Lessons from the evaluation of a theory. *Organizational Behavior and Human Decision Processes, 73*(2–3), 105–115. https://doi.org/10.1006/obhd.1998.2756

Chapter 3
The Mental and Interpersonal Mechanisms of Groupthink Maintenance

David M. Allen

One of the defining characteristics of groupthink is something called "willful blindness" (Heffernan, 2011). This term was originally used as a legal concept in the nineteenth century. People often know things, or at the very least should know things, but choose to pretend that they do not, in order to fit in with larger social groups. They will refuse to look at any sources of information that might call into question any beliefs that help them to "convey and conform to" (p. 3) the needs of the various groups to which they belong. The paradox of such willful ignorance is that in cases in which you are motivated to avoid looking at something, you have to know where not to look! In other words, you did see it. We often see what we are not supposed to but look away, and then lie to ourselves about what we know or do not know. We do this to promote what we perceive to be the interests of our significant others or to enforce group harmony.

The reason that we all do this has to do with a significant characteristic of natural selection that was operative during our biological evolution. Conforming to the values and requirements of our kin group or our tribe has high adaptive value. Genes that contribute to the survival of the tribe or clan to which we belong, as opposed to those that only benefit individuals, are highly likely to be passed on. Other adaptive genes are likely to be lost if only one individual has them. This process is known by evolutionary biologists as *kin selection* (Wilson, 1998), a significant component of a more inclusive concept called *multi-level selection* (Sober & Wilson, 1998). The concept of kin selection goes all the way back to Darwin, but only a minority of modern-day evolutionary biologists will discuss it because of political fears that it will be misused to promote a "survival of the fittest" political agenda.

While sacrificing oneself for a group – such as the widespread willingness to die for one's country in a war – is not great for individual survival, it does contribute significantly to group survival. Nonetheless, it can sometimes actually harm a

D. M. Allen (✉)
Department of Psychiatry, University of Tennessee Health Science Center, Memphis, TN, USA
e-mail: dallen49@comcast.net

D. M. Allen, J. W. Howell (eds.), *Groupthink in Science*,
https://doi.org/10.1007/978-3-030-36822-7_3

group's interests in the long run. The term *pathological altruism* (Oakley, Knafo, Guruprasad, & Wilson, 2011) has been used to describe situations in which this tendency to self-sacrifice backfires and harms not only the individual making the sacrifice but his or her group as well.

Another major characteristic of functioning groups is the usual presence of a pecking order, with leaders of the group who tend to set agendas and who mentor more junior group members. Because of this, group leaders are far less likely to be challenged by the rest of the group, even when they seem to be wrong. In scientific circles, this can lead to situations in which misleading studies and conclusions from those studies get published. Once again, willful blindness becomes operative.

Many mental mechanisms and tricks have evolved to help us lie to ourselves to achieve these purposes. Interestingly, we also tend to assist our fellow group members in using these tricks on themselves. Groups as a whole also have a variety of mechanisms for keeping certain information censored. The mechanisms at both levels are the subject of this chapter.

For almost all of us, it is generally more important to look right than to be right (Haight, 2012). The use of our reasoning skills for this purpose appears at the level of the individual, where they are called either *defense mechanisms* by psychoanalytically oriented psychotherapists or *irrational beliefs* by cognitive behavioral (CBT) psychotherapists. They also appear at the level of the family or kin group, where they are called *family myths*. They also exist at the level of cultural groups, where they are called *theology*, or when they are not your own particular brand of theology, *mythology*. In science, they appear as part of such phenomenon as confirmation bias, the use of logical fallacies in discussions of research findings, and the ignoring of important contextual factors in evaluating experimental phenomena. The chapters of this book will go into the details of how these different mental and interpersonal groupthink mechanisms operate, with an emphasis on how they affect the scientific enterprise.

Groupthink Mechanisms Within Individuals

Defense Mechanisms

Defense mechanisms (Freud, 1966) were originally defined as mental processes, typically at a subconscious level, employed by individuals to avoid ideas or impulses that are unacceptable to their own value personal system (*superego* or conscience), and to avoid the anxiety that those ideas or impulses therefore create. Notice, however, that these mechanisms do not just serve an internal purpose within our mind, but an interpersonal one as well. We may, for example, compulsively try to act in the opposite way that an impulse that is unacceptable to our group would dictate (*reaction formation*), or *displace* our anger at one person within our kin group onto another outside person to avoid tension within our group. We may *repress* or push out of our awareness impulses or thoughts unacceptable to our cohort, or *project* them on to outsiders.

Thusly, we are all at times highly motivated to screen out and avoid revealing to the others beliefs and impulses that are not accepted by a group to which we belong, and which might cause us to get into trouble. Someone engaging in these defenses in scientific circles may do so in order to fit in, to curry favor with other group members, to avoid angering group leaders, to increase their chances at getting tenure, to appeal to funding sources that are enamored with a particular scientific viewpoint or theory, or to help other members of groups with a theoretical bent or school of thought similar to the person's own group through providing favorable peer review of their research output.

Irrational Thoughts

The irrational thoughts that have been catalogued by CBT therapists (Ellis & Grieger, 1977), although not conceptualized by CBT therapists in the same way as defense mechanisms, in fact also function in much the same way. They are often *automatic* in that they come to us without any conscious effort in response to an environmental event, and they quickly lead to specific behavior patterns. They are often said to be *subliminal*, which is a similar concept to subconscious. If you, for example, *catastrophize* (imagining every single thing that could possible go wrong if you did something, no matter how unlikely) about your engaging in a course of action not condoned by your group, you will indeed scare yourself away from engaging in it.

Group norms are often internally policed by unquestioned thoughts that start with "I *should* or *must*" do or think this or that. If you had contrary thoughts in the past that turned out to be wrong, you might *overgeneralize* by thinking that all the thoughts related to the earlier ones are always going to be wrong as well. Another way to do this is to tell yourself that you just will not be able to *stand it* if you ever are proved incorrect again, or that you are a terrible person for even having thought of something in the first place. These sorts of self-negating thoughts can be used when willful blindness seems to fail. If a scientist finds that he or she is unable to pretend that anomalous data or other findings do not exist, they can instead dismiss them as irrelevant, unimportant, immoral, or merely invalid. The end result is the same: important scientific ideas are quashed.

Irrational thoughts may be conceptualized as *self-invalidation,* but once again the reason one engages in it is interpersonal in nature. To better understand this, let us now examine behavioral and mental mechanisms for maintaining group cohesion.

Mechanisms Within Groups

Group Mythology

In order to operate as an integrated unit, groups with a common purpose also have mechanisms that they use to enforce conformity of thought within their numbers, as well as having its members employ various strategies to invalidate any competing ideas with which they might be challenged. Once again, group cohesion has its advantages; it often maximizes the group's chances of success, but these mechanisms can also backfire severely.

Family therapists have studied groupthink phenomena within families, but similar ones are used by other groups as well. An individual's family often acts as if they all share a set of beliefs, and they all seem to live by them almost compulsively. While some of these beliefs can be applied only to certain individuals within the family (for example, ideas about what one family member is "really" like and who within the family he or she is supposed to be closest to), others apply to all family members. The latter ideas are referred to as *family myths*. They justify and support a set of rules which dictate how each family member should behave, and what family roles each must fully and habitually play, in order for the family to function in a predictable way *(family homeostasis)*.

The myths also function as a belief system which the family uses, often defensively, to explain its experience to itself. They are sometimes not verbalized explicitly so as to avoid any challenges to them. They can be taught implicitly through various forms of acting out and family rituals. However, they may frequently take the form of oft-verbalized adages or slogans. One good example of this was seen in a family that strongly believed in fatalism – the idea that people are powerless to change their world so should make the best of that which already exists. They all spouted three different proverbs on numerous occasions that expressed and reinforced within the group a warning about what happens to anyone who tries to take charge of their lives: "The grass is always greener on the other side of the hill;" "The devil you know is better than the devil you don't know;" and "You've made your bed so now you have to lie in it."

In scientific groups, related strategies are employed by speakers after their presentation at a scientific conference in response to arguments and critiques by audience members. One common one is that they often employ clear logical fallacies in order to advance their agenda and to invalidate anything that might sound to the general audience like disconfirmation of the viewpoint that they are advancing.

A common example is the use of post hoc reasoning, which assumes wrongly that if event A is quickly followed by event B, then it is probably true that A caused B. A common intriguing variation of this common fallacy is often seen in discussions about epidemiological studies. The fallacy is based on the fact that the odds that two variables will have identical prevalence in any two populations is next to zero (Ellenberg, 2014). This means that the two variables will always appear to be either positively or negatively correlated, even when they are mostly or even completely unrelated. This happens because the number of possible confounding variables is so high that it impossible to control for them all.

Similar misleading interpretations of data occur when scientists look at risk factors for characteristics of people when both the risk factor and the characteristic are both normally distributed in a given population – say human weight and dietary protein intake, for example. Assuming that high protein intake is indeed a risk factor for obesity, whether it appears as necessary, sufficient, or both in creating a disorder depends entirely upon where the experimenter draws the line between "high" and "low" for both weight and intake with their subjects (Cook & Campbell, 1979).

A few other examples rampant in science that may characterize debates in my field of psychiatry are:

(a) Black-and-white, or all-or-none thinking. Some "biological" psychiatrists seem to think that everything in the diagnostic manual is a brain disease, whereas psychoanalysts used to believe that almost none of them are. Alternately, some therapists advance the idea that, because some of Freud's ideas were totally off-base (like "penis envy" and his theories about homosexuality), that therefore *all* of his ideas are wrong (including such obviously real things as intrapsychic conflict and defense mechanisms).
(b) Stating facts about the results of studies without describing certain contextual elements that put those facts in a different light. A great example was described by Carl Hart (2013). Speakers for the National Institute on Drug Abuse speak about experiments with monkeys that show them continuing to pull a lever to get cocaine until they die. They did not mention, however, that the animals were in solitary confinement during the experiment with nothing else to do, and when that was not the case, they behaved very differently.
(c) Conflating the issue of how a phenomenon arises or what it means with the issue of whether the phenomenon even exists at all. For example, some CBT'ers deny that the concept of resistance – a psychoanalytic idea that states that people are often highly invested in their psychological symptoms and resist change – is a real phenomenon. All the while, they failed to report in their case studies that noncompliance with CBT homework assignments by their patients in treatment is highly prevalent.
(d) Conflating another scientist's conclusion about the significance of a clinical anecdote with the *description* of the anecdote, or not considering several different possible explanations in theorizing about what anecdotal situation might actually mean.
(e) The ecological fallacy, in which an average on a continuous variable within a group (such as how impulsive individuals with a certain psychiatric diagnosis tend to be) is applied automatically to *any* individual with said group. Making this assumption ignores the fact that almost all such variables exist in a so-called normal distribution (the bell-shaped curve) within the members of any group.
(f) Scientism: the idea that randomized placebo-controlled studies are the end-all and be-all of science, and that everything else is just anecdotal and not science at all. Someone made fun of this argument by asking for volunteers for a randomized placebo-controlled study on whether parachutes reduce the incidence of deaths and injuries during falls from airplane flights.

Another groupthink strategy employed during question and answer periods following a presentation at a scientific conference is a version of, "My mind is made up; don't confuse me with the facts." A valid argument against a proposition is just ignored, dismissed out of hand with no explanation (*begging the question),* offering a related but tangential argument, or smoothly and insidiously changing the subject altogether. Yet another common strategy is for a speaker to focus exclusively on some trivial aspect of the audience member's statement or question while completely ignoring inconvenient truths also contained therein, and then not allowing a follow-up question before going on to recognize the next audience member in line at the microphone.

Scientists will often accuse other scientists of doing these things while doing them themselves. This is the defense mechanism of projection. These mental mechanisms are so pervasive in human beings that we are quite likely to find at least some of them in any ongoing scientific discussion.

Within-Group Mechanisms for Enforcing Groupthink: Disqualification and Invalidation

When potentially controversial topics are debated *within* a group advancing a particular scientific viewpoint, individuals can, when seemingly necessary, use two related mechanisms to obfuscate their own beliefs. This is done so that if later said beliefs are rejected, they do not appear to have been the ones who had advanced them in the first place. These tactics are called *disqualification* and *invalidation*. Disqualification is a strategy used to make one's own position on an issue ambiguous. When someone does this, other members of the group cannot say for certain what it is that the person actually believes, so that the person cannot be held to account if the group eventually objects to the idea. When the other people ask for clarification, they are basically told that they are misperceiving the person they are asking in some way. Doing this is invalidation.

Someone who is disqualifying themselves may *seem* to address an issue but really is not addressing it all, while in the process leaving others stymied as to where to go next. The answers they give may sound definitive, but they are really ambiguous. Linguists have learned that ambiguity is a core feature of all languages (Allen, 1991). Anything that is said can be interpreted in different and sometimes in completely opposite ways.

Said another way, in terms of what we are discussing here, ambiguity is used by those who have internal conflicts over group ideology in order to accomplish two goals:

1. Making their conflicted feelings, beliefs, and motivations unclear to other people.
2. Keeping those things unclear to even themselves in order to avoid anxiety over potentially problematic thoughts and ideas.

As described by Watzlawick, Beavin, and Jackson (1967, p. 76), "Disqualifications cover a wide range of communicational phenomena, such as self-contradictions, inconsistencies, subject switches, tangentializations, incomplete sentences, misunderstandings, obscure style or mannerisms of speech, the literal interpretation of metaphor and the metaphorical interpretation of literal remarks, etc."

If group members happen to call out the person on being thusly ambiguous, a common reaction is for the disqualifier to turn the criticism around onto the persons making the call. They are told in so many words that they are being somewhat dense because the speaker was perfectly clear, misinterpreting the speaker's words, or just not thinking straight. As mentioned, being told these things is invalidation. Invalidation is not merely disagreement, but a statement that says or implies that a person is irrational, ignorant, stupid, overly sensitive, or even completely insane.

When Groupthink Backfires and Harms the Group: An Illustrative Example

Jerry Harvey (1974) identified an example of a process in which a group decides collectively on a course of action which none of them really thinks is a good idea. They all mistakenly believe that all the *others* do think it a good idea, and go along with this misperception in order to help the group remain cohesive. He called it the *Abilene Paradox* because it was based on a personal experience in which his family all agreed to travel over 50 miles in extreme heat and in an uncomfortable, non-air-conditioned vehicle in order to eat at a restaurant in Abilene, Texas. In reality, not a single member of the family actually wanted to take this trip when someone had suggested it. However, every single one of them mistakenly believed that all the *other* family members were in favor of going. And so they all went, and of course absolutely no one had a good time.

More commonly, an individual who has reservations about a group decision goes along with a group on some idea or project when the other members all, in fact, *do* think it is a good idea. The end result in either case is of course identical: everyone goes along with the idea. In many such cases, the altruistic intention backfires and ends up harming everyone.

Going along to get along in a business atmosphere can eventually lead to the demise of an entire business (Senge, 1990). In a scientific group, it can lead to a situation in which a group sticks with an incorrect idea for far too long, even as the evidence against it piles up, leading their group to become marginalized or completely irrelevant in their field.

I described at the beginning of this chapter how our evolutionary past has conditioned us to participate in groupthink, but clearly, some people are able to override this tendency and persist with an idea that is highly unpopular or even completely dismissed by the overall community of members of their scientific field. We will discuss some impressive examples of this in Chap. 5. While this is indeed the case, defying one's group's ideas and rules is something that is extremely difficult for many people to do. So, how does our evolutionary past directly affect us at the individual level? This is the subject of the next section.

Existential Groundlessness

Every so often, almost everyone is overcome by a sense of doubt about who they are and the choices they have made, as well as an existential sense of the meaninglessness of all of it. However, because most of us will go to any length to avoid feeling that way – let us call this feeling *groundlessness* – the feeling usually does not last very long. So in spite of its universality, many people think the feeling is something that is imagined, unimportant, or is only the concern of pointy-headed intellectuals like Jean-Paul Sartre.

In psychotherapy, however, when we try to help patients follow their own muse, so to speak (*self-actualize),* they often find themselves at odds with a set of rules that they had learned in their families of origin (Allen, 1988). And when they begin to experiment with breaking *those* rules and striking out on their own, a terrifying sense of groundlessness begins to manifest itself. The feeling is so distressing that patients may think they are getting worse, and may even start to seriously contemplate suicide.

When we start to defy a group to which we are highly attached, the feeling of groundlessness arises, and we are sorely tempted to force ourselves to get back in line. This strong internal, genetic tendency is how the evolutionary forces of kin selection express themselves within an individual's brain as the individual operates in a social context.

One important characteristic of groundlessness was described by Yalom (1980). He called it *defamiliarization*. It is a disturbing feeling that all is not well, that the meaning and purpose of the outside world, which once seemed so clear to us, is all a charade. Previously, we felt at home in the world. Things, people, roles, values, ideals, symbols, institutions, seemed comfortably real, familiar, and meaningful. While a sense of meaningfulness is to some extent personal, it is more primarily collective. We share much of our sense of meaning with others within the particular systems in which we operate. When we buck them, suddenly life begins to seem absurd and pointless.

So why is it that some people can endure this unnerving feeling and persevere in challenging their profession with new and unpopular ideas, while others cannot? In the opinion of this author, that question at present has no clear answer.

References

Allen, D. (1988). *A family systems approach to individual psychotherapy (originally titled unifying individual and family therapies)*. Northvale, NJ: Jason Aronson.

Allen, D. (1991). *Deciphering motivation in psychotherapy*. New York: Plenum.

Cook, T., & Campbell, D. (1979). *Quasi-experimentation: Design and analysis issues for field settings*. Boston: Houghton Mifflin.

Ellis, A., & Grieger, R. (1977). *Handbook of rational emotive therapy*. New York: Springer.

Freud, A. (1966). *The ego and the mechanisms of defense* (Rev. ed.). New York: International Universities Press.

Haight, J. (2012). *The righteous mind: Wy good people are divided by politics and religion*. New York: Pantheon Books.

Hart, C. (2013). *High price*. New York: Harper.

Harvey, J. (1974). The Abilene paradox: The management of agreement. *Organizational Dynamics, 3*, 63–80.

Heffernan, M. (2011). *Willful blindness: Why we ignore the obvious at our peri*. New York: Bloomsbury.

Henriques, G. (2020). Groupthink and the evolution of reason-giving. In D. Allen & W. Howell (Eds.), *Groupthink in science*. New York: Springer.

Ellenberg, J. (2014). *How not to be wrong: The power of mathematical thinking*. New York: Penguin Press.

Oakley, B., Knafo, A., Guruprasad, M., & Wilson, D. (Eds.). (2011). *Pathological altruism*. Oxford, UK: Oxford University Press.

Senge, P. (1990). *The fifth discipline: The art & practice of the learning organization*. New York: Doubleday.

Sober, S., & Wilson, D. (1998). *Unto others: The evolution and psychology of unselfish behavior*. Boston: Harvard University Press.

Watzlawick, P., Beavin, J., & Jackson, D. (1967). *Pragmatics of human communication*. New York: W. W. Norton.

Wilson, E. (1998). *Consilience: The unity of knowledge*. New York: Alfred A. Knopf.

Yalom, I. (1980). *Existential psychotherapy*. New York: Basic Books.

Chapter 4
False Beliefs and the Social Structure of Science: Some Models and Case Studies

Cailin O'Connor and James Owen Weatherall

Introduction

Humans are inherently social animals. It should come as no surprise that our systems of knowledge formation are social as well. We pass information and evidence from person to person via testimony. As a result, for each of us, the majority of things we believe were learned from other people. This is an enormously powerful and successful ability, in general. Human culture and technological innovation would not be possible without the social spread of knowledge. But the social spread of knowledge opens us up to a potential problem - when we trust the testimony of others, we will sometimes trust false things as well as true ones.[1]

In this paper, we consider how the social spread of knowledge happens, especially in scientific communities and regarding scientific beliefs. In particular, we will use a set of agent-based models, drawn from what is called the network epistemology framework, to illustrate how the social aspects of science can influence theory adoption and lead to potential problems. The second section introduces this framework and makes clear how it can be used to represent the spread of scientific beliefs. The third section is the heart of the paper, where we discuss a number of historical cases in science where (1) social factors influenced outcomes and (2) network epistemology models can help us understand how. As it will become clear, these models can be applied both to cases where aspects of social psychology influence belief spread, and to cases where pernicious influencers or propagandists attempt to shape scientific belief. The last section concludes by briefly discussing some social and political issues that arise as a result of the persistence of false scientific beliefs.

[1] For a nice discussion of this trade-off, see (Mayo-Wilson, 2014).

C. O'Connor (✉) · J. O. Weatherall
Logic and Philosophy of Science, University of California Irvine, Irvine, CA, USA
e-mail: cailino@uci.edu

D. M. Allen, J. W. Howell (eds.), *Groupthink in Science*,
https://doi.org/10.1007/978-3-030-36822-7_4

Network Epistemology Models of Science

Mathematical models are commonly used in the social sciences as a tool to understand human interaction. These models are especially useful in cases where it is difficult to fully investigate a group of people empirically. In the case of information spread and theory change, scientific communities often adopt a new theory slowly over the course of many years, and as a result of thousands of interactions between scientists and dozens of experiments. Although we cannot directly observe each of these interactions, we can use a combination of empirical observation and modeling work to develop an understanding of how these processes occur. The network epistemology framework was first introduced by economists Bala and Goyal (1998) to model the spread of social knowledge.[2] *Epistemology* refers to the fact that these models are about knowledge and belief formation. More recently, they have been used to directly model scientific communities, starting with the work of the philosopher of science Kevin Zollman (2007, 2010b). Since then, this framework has been used widely to model scientific consensus and the spread of scientific belief.[3]

How does this sort of model work? Here, we will give a relatively nontechnical description, as is appropriate for an interdisciplinary book. There are two features of these models – a decision problem and a network. Let us first discuss the decision problem. In all of the models we consider, agents face a two-armed bandit problem. A "bandit" is another name for a slot machine. The idea is that they face a problem analogous to choosing one of the two arms on a slot machine, where one arm pays out more often than the other. We use this problem to represent situations in science where agents are considering two possibilities – say, two theories, or two medical treatments – that may be more or less successful, and attempting to choose the best one. In what follows, we will refer to the two possible actions/theories as "Arm A" and "Arm B," in keeping with the two-armed bandit metaphor; in general, Arm B will refer to the more successful of the two actions (B is for "better").

How do agents choose? These models assume that agents have a belief about which arm is best, that they can gather evidence by actually testing the world, and that their belief is sensitive to the evidence gathered. Belief is represented by a credence – this is a number between 0 and 1 reflecting a degree of belief in something. For example, suppose that Karen thinks there is a 60% chance that arm B is better than arm A. We can say she has credence.6 that arm B is best. As mentioned, credences are sensitive to the evidence that agents gather from the world. Typically,

[2] There is another, highly influential, framework for modeling the spread of belief that treats beliefs like viruses in a contagion (Rogers, 2010). We focus on network epistemology as a better modeling framework for science because agents can gather and share evidence from the world to support belief.

[3] For more on the use of this framework in philosophy of science, see Zollman (2010b, 2013); Mayo-Wilson, Zollman, and Danks (2011); Kummerfeld and Zollman (2015); Holman and Bruner (2015, 2017); Rosenstock, Bruner, and O'Connor (2017); Borg, Frey, and Seselja (2017); Frey and Seselja (2017a, 2017b); Weatherall and O'Connor ((forthcoming), 2018); Weatherall, O'Connor, and Bruner (2018); O'Connor and Weatherall (2018, 2019).

these models start with agents who have random credences about whether A or B is better. In each round, agents decide to make a test. They can either pull arm A or arm B. A common assumption in these models is that their beliefs guide their choice – if a scientist thinks B is the better theory, she is more likely to test it. Then, based on the evidence they gather, they change their credence. Suppose an agent pulls arm B, and it is very successful. That agent's credence that B is better should go up. If arm B fails, this credence goes down. Many of these models assume agents change their beliefs using some version of Bayes rule, which probability theory tells us is the rationally best way to change beliefs in light of evidence. From model to model, there are variations on exactly how beliefs are represented, evidence is gathered, and beliefs are updated.

Now, let us turn to the network aspect of the model. Agents are part of a network where each node is an individual, and each edge is a social connection. Agents in this sort of model share the evidence they gather with their neighbors in the network. In this way, beliefs can spread throughout a network. How does this work? Suppose a community is settled on some theory, represented by arm A. This could be "cigarette smoking is safe." Now, one scientist develops a different theory, represented by arm B, "cigarette smoking causes cancer." This new belief leads the scientist to change behaviors. Now that they think cigarettes might be dangerous, they begin to gather data about whether this is indeed the case. If their evidence is persuasive, as they share it with their peers, these peers will also become convinced and begin to change their own behaviors to reflect the new belief. Over time, the entire network may switch to the new, successful theory. For this reason, a common endpoint of these models is that all agents have settled on a correct consensus.

This is not what always happens, though. Social influence can also lead the entire group to settle on incorrect beliefs. For instance, a few pieces of spurious evidence in favor of a false belief, if shared widely, may be enough to convince an entire community of something incorrect. In the next section, we will discuss this possibility at more length. And we will discuss what sorts of conditions make false consensus more or less likely in a scientific community.

Cases and Results

The models described in the last section have been widely used to study the spread of scientific beliefs. They have been used to ask: what is the best communication structure for science? Is there true wisdom of the crowds? Is experimentation good for scientific communities? How does cognitive diversity benefit science? In this section, we will briefly go through some variations in the model, connecting them with real cases from science.

Ulcers and the Zollman Effect In the early 1900s, scientists were divided on the topic of stomach ulcers. Some thought that ulcers were caused by bacteria, and others that the cause was stomach acid. There was evidence supporting both theories. But in 1954, the gastroenterologist E.D. Palmer, upon biopsying the stomachs of over 1000 patients, found no evidence of bacterial life at all (Palmer, 1954). Of course, stomachs do, in fact, have bacteria in them. Palmer's findings were misleading. But they were so influential that an entire generation of scientists turned away from the bacterial theory of ulcers and focused on treatments for stomach acid. It was not until 30 years later that researchers Robin Warren and Barry Marshall revived the bacterial theory. They did so in dramatic fashion. After encountering skepticism from the scientific community, Marshall downed a Petri dish of H. Pylori, the bacteria that cause stomach ulcers, developed a case of ulcers, and cured himself using antibiotics (Kidd & Modlin, 1998). In 2005, their work earned them a Nobel Prize.

Zollman (2007, 2010b) made a curious discovery about epistemic network models. One might think that in general communication among agents is a good thing. Each agent is gathering real evidence by testing the bandit arms. If each agent receives more of this good evidence from neighbors, surely they are better able to draw accurate conclusions. As it turns out, though, this is not always the case.

Scientific evidence is probabilistic, which means that sometimes it is misleading. For instance, many individual studies on the dangers of smoking find no link between tobacco and cancer. This is because not everybody who smokes gets cancer, and some people get cancer who do not smoke. If we do enough studies, some, by chance, will fail to detect the increased risk that smoking causes. Likewise, agents pulling arms on a bandit will sometimes get spurious results. Suppose arm A is successful 50% of the time, and arm B 60% of the time. An agent who tests arm B 10 times may find that it is successful in only four of these tests. These data make B look worse than A. In these models, sometimes a single set of misleading results of this sort will be enough to convince an entire network, or a large portion of it, of a false belief. In other words, too much connectivity can be a problem.

Here is another way to put the issue: some transient disagreement in beliefs is generally a good thing for a scientific community. Without diversity of belief, a community might fail to ever investigate a promising theory. A community that is too united, and communicates too much, may fail to maintain enough diversity of opinion to settle on the best option.

Zollman finds, in particular, that well-connected groups of researchers tend to come to consensus quicker in network epistemology models. But sparsely connected networks are more likely to settle on a true consensus, rather than a false one. This has since been called the Zollman effect.[4] Something like this is arguably what happened in the H. pylori case. Palmer's findings were too influential, and they led an entire community to prematurely settle on a false consensus. If a subcommunity had continued to test the bacterial theory, they may have managed to convince the larger community of the truth with the evidence they gathered.

[4]Though, as Zollman (2013) and Rosenstock et al. (2017) point out, this finding is sensitive to parameters in the model. For many parameters, there is no such effect (though it never seems to reverse). See also Frey and Seselja (2017a) for critiques of the robustness of these models.

Smallpox and Conformity Lady Mary Whortley Montague was a British aristocrat born in the late seventeenth century.[5] As a young woman, she suffered a bout of smallpox. While she survived, she lost a brother to the disease and she was permanently scarred. A few years later, Montague traveled to Turkey with her husband. While there, she encountered the practice of smallpox variolation. Similar to vaccination, this involved exposing patients to pus from smallpox pustules via a scratch on the arm. The subsequent infection tended to be mild, and to prevent further, more virulent infection. With a Turkish nurse and an English physician named Charles Maitland, she had her own son variolated before returning to England.

Upon her return in 1721, Lady Montague attempted to spread the practice, but met with resistance from English physicians. They were not particularly interested in a practice performed by Turkish women and advocated for by an English woman. Even Charles Maitland was unwilling to perform variolations once under the eye of his English peers.

Montague managed to get around their resistance in a particularly clever way. She was friends with Princess Caroline of Ansbach, who was married to the Crown Prince of England. Montague convinced the princess to publicly variolate her own two daughters. After this, the practice spread quickly among the nobility, especially those with personal connections to the princess and Lady Montague.

In O'Connor and Weatherall (2019), we argue that the spread of variolation in this case ultimately had relatively little to do with evidence and belief. Instead, it was a largely social phenomenon. Experimental psychologists, starting with Asch and Guetzkow (1951), have shown that humans have tendencies toward social conformity. We do not like to stick out from the crowd, and this leads to behaviors like publicly avowing a belief, even if we have good reason not to hold it (Bond & Smith, 1996). In the case of smallpox variolation, English physicians were likely influenced by conformist tendencies in assessing whether variolation might be a good practice. This is especially notable in the case of Maitland who was perfectly happy to perform a variolation in Turkey, but was hesitant to do so in England.

This tendency hurt the belief state of English physicians, but in this particular case conformity bias also ended up playing a positive role. Lady Montague made use of the desires of English nobility to conform to the practices of the most respected and influential members of their society. This desire helped convince many people to variolate once the princess did so.

In Weatherall and O'Connor (forthcoming), we consider what happens in epistemic network models when actors have a tendency to conform. We do this by supposing that they weigh two desires. The first is a desire to take the action best supported by their beliefs. The second is a desire to conform, by testing the theory that their network neighbors also test. Actors balance these desires in deciding which arm to pull.

In these models, the tendency toward conformity means that communities no longer necessarily converge to a consensus. Instead, sometimes there are cliques

[5] This history is drawn from Grundy et al. (1999).

that hold stable, opposing beliefs. Imagine if one clique settles on one action (variolating) and another on a different action (not variolating). Some members of the nonvariolating clique will learn the truth via evidence that comes from the other clique. But their desire to conform means that they never test the better action themselves, and thus they fail to spread evidence of its success to their network neighbors.

In general, the greater the tendency of actors in these models to conform, the worse the beliefs and practices of the agents. Conformity stops the natural spread of good practices to new parts of a social network. There are conditions that make these effects more or less serious, though. In particular, the models predict that conformity will be less of a problem when there is a big difference in the success of the theories under consideration. For instance, even strong social pressures will not protect a belief like "it is safe to drink cyanide" from disconfirmation. The negative consequences will outweigh the desire for social conformity. But we might expect conformity to play a big role in the spread of something like evolutionary theory. For most people, there are few consequences one way or another to believing in evolution. Thus, social pressures tend to determine what they espouse.[6]

Lyme Disease and Polarization Polarization is a popular political buzzword. It usually refers to situations where groups of individuals fail to achieve consensus, or even move further apart in belief/opinion over the course of interaction. Typical cases of polarization happen along political lines and involve differences in social and moral values. Consider, for instance, debates in the USA about gun control or abortion. In some cases, though, polarization happens over matters of scientific fact, and among groups of individuals who share values.

In the mid-1970s, rheumatologist Allen Steere identified Lyme disease as a new tick-borne illness. The symptoms of Lyme disease are many and varied, but typically involve joint pain, nerve pain, headaches, fatigue, and brain fog. Because Lyme is caused by a spirochete, it can be treated by antibiotics. This discovery thus radically improved the lives of thousands of sufferers whose symptoms were reduced or eliminated by antibiotic treatment. Despite this apparent success, however, by the late 1990s Steere was receiving death threats from Lyme patients.

In the early 1990s, Steere became concerned that Lyme was being treated as a catchall diagnosis for anyone suffering from pain and fatigue. He worried that the long-term antibiotics these sufferers were prescribed were causing unnecessary harm, and began to advocate for stricter standards in Lyme treatment. This was the beginning of what is now called the "Lyme wars." At the heart of this debate is the question of whether Lyme is always cured by a short dose of antibiotics, or whether it sometimes persists in a chronic form that requires long-term antibiotic treatment.

---

[6]Others have used different versions of network models to consider the role of conformity in belief. Zollman (2010a) points out that in cases where agents do not have better ways to combine data, conformity can play a beneficial role. Mohseni and Williams (2018) look at an epistemic network model where agents have expectations about how conformity influences their peers, and these expectations can change their social trust. They find that conformity bias hurts the ability of the network to develop accurate beliefs.

What is striking about this debate is that the physicians involved seem to share goals and values. They want to learn the truth, and they want to successfully treat the Lyme patients they see. Nonetheless, the two sides of the "war" are highly polarized. There is an enormous amount of mistrust. The physicians and patient groups who believe in chronic Lyme accuse the establishment camp of being influenced by money from insurers who do not want to pay for long-term treatment. The establishment physicians accuse doctors who treat chronic Lyme of taking financial advantage of vulnerable patients, and have often attempted to revoke their medical licenses.

In O'Connor and Weatherall (2018), we use epistemic network models to ask: how might a scientific community end up in such a polarized state? And might this happen without the influence of money or bad actors? There is a long literature using models to explore polarization, but these models are usually not well tuned to scientific communities. In previous polarization models, actors' opinions are typically determined solely on the basis of social influence, rather than evidence from the world.[7] And they usually change opinions in non-rational ways. Our goal is to consider agents who (1) collect evidence, (2) use this evidence to shape beliefs, and (3) share this evidence within their communities, but who nonetheless end up polarizing.

The key modification we make to the standard epistemic network model is to add a component of social trust. In particular, we assume that agents treat the evidence they receive as uncertain. If they see some set of data, they think there is some chance that these data are valid, and some chance that they are not. Furthermore, their level of uncertainty is determined by how close their beliefs are to a peer in the network. So, if two agents have very similar beliefs (both support chronic Lyme, say), they trust the evidence shared by the other. If two agents have disparate beliefs (one believes in chronic Lyme and one does not), they treat each other's evidence as uncertain. There is something reasonable about this – scientists should not treat all data as totally trustworthy, given the presence of quacks in scientific communities.

What we find is that this uncertainty can lead to stable polarization. When this happens, two groups form. One group has good beliefs, and takes the more successful action. The other group has worse beliefs, and takes the less successful action. But because this second group does not trust evidence coming from the first group, they never learn about the better action.

It is interesting to note that polarization can appear in the conformity models discussed above, as well. In that case, polarization arises when networks exhibit a certain "clique" structure, where there exist tightly knit groups that are only weakly connected to one another. In such cases, members of different cliques come to conform only with members of their own group, preventing outside information from coming into the clique. This mechanism is importantly different from the one that arises in the social trust models now under consideration. Consider how one might eliminate polarization in each case. If polarization arises from clique

[7] We do not review this literature here for space reasons. See O'Connor and Weatherall (2018) and Bramson et al. (2017) for reviews.

structure and conformity, increasing the degree of social connectedness of a community should lead to less polarization, because now information may flow more freely. But if social trust is responsible for polarization, new social connections will make no difference – unless agents have some reason to trust their new neighbors.

Across the polarization models we explore, we find that this sort of mistrust makes the community as a whole worse at forming beliefs. In particular, many more individuals end up with bad beliefs, because they ignore the best data available to them.[8]

Industrial Selection In the last two parts of this section, we will describe models that consider how outside forces, especially those from industry, can influence scientific beliefs.

In the late 1970s, medical researchers began to explore the arrhythmic suppression hypothesis, which states that because heart arrhythmias often precede a heart attack, suppressing arrhythmia might work to prevent them.[9] Bernard Lown, who first proposed this hypothesis, pointed out that it was not clear whether arrhythmia suppression would have the desired effect. He advocated for testing anti-arrhythmic medications by looking at whether they reduced heart attack deaths. Other researchers, though, tested the efficacy of these drugs by looking simply at whether they were successful at reducing arrhythmia. Pharmaceutical companies funded researchers only in the latter camp, and the results of this research led to the widespread prescription of anti-arrhythmics.

The problem was that these drugs in fact increased heart attack deaths, rather than preventing them. It was not until the late 1980s that the large-scale Cardiac Arrhythmic Suppression Trial showed this conclusively. It has been estimated that upwards of one hundred thousand deaths may have been caused by anti-arrhythmic medications in the intervening years.

There is a widespread idea that the way industry influences science or scientists is by paying scientists to get certain outcomes – that is, by scientific fraud. But as Holman and Bruner (2017) emphasize, the pharmaceutical industry did not need to buy off or even influence researchers in this case to have serious effects on the progress of science. Instead, they simply selected who was to receive funding. Holman and Bruner use the network epistemology framework to explore how industrial influence might shape a community in cases like this. In their model, not all scientists draw from the same bandit arms. Instead, the assumption that scientists use different methods means that some scientists pull arms that are biased in one direction or another. They assume that arm B is better than arm A, and most studies reflect this fact, but when some scientists pull arm B their payoffs are worse than

[8] In Weatherall and O'Connor (2018), we consider similar models but where actors consider multiple arenas of belief, and ground trust in all of these. For instance, in deciding whether to trust evidence about the safety of vaccines, an individual might compare beliefs about vaccines, but also about the safety of genetically modified (GMO) crops in deciding whom to trust. We find that groups holding multiple, polarized beliefs can endogenously emerge in these models.

[9] For the history of this episode, see Moore (1995).

A. Furthermore, the model assumes that funding levels influence the productivity of scientists, and that industry can shape these funding levels. In particular, industrial agents choose to fund only those scientists whose results tend to support A.

As they show, this can create a situation where results supporting the worse belief flood the community and convince many other researchers of the wrong thing. In addition, as they point out, various feedback loops can exacerbate the effect. Successful scientists who have received large grants are often better at placing students, and these students tend to use their (in this case, faulty) methods. They are also more likely to get independent government grants to support their research. The result is a community with widespread beliefs in the worse theory.

What is striking about this model, and the historical case, is that the pharmaceutical industry did not do what we typically think of when it comes to industry influence on science. They did not change the research practices that individual scientists were engaged in. There was no corruption or fraud. Instead, they made use of the natural variation within a community to shape outcomes in a much more insidious way. In the next section, we will discuss another set of models looking at subtle and surprising industry influences on scientific belief.

The Tobacco Strategy

The historians of science Oreskes and Conway (2011) painstakingly document how, starting in the 1950s, tobacco companies managed to spread public doubt about the growing consensus that cigarettes were dangerous. Their strategy, which Oreskes and Conway call "The Tobacco Strategy," involved fighting science with science for the first time. There were various components to this strategy. In Weatherall et al. (2018), we use models to explore the workings of several of these components.[10]

In 1954, six major US tobacco companies started an organization called The Tobacco Industry Research Committee, which was headed by a prominent geneticist. The ostensible goal of the committee was to fund research into whether tobacco smoking was dangerous to health. In fact, the group was a propaganda machine. In 1957, for example, they produced a pamphlet called "Smoking and Health" that emphasized independent research finding no link between tobacco and cancer while downplaying research that did find such a link. This pamphlet was distributed to hundreds of thousands of doctors and dentists.

We describe this sort of case as one of selective sharing. Industry propagandists were not producing biased research, and, in this particular case, were not even intervening in the scientific community in any way. Instead, they were taking advantage of the fact that scientific evidence is probabilistic. Remember, some studies on the link between cancer and cigarette smoke will not find any connection. Industry actors can widely publicize just these studies, while failing to mention the larger body of data supporting a link between smoking and cancer.

[10] See also Lewandowsky et al. (2019).

In our model, we supplement the basic network epistemology model with two new sorts of actors. The first we call observers. These actors do not test the world themselves, but they have credences, and they update these credences on the basis of evidence. They correspond to members of the public who are interested in developing true beliefs, but do not have the tools to gather evidence. Second, we add a propagandist. This agent scours the scientific community and in each round of the model shares only data that spuriously suggest arm A is better to each of the observers. In this way, they engage in selective sharing, and bias the total body of data seen by each observer toward the worse belief.

We analyze these models and ask: when the scientific community settles on successful beliefs, do the observers as well? Can the propagandist confound them simply by sharing real, independent data from the community? What we find is that for many parameter settings the propagandist can, indeed, convince the public of the worse belief. The problem at hand and the behaviors of the scientists, though, determine how easy it is for the propagandist to do this.

In particular, we focus on the role of sample size in this process. In the model, as discussed, agents can gather different amounts of data each round. They could pull arm B 10 times, for example, or 1000. Less data correspond to real-world studies that are lower powered. For these smaller studies, it is more likely that each one happens to support the worse theory. A large study, on the other hand, is very likely to support the better theory. What this means is that in communities where scientists run studies with small samples, propagandists have more material to work with, and are better at deceiving the public. The take-away is that when public belief is at stake, scientists should maintain high standards.

This observation also tells us something about the best strategies for propagandists. Suppose that the tobacco industry was funding research themselves, but that the scientists involved were unwilling to commit fraud. The smaller their studies, the more likely they are to generate a spurious result that industry can use in their best interests.

Conclusion

In this short piece, we have outlined some of the ways the network epistemology framework has been used to explore the workings of scientific communities. In particular, there are a number of lessons here about false belief and how scientific communities can go wrong. Biases toward conformity and an inclination to ground scientific trust in shared belief can hurt the knowledge producing capacity of a community. In addition, pernicious influencers, such as industry propagandists, can make use of subtle strategies that do not subvert the norms of science, but nonetheless mislead.

In general, this overview shows some of the reasons that formal models are useful in studying scientific communities. First, they allow us to represent and explore processes that, in the real world, are very hard to get empirical access to because of how large and extended they are. Second, they allow us to engage in interventions that tell us something about causal effects. We can add more conformity to the model, and observe that actors do worse. Or we can see what happens when study power goes up, to figure out how study power is linked to outcomes. It is typically impractical to make interventions like these in real communities of scientists. Last, the models allow us to gain understanding about causal processes by removing factors that are at play in the real world. For instance, real-world actors have many psychological biases and are sometimes bad at reasoning. In the real world, conformist biases and aspects of social trust are at play at the same time. By stripping away such factors, the models let us focus on just one aspect of the problem at a time.

Of course, stripping away factors that are important in the real world can also be dangerous in a model. It could be that other causal factors interact with things like conformity bias, or industrial selection, to negate, or seriously alter their consequences. For this reason, social modeling results like those discussed here must always be taken with a grain of salt and supplemented with historical and empirical work.

References

Asch, S. E., & Guetzkow, H. (1951). Effects of group pressure upon the modification and distortion of judgments. In *Groups, leadership, and men* (pp. 222–236). Pittsburgh, PA: Carnegie Press.

Bala, V., & Goyal, S. (1998). Learning from neighbours. *The Review of Economic Studies, 65*(3), 595–621.

Bond, R., & Smith, P. B. (1996). Culture and conformity: A meta-analysis of studies using Asch's (1952b, 1956) line judgment task. *Psychological Bulletin, 119*(1), 111.

Borg, A., Frey, D., & Seselja, D. (2017). Examining network effects in an argumentative agent-based model of scientific inquiry. In *International Workshop on Logic, Rationality and Interaction* (pp. 391–406). Berlin, Heidelberg: Springer.

Bramson, A., Grim, P., Singer, D. J., Berger, W. J., Sack, G., Fisher, S., et al. (2017). Understanding polarization: Meanings, measures, and model evaluation. *Philosophy of Science, 84*(1), 115–159.

Frey, D., & Seselja, D. (2017a). *Robustness and idealizations in agent-based models of scientific interaction*. philsci-archive.pitt.edu/14508/.

Frey, D., & Seselja, D. (2017b). *What is the function of highly idealized agent-based models of scientific inquiry?* https://journals.sagepub.com/doi/abs/10.1177/0048393118767085.

Grundy, I., et al. (1999). *Lady Mary Wortley Montagu*. Oxford, NY: Clarendon Press.

Holman, B., & Bruner, J. (2017). Experimentation by industrial selection. *Philosophy of Science, 84*(5), 1008–1019.

Holman, B., & Bruner, J. P. (2015). The problem of intransigently biased agents. *Philosophy of Science, 82*(5), 956–968.

Kidd, M., & Modlin, I. M. (1998). A century of helicobacter pylori. *Digestion, 59*(1), 1–15.

Kummerfeld, E., & Zollman, K. (2015). Conservatism and the scientific state of nature. *The British Journal for the Philosophy of Science, 67*(4), 1057–1076.

Lewandowsky, S., Pilditch, T. D., Madsen, J. K., Oreskes, N., James, S., & Risbey, J. S. (2019). Influence and seepage: An evidence-resistant minority can affect public opinion and scientific belief formation. *Cognition, 188*, 124–139.

Mayo-Wilson, C. (2014). The reliability of testimonial norms in scientific communities. *Synthese, 191*(1), 55–78.
Mayo-Wilson, C., Zollman, K., & Danks, D. (2011). The independence thesis: When individual and social epistemology diverge. *Philosophy of Science, 78*(4), 653–677.
Mohseni, A., & Williams, C. R. (2018). Truth and conformity on networks. *Erkenntnis*. 1–22
Moore, T. J. (1995). *Deadly medicine: Why tens of thousands of heart patients died in America's worst drug disaster*. New York: Simon and Schuster.
O'Connor, C., & Weatherall, J. O. (2018). Scientific polarization. *European Journal for Philosophy of Science, 8*(3), 855–875.
O'Connor, C., & Weatherall, J. O. (2019). *The misinformation age: How false beliefs spread*. New Haven, CT: Yale University Press.
Oreskes, N., & Conway, E. M. (2011). *Merchants of doubt: How a handful of scientists obscured the truth on issues from tobacco smoke to global warming*. New York: Bloomsbury Publishing.
Palmer, E. D. (1954). Investigation of the gastric spirochetes of the human. *Gastroenterology, 27*, 218–220.
Rogers, E. M. (2010). *Diffusion of innovations*. New York: Simon and Schuster.
Rosenstock, S., Justin Bruner, J., & O'Connor, C. (2017). In epistemic networks, is less really more? *Philosophy of Science, 84*(2), 234–252.
Weatherall, J. O., & O'Connor, C. (forthcoming). Conformity in scientific networks. *Synthese*.
Weatherall, J. O., & O'Connor, C. (2018). Endogenous epistemic factionalization: A network epistemology approach. *SSRN Electronic Journal*. https://doi.org/10.2139/ssrn.3304109
Weatherall, J. O., O'Connor, C., & Bruner, J. (2018). How to beat science and influence people. *British Journal for Philosophy of Science*. https://doi.org/10.1093/bjps/axy062
Zollman, K. J. S. (2007). The communication structure of epistemic communities. *Philosophy of Science, 74*(5), 574–587.
Zollman, K. J. S. (2010a). Social structure and the effects of conformity. *Synthese, 172*(3), 317–340.
Zollman, K. J. S. (2010b). The epistemic benefit of transient diversity. *Erkenntnis, 72*(1), 17.
Zollman, K. J. S. (2013). Network epistemology: Communication in epistemic communities. *Philosophy Compass, 8*(1), 15–27.

Chapter 5
Seven Cases: Examples of How Important Ideas Were Initially Attacked or Ridiculed by the Professions

David M. Allen and Elizabeth A. Reedy

Introduction

Scientists are generally both skeptical of new ideas and taught not to rush headlong into scientific fads that may later turn out to be wrong or partly wrong due to misinterpretations of scientific evidence. Given the history of the field, and examples such as phrenology or the use of leeches in medicine, this is, of course, the way scientists should be. It is the primary reason that replicating studies and examining and re-examining all the data produced as well as considering alternate explanations for any legitimate findings are all essential to the scientific enterprise. This sort of skepticism is often *under*employed if anything.

However, sometimes, scientific skepticism is acted out in ways that are counterproductive to the advancement of science. The usual culprit is herd behavior that is created by the interests of various groups that have an ideological, economic, or political stake in whether these new ideas become widely adopted. As this volume discusses, new ideas are often ridiculed; publication of important papers is blocked; research does not get funded, tenure requirements are not met, this leads to major damage to scientific careers.

Some scientists are able to break through, and their ideas eventually become the new conventional wisdom, while others fail miserably. The ideas and discoveries of those who fail are often "rediscovered" decades later. What distinguished those scientists who are able to break through group resistance from those who are not? This is an open question. For some, it seems that the character trait of being doggedly persistent is one necessary factor, but not in and by itself. Often, it also takes another

D. M. Allen, M.D. (✉) ·
Department of Psychiatry, University of Tennessee Health Science Center,
Memphis, TN, USA
e-mail: dallen49@comcast.net

E. A. Reedy
Penn State University, College of Nursing, University Park, Memphis, TN, USA

D. M. Allen, J. W. Howell (eds.), *Groupthink in Science*,
https://doi.org/10.1007/978-3-030-36822-7_5

person in the field who takes an interest, or an interested entity that has its own separate economic interests that provides funding for further research or even provides needed lab space. And often, plain old dumb luck seems to be in the mix as well. These phenomena are illustrated in the case examples that follow.

Stanley B. Prusiner, M.D., and Prions

As described in his book (2014), Stanley Prusiner won the Nobel Prize in 1977 for his discovery of prions, which are self-replicating and infectious agents composed entirely of proteins and containing neither DNA or RNA or any nucleic acid whatsoever. The virology community found this idea so difficult to process that they fought his ideas tooth and nail for many years—and he was still widely criticized by virologists even after winning the Nobel. In fact, when the prize was awarded, he was attacked in an article in *The New Yorker* entitled "Pathological Science" which said that it was highly likely that he would eventually be proved wrong, and that the Swedes had made a huge error.

Prusiner had at first started working on finding the cause of a disease called scrapie. That disorder, along with other conditions like Creutzfeldt–Jakob disease, was thought to be caused by something called a "slow virus." What he found instead were certain proteins that had been split up by an enzyme, and which made copies of itself.

The uproar in this field caused by the prion concept was similar to another one, although the earlier one did not last nearly as long. It was created by geneticist and neurologist Howard Temin. He, along with another scientist named David Baltimore who was working independently, showed that certain tumor viruses carried the ability to reverse the flow of information from RNA back to DNA using an enzyme called reverse transcriptase. At the time, this discovery upset a widely held belief by biologists including Francis Crick, who was one of the co-discoverers of the structure of DNA. That belief was that sequence information flows in only one direction from DNA to RNA to protein. Temin and Baltimore received the Nobel Prize in 1975. Their work was then widely accepted. Not so with Prusiner's initial efforts.

Prusiner's work was based on a body of knowledge that he had obtained through a long, arduous, and expensive process of testing and retesting. When his findings were attacked by his critics, he typically responded by going out and getting even more data. He was able to do this in spite of the fact that his research was very expensive. What made obtaining funding even more of a problem than it might have been otherwise is because his results were contradicting a well-accepted body of scientific knowledge. He had issues obtaining funding and lab space and even getting tenure at his university medical school so he could continue his work. With the help of a few colleagues, he managed to overcome them all.

He persevered even though he admittedly was not prepared to be the target of attacks by the scientific community that were at times quite personal and which continued over more than 10 years. Some attacks were done in person during scientific meetings. Prusiner seemed to be a highly competitive person, which was a major factor in his ability to persist. He really wanted to be the first to isolate and define the scrapie agent.

According to Prusiner (2014), other scientists would not even look at his findings. He was told to keep repeating the same negative experiments as long as necessary because they just *had* to reveal an agent with nucleic acids. He persisted even when fellow scientists came out in public saying a paper he published should never even have been accepted by the journal that printed it. One British scientist bemoaned the fact that his own funding was being cut whenever Prusiner made a discovery.

Prusiner also had a contentious relationship with the popular press. The controversy seemed to him to be more interesting to the press than the actual science, and journalists frequently made him look bad to the public. For this reason, he often refused to talk to them at all. Particularly damaging was an article in *Discover* which basically accused him of putting his own desire for fame over good science. His naming of the infectious agent as a *prion* was described as a publicity stunt, as the first two letters were the same as those of his last name. Another scientist used the *Discover* article to attack his character at a meeting of the CIBA foundation in London in 1987. Prusiner was there to receive an award from the prestigious Albert Lasker Foundation for basic medical research; a newspaper article made it sound as if the foundation had been duped.

Through his ability to network with colleagues and make valuable connections, the backing of the dean of his medical school, and sometimes just dumb luck, he was able to regain both funding and lab space when sources of both suddenly dried up. Much of his early research at the University of California San Francisco Medical Center was funded by the Howard Hughes Medical Institute; this funding was suddenly withdrawn just when he was about to be up for promotion and tenure. Furthermore, the neurology faculty at his school was often unsupportive and often discouraged graduate students from working with him. With the help of his Dean, however, he was able to secure continued funding—from a Tobacco company!

He related an incident in his book in which he said he felt that the editor of the prestigious journal *Science* was dragging his feet on publishing one of his papers, even though it had already been accepted. Prusiner thought the editor was hoping against hope that a nucleic acid would somehow turn up in the work of some other researcher.

E.O. Wilson and Kin Selection

E.O. Wilson was an entomologist (the study of insects) who was fascinated by the behavior of worker ants, who seem to be sacrificing their own reproductive success in order to enhance the reproductive success of their queen. He later wrote a groundbreaking volume about the relationship between evolution, group behavior, and individual behavior in various species. The book (1974) was *Sociobiology: A New Synthesis.* He made the political mistake of including a final chapter that had the audacity to describe, somewhat speculatively, his ideas about the possible relationships between genes and culture in human beings.

He employed the concept of *kin selection*, an old idea that was somewhat popularized by William Donald Hamilton and others in 1964. It refers to ideas that Charles Darwin himself had considered: the idea that organisms might, under certain environmental conditions, have a tendency to sacrifice themselves in order to ensure the survival of closely related kin. This tendency would be a powerful one because the probability of genes being passed down is increased by their presence in several organisms rather than if they are present in only one. An individual may have a great adaptive gene, but if it is killed off before the organism reproduces, that gene will be lost. Therefore, organisms with this tendency would be more likely to survive because of natural selection. Wilson discussed what this might mean in the case of human beings, and in particular, what it might say about the culture of groups.

The chapter on humans was only 30 pages long and consisted mostly of speculation about possible roles for genes in aspects of human culture that are characteristic of many societies all over the world. He spoke of how genes and culture *co-evolve*. Despite the obvious omnipresence of tribalistic behavior of various sorts that is quite similar in cultural groups all over the world, he was immediately attacked by leftists, including two Marxist biologists in his own University Department, Stephen J. Gould and Richard Lewontin (Campbell, 1986). According to Ed Douglas (2001), Wilson was accused of racism and misogyny, of suggesting that some human beings are genetically superior to others, and of echoing the doctrines of eugenics that helped lead to the rise of Nazi Germany. Wilson and his ideas were featured on the cover of *Time* and the front page of *The New York Times*.

Richard Dawkins opined that part of the reason for the viciousness of the attacks against him was that Wilson was talking about scientific issues that had been the exclusive province of sociologists and anthropologists, and he was perceived as "trying to move in on their territory." This, of course, was a bit of tribalism itself, exhibited by the critical scientists. Additionally, a large part of the furor over Wilson was political and not scientific at all.

Things came to a head, literally and figuratively, with two events: an article published in *The New York Review of Books* in November of 1975, and an incident in which a group of radical students poured a pitcher of ice water on his head while he was giving a talk at a meeting of the American Association for the Advancement of Science in February of 1978.

Fifteen scholars in the Boston area, including Gould and Lewontin, had formed the Sociobiology Study Group. The group believed that the main purpose of science was to promote socialism and saw sociobiology as right wing and deterministic. The article they wrote in 1975 accused Wilson of saying or implying many things he never actually said or implied, as he pointed out in a rebuttal of his own in *Bioscience* in March of 1976. They said he believed that deviant behavior was genetically based and that he was giving a genetic justification for the status quo. Even worse, they mischaracterized his position as advancing the notion that anything that is adaptive is good, and so his ideas justified *any* existing social order. They also made the odd case that an understanding of behavior of animals is in all cases irrelevant to understanding the behavior of people.

Wilson replied that he was indifferent to determinism and that he did not believe that human behavior was either infinitely malleable or completely fixed. He actually thought environment was more important than genetics in determining human behavior, not less. He made the case that the last chapter of *Sociobiology* was intended as a beginning of the discussion, not the final conclusion—it described working hypotheses, not facts. He accused his attackers of misstating what he believed about the rate that the evolution of human culture occurs. Additionally, he made the point, now generally accepted, that any genetic influences on behavior do not come from single genes, but result from the product of the interactions of a large number of genes operating within a specific environment.

Three years after the Sociobiology Study Group article, Wilson was assaulted during a speech at the annual meeting of the American Association for the Advancement of Science. The demonstrators were affiliated with the International Committee Against Racism, a front group of the Marxist Progressive Labor Party. They carried anti-sociobiology signs—one displaying a swastika—and chanted "Racist Wilson you can't hide, we charge you with genocide!" The demonstrator who dumped the ice water yelled out, "Wilson, you're all wet!" Wilson went on to give his talk despite the attack, and in spite of the fact that the police were not called and the protestors were not even asked to leave the hall.

This whole fiasco was emblematic of a particular viewpoint in many fields of scientific inquiry that wants to stop the research or even discussion about any scientific fact that *might* be used as ammunition by certain political or social groups to advance a nefarious or destructive cause. Even today, many evolutionary biologists reject kin selection not because of a lack of evidence for it, but because some group or other might use it to justify politics based on social Darwinism.

Clair Patterson and Lead in Gasoline

The story of Clair Patterson clearly illustrates how groups with economic interests can hire scientists to spread confusion about scientific issues. In the new, 2014 edition of the PBS series *Cosmos* with Neil DeGrasse Tyson, the story of Cal Tech geochemist Clair Patterson and his battles with the oil industry over the toxicity of lead in gasoline was reviewed in some detail. The story was also covered in an article by Needleman (1998).

Patterson (1965), in a paper published in the September issue of *Archives of Environmental Health*, refuted the scientific belief, which had come mostly from scientists in the fossil fuel industry such as Robert Kehoe, that industrial and natural sources contributed roughly equal amounts of lead to the environment that people might ingest and absorb, and that the total level they absorbed was safe.

Patterson originally had been working on an unrelated problem: trying to measure the age of the earth, which had yet to be established. In this effort, he had been trying to measure the lead—a product of the radioactive decay of uranium—in certain crystals, but kept getting wildly different results. After 6 years of trying to find a way to work in a super clean laboratory, he came to understand that there was significant lead contamination in the environment and that it mostly originated not from the natural environment but from the burning of automobile fuel that contained lead.

Lead had long known to be poisonous. It had even been considered by the US War Department for use in poisonous gases in weapons prior to chemical weapons being "outlawed" by the 1925 Geneva Protocol. We now know that even trace amounts of lead are not safe in human beings. It displaces from cells important and useful minerals like zinc, and it interferes with electrical transmission in nerve cells. The latter is particularly problematic in the developing brains of children.

Nonetheless, lead has useful properties used in such things as paint and gasoline. Advertisements, ran by manufacturers of paints, even tried to portray lead as child friendly. In the early 1920s, tetraethyl lead was added to gasoline to stop engine "knock." This substance is particularly problematic because it is fat soluble and easily penetrates human skin. Workers involved in its production within the Ethyl Corporation, which began manufacturing the substance, quickly gave it the tag "loony gas" because anyone who spent much time handling the additive showed stunning signs of mental deterioration, from memory loss to loss of coordination to sudden twitchy bursts of rage. In October of 1924, workers began collapsing, going into convulsions, developing hallucinations, and babbling incoherently.

The petroleum and chemical industries hired a scientist named Robert Kehoe to put to rest potential public concern by sewing doubts about lead's dangers. He made the case that the industry could handle the problem of poisoning of the lead workers and that, outside of those involved in manufacturing, there was no threat to consumers. He was not challenged on this for decades. Highly relevant was the fact that almost all funding for studying lead came from industry sources and was directed to Kehoe—for the next 50 years. He, therefore, had a sort of monopoly on relevant information.

Oddly, Clair Patterson's work on measuring lead had also been originally financed by a grant from the American Petroleum Institute. He, like most people at the time, assumed that the contamination in his lab was occurring naturally. Just to be certain, he used the grant to measure lead concentrations in seawater at the surface and in deeper water, and he was surprised to learn that the surface water contained lead levels hundreds of times greater than the water below. Since he also knew how slowly lead could mix in solutions, he realized that this could not have happened naturally.

He published his findings in the journal *Nature*. Very soon afterward, the American Petroleum offered him a lot of grant funding but only if he would switch the focus of his studies from lead to other trace elements. When he refused, his funding vanished, and they even tried to get him fired from his research position. In 1971, he was excluded from a National Research Council panel on atmospheric lead contamination even though he was considered the foremost expert on the subject. Patterson's research also lead to outrage from the toxicological establishment because Patterson had the nerve to step outside of his field and talk about people instead of minerals.

In 1966, the issue came before a congressional subcommittee chaired by Senator Edmund Muskie. The hearing was scheduled, perhaps knowingly, when Patterson was away in Antarctica, studying whether or not his findings with ocean water would also be relevant to lead levels in the ice sheets. Nonetheless, after a few days, he was able to make a surprise appearance before the Committee.

Kehoe had already testified regarding his own scientific conclusions. He cited studies of the environment around Cincinnati that seemed to show that the amount of lead had actually *decreased*. He neglected to mention that those studies were biased by the fact that the later ones took samples from far fewer industrial sites than the earlier ones. He nonetheless argued that the levels of lead present in the general environment were about the same everywhere, so therefore they were "typical" and somehow therefore "safe."

Some of the actual numbers concerning amounts of lead in the environment used by Patterson to come to a different conclusion were actually the same as the ones Kehoe had cited. Patterson argued that just because these levels were common, that hardly proved they were safe. Kehoe seemed to be arguing that lead poisoning is either present or absent rather than that the amount of lead one has in one's system leads to different degrees of being poisoned.

Patterson had to fight industry for another 20 years before lead was finally banned in consumer products in the United States. Luckily, there were people in the military, the Atomic Energy Commission, and the National Science Foundation who were concerned enough to continue funding his work.

The National Research Network funded two studies under the Environmental Protection Agency. The first was released in 1972. Neither the committee members nor its consultants had personally worked on airborne contamination, while Patterson and three other highly qualified scientists were excluded. There was heavy industry participation. However, a second report was commissioned in 1980, and this time Patterson was included. Still, he had to have a separate entire chapter in the report discussing a dissenting opinion from the one expressed in the Network's conclusions.

Amazingly, Patterson finally prevailed. In 1990, in amendments to the Clean Air Act, lead was banned from gasoline. The measure was to take effect in 1995, giving gasoline companies five more years to completely phase out lead. Later studies revealed that after lead was removed, blood levels of lead in both children and adults fell by 80%.

J. Robin Warren, Barry Marshall and Peptic Ulcers and the Helicobacter Bacteria

Although a spiral-shaped bacterium (later called Helicobacter) had been described as present in the lining of the stomach by a doctor in 1893, because the bacteria could not be cultured at the time, these findings were ignored for decades by the medical and scientific establishment. The story of their re-discovery was told by Tanenbaum (2005), Altman (2005), and in an interview with Barry Marshall by Jennifer Abbasi (2017).

Ulcers were serious medical problems and could sometimes lead to death. You would think doctors and the public would be overjoyed at the prospect of an effective cure, but such was not the case. In 1979, Dr. J. Robin Warren, a pathologist, again noticed the spiral-shaped bacteria in the stomach biopsies in a hospital in Perth, Australia, and thought it might be the cause of peptic ulcer disease (PUD). This idea was met with profound skepticism from most of his colleagues. The prevailing view was that the stomach was too acidic to possibly harbor any bacteria, and that stress was the primary cause of stomach and duodenal ulcers. In April of 1982, Dr. Marshall, a gastroenterologist, cultured *Helicobacter pylori* from patients with gastritis (inflammation of the stomach lining). By 1983, the two doctors were almost certain that the bacteria were also the cause of PUD.

Part of the reason they were certain that they were on the right track was because existing treatments like antacids and histamine blockers such as Tagamet did not cure the disease—the ulcers would return soon after they were discontinued. With certain antibiotic treatments, however, a large percentage of patients not only got better much more quickly with antibiotics but seemed, in fact, to be cured completely.

Nonetheless, it took a good 10 years before their treatment became widely accepted, with pockets of resistance persisting well into the late 1990s. In 1982, the Australian Gastroenterological Society rejected as unimportant a study by Marshall that was later published in the *Lancet.* In July of 1984, Marshall even took the somewhat unusual and perhaps even foolhardy step of serving as his own research subject. He ingested a pure culture of *H. pylori.* Although he did not develop a peptic ulcer, he did, not surprisingly, develop gastritis. Endoscopy and a biopsy demonstrated that the bacteria were abundant in the inflamed portions of his stomach.

A 1994 National Institute of Health report made the recommendation that antibiotics, combined with drugs that reduced stomach acid (proton pump inhibitors like Omeprazole which increase the effectiveness of the antibiotic treatment), should be used in all infected cases of PUD. About 19 of 20 patients with duodenal ulcers, for example, had such infections. Even after that report, doctors challenged the research on which the recommendation was based, with a popular argument being that the bacteria that was seen was not the actual cause of the disorder but merely an opportunistic bug that was able to survive within preexisting ulcers. It was not until 2005 that Warren and Marshall's incredible discovery was rewarded, as with Stanley Prusiner, with a Nobel Prize—this time in physiology and medicine.

There were myriad reasons why the idea of ulcers being causing by an infection had such a hard time becoming accepted. Oddly, the usual groupthink involved in the competition and professional hubris between various medical specialties or academic research was in one aspect partly backward. Marshall was a gastroenterologist, but it was his fellow gastroenterologists who resisted him the most strongly of all the specialists. Infectious disease doctors were much happier to come on board with him.

Doctors from a couple of other specialties also became critics, primarily due to economic concerns. Surgeons often made considerable sums removing parts of the stomach from patients with serious bleeding or chronic symptomatology from ulcers. Then, there was the prevailing wisdom that stress was a cause of ulcers, which led psychiatrists and psychologists to want to treat sufferers for that. Naturally, drug companies had a significant financial stake in existing treatments, as drugs like histamine blockers had to be taken indefinitely, whereas curing the patients with antibiotics only involved short-term use of medications—and usually only once. Tagamet had been the first drug to reach $1 billion dollars in annual sales due primarily to long-time use by ulcer sufferers.

Other factors that delayed general scientific approval was the location of the researchers in far off Western Australia and the difficulty getting grant funding for innovative ideas due to financial limitations at the American National Institutes of Health. In an interview (Abbasi, 2017), Marshall also described the usual publication biases against articles that were at odds with conventional thinking on a subject. Luck was on the side of Warren and Marshall because Hill and Knowlton, a public relations firm who also represented the makers of Pepto-Bismol (which also increased the effectiveness of antibiotic treatments in the acidic stomach), managed to obtain coverage in popular lay publications such as *Reader's Digest*.

Alfred Wegener and Continental Drift

Any child in grade school looking at a world map for the first time can notice right away that the east coast of South America and the west coast of Africa seem to fit together like pieces of a jigsaw puzzle, and perhaps wonder about it for a while. It is that obvious. If anything, they might think it an odd coincidence.

Between 1911 and 1915, A German meteorologist named Alfred Wegener found additional evidence that the two continents might actually have been joined together at some time in the distant past. Later it was found that he was indeed correct (University of California Museum of Palentology, n.d.). His story was told by Burke (1985) and the PBS televisions series, *The Day the Universe Changed.*

Wegener had noted that the geology of the areas near the two coastlines was unmistakably similar, and that many fossils in both areas that came from the Paleozoic Era, but none that came from later time periods, were identical. Although he did not know exactly how, it appeared to him that the continents may be drifting apart. Perhaps they were floating in some way on heavier materials on the ocean floor. He then noted striking similarities between large-scale geological features further north. For example, the Appalachian Mountains of eastern North America matched with the Scottish Highland. In 1915, his theories were outlined in the first edition of *The Origin of Continents and Oceans,* in which he claimed that about 300 million years ago, the continents formed a single mass which he called Pangaea which then split, with the pieces moving apart from each other ever since.

Geologists thought he was crazy—especially since he was not even a geologist. In order to explain the fossils, they had actually hypothesized that there must have been some sort of now-sunken land bridges (of which there is no evidence) between the two continents. This, despite the fact that, at their closest, South America and Africa are approximately 1,770 miles, apart! Since there were also some flaws in Wegener's original theory, as one might expect, these also led to scathing criticism. How could the continents be able to move without the sheer forces involved distorting them beyond all recognition? The American Association of Petroleum Geologists had a whole symposium opposing the whole idea of continental drift after an English version of Wegener's work was published in 1925.

It took another 30 years before other scientists began to take Wegener's ideas seriously. In the 1950s, newly invented magnetometers showed evidence that rocks retain their original magnetic orientation, yet that orientation seems anomalous in many samples. A decade later, oceanographers found that they had to alter their original views about the seabed on which the continents seem to rest, because there was unmistakable evidence of continued movement. The seabed was also found to be younger and considerably thinner than previously thought. In 1966, magnetic profiles were used to demonstrate that the seabed was spreading outward from ridges, literally pushing the continents apart. By then, the theory of *plate tectonics* was well supported by geologists everywhere.

Joseph Altman, Michael Kaplan, Fernando Nottebohm, Elizabeth Gould and Neurogenesis in Birds and Mammals

For many decades, a given in neuroscience was that very few new brain cells are present after birth in both birds and mammals, including human beings, and that adult brains make no new ones at all. No stem cells created any new circuits, and new cells were not required for any functions of the adult brain. When findings started to come out that challenged this idea, resistance was high, particularly from a leader in the field, Pasko Rakic of Yale. The saga of this dispute was recounted by Robert Sapolsky in his book *Behave* (2017), and in the popular press in an article by Michael Spektor (2001) in *The New Yorker.*

An associate professor named Joseph Altman and his collaborator, Gopal Das, found in 1965 the first evidence of adult neurogenesis. They used new laboratory techniques that involved radioactive tagging of DNA molecules which were then injected into adult rats. While his results were published in respectable journals, the finding was rejected by leaders in the field. Because he was not tenured at the time, his academic career was negatively impacted. He eventually failed to get tenure, he had to move to another university, and his funding for adult neurogenesis studies dried up.

Ten years later, another scientist named Michael Kaplan found new evidence for Altman's findings using even newer techniques. Just as with Altman, he experienced the reception of negative reactions by leaders in the field, most notably Rakic, who said he had looked for new neurons himself and they simply did not exist. This rejection turned out to be poison for Kaplan's academic career, and in frustration, he eventually left it behind altogether.

Still another 10 years elapsed before yet another scientist, Fernando Nottebohm, unexpectedly found more evidence of adult neurogenesis—in birds. He found that if you gave testosterone to a female canary, the brain nuclei responsible for its song doubled in size. He later found new neurons in those birds that learn new songs every year. He, unlike his predecessors, was highly respected, and as Sapolsky describes him, "…As good an old boy as you get" (p.148). At first, even his findings were pooh poohed; what about mammals, let alone people? And how could he be sure that the new cells were actually neurons, or that they were really new?

Luckily, even newer laboratory techniques were being developed that helped a behavioral scientist named Elizabeth Gould, described as "driven" by Specter, to demonstrate neurogenesis in the brains of rats. She embarked on this work after she noted that, in rats, when large numbers of neurons in the part of the brain called the hippocampus died off due to destruction of a certain gland, there seemed to be no corresponding decrease in their total number soon afterward. She then started looking into whether there was any evidence that new cells might be being produced, and happened upon the work of Altman. She later discovered neurogenesis in monkeys. Soon, even Rakic started to find adult neurogenesis, but protested that the new cells were few and far between, and did not occur in the higher center of the brain, the cerebral cortex. In Spektor's article, Nottebohm reluctantly remarked that in his opinion, Rakic had single-handedly held the field of neurogenesis back for about a decade.

We now know that neurogenesis and the incorporation of new neurons into existing circuits is quite prominent in a part of the brain called the hippocampus that is important in incorporating some types of new learning, and that there also is, in fact, some neurogenesis in the cortex. Neurogenesis can be stimulated by a wide variety of physical activities and factors, including exercise and antidepressant drugs. Unfortunately, although brain injury can stimulate neurogenesis, it is not enough to lead to actual improvement in brain functioning, and in some cases actually might make the damage worse rather than better (Sapolsky, 2017).

Saving the strangest case for last in this chapter, the last section of the chapter tells the story of one doctor who literally had to set up shop in a New York City amusement park and charge admission to his "ward."

Hatching Babies? Martin Couney and the Rise of the Infant Incubator

In the twenty-first century, prematurely born babies are cared for in neonatal intensive care units around the world. These units are located in big cities and rural areas, large hospitals and small hospitals. Upon birth, many of these babies are placed in infant incubators designed to monitor their temperature and provide the warmth necessary for survival. Some babies spend weeks and months in the incubators, removed only for parental bonding, medical procedures, and sometimes for feeding. This type of care is expected and accepted by the general public and the general medical community. However, it was not always so.

Toward the end of the nineteenth century, physicians and scientists "discovered" prematurely born infants. Naturally, babies born prematurely were not a new phenomenon, but previously were not generally thought about, other than that they were an unfortunate burden on the family and potentially on society at large. Many people simply referred to premature babies as weaklings (Baker, 1996).

But parents tried to help their newborns. Wrapped in blankets, feathers, or even leaves for warmth and fed carefully; some survived and prospered (Ackerknecht, 1946). It took the advent of new considerations for the plight of all babies and children in the industrial age to bring outside attention to the "preemies." Beginning in France in the 1870s and spreading across Europe to the United States by the 1890s, preemies caught the attention of a slowly increasing number of physicians and the general public. Displayed in incubators at world, national, and regional fairs and exhibitions, they were the darlings of the Midway.

The first incubator exhibits were set up in France by Alexandre Lion, an early proponent and inventor of incubators. These exhibits typically were set up in store fronts in cities, including Paris, Bordeaux, Lyons, and Marseilles in the early 1890s. The general public was charged admission to view the premature babies being cared for in the incubator. The success of these exhibits led to incubator shows at fairs and exhibitions on an increasingly large scale. Martin Couney, a physician originally from Europe, brought the concept of the incubator show to America in 1898 at the Trans-Mississippi and International Exposition. Later, national exhibitions took place at the Pan-American Exposition in Buffalo in 1901, the Louisiana Purchase Exposition in St. Louis in 1904, and the Chicago Century of Progress exhibition in 1933–1934, among others. Yearly exhibitions took place on Coney Island and the Boardwalk in Atlantic City, New Jersey. For his efforts, he was routinely ignored and vilified by the traditional medical establishment for promising that a machine could help save these babies. In 1906 and again in 1911, the New York Society for the Prevention of Cruelty to Children tried to pass legislation outlawing incubator shows. Although unsuccessful, efforts like these added to the belief among medical professionals that the incubator shows were spectacle at best and potentially dangerous at worst (Editor, 1898; Silverman, 1979) (Baker, 1996; Reedy, 2003).

The incubators of the time were far from the high tech wonders of today. Most did not accurately regulate temperature within the infant compartment and all required frequent maintenance to work at all. Some became too hot and others too cold, and many premature babies still died despite incubator use (Baker, 1996). But Couney's incubator shows provided some hope for parents who felt they had nowhere else to turn. That Couney was a showman is not disputed. He did claim he was providing "propaganda for the preemies" (Liebling, 1939), and he did charge admission to those who wanted to view his patients in the incubators. His shows were not accepted in the scientific and technological areas of world's fairs and exhibitions, but were relegated to the Midway with the other carnival style shows. His incubator shows at Coney Island and the Atlantic City Boardwalk every summer among the rides and amusements of the boardwalk only added to his negative perception among the learned men of science (Baker, 1996) (Reedy, 2003).

Another issue for which Couney was roundly criticized was that the babies remaining in the incubator shows at the end of the Fair, or the end of the summer season on the boardwalk, were often sent home with no potential for continuing or follow-up care. This began to change with the Chicago Century of Progress exhibition in 1933 and 1934. In 1922, Julius Hess, MD, established the first, permanent Infant Incubator Center (the precursor to the NICU) at the Michael Reese Hospital in Chicago. There, nurses under the direction of Evelyn Lundeen, RN, provided premature-specific care to babies in incubators which were often designed by Hess himself. Babies born prematurely at home, at other area Chicago hospitals, and at Michael Reese were routinely admitted and provided warmth, nutrition, and infection prevention. It should be noted that not all babies cared for in incubators survived, whether in the hospital or at an exhibition. Those who could not breathe died as infant ventilators would not be available until the 1960s and 1970s, but the acceptance of incubator use was growing, at least in Chicago, throughout the 1920s and early 1930s. Once Couney agreed to set up an exhibit at the Century of Progress in 1933, he turned to his friend Hess, often considered the "Father of American Neonatology," for assistance. Hess transferred babies from the Infant Incubator Center at Michael Reese Hospital to Couney's exhibit for the duration of the fair in 1933 and 1934. Nurses from Michael Reese were assigned to care for these babies. At the end of the fair each autumn, the babies still remaining in the incubators were returned to the hospital (Baker, 1996).

The incubator shows were a hit with the general public. The shows were well attended, and their popularity is evidenced by the location of the Century of Progress's exhibit close to one of the major entrances to the fair. Babies who might have died were saved, and the gratitude of parents everywhere they ran was evident. In the process, Couney demonstrated this new, if imperfect, manner of caring for the prematurely born to the masses. The earliest incubators were soon replaced by newer models and new procedures. The birth of the Dionne quintuplets of Quebec, Canada, at the start of the 1934 season in Chicago brought further attention to the plight of premature babies and the role of incubators.

Couney continued his displays until just after America's entrance into World War II although it was not until the postwar era that incubators became a standard of care within hospital nurseries. It is still tempting today to write off Couney's efforts as pure sensationalism and the evidence is clear that incubator technology developed and improved throughout his career and probably would have done so without the influence of the shows and exhibitions. The location of the incubator shows among the side show madness of the Midway in the national fairs and exhibitions and along the Boardwalks of Coney Island and Atlantic City perpetuated the view of the shows as purely entertainment and made it easy for physicians and scientists to ignore.

Thus, while Couney was widely viewed as nothing more than a showman, his "propaganda" did result in increased attention to a machine that would revolutionize the care and survival of babies born too soon. The general public came to expect and even demand that prematurely born infants not be ignored any longer and sought out physicians and hospitals who would honor that demand. Couney was afforded some accolades from the medical profession toward the end of his career. Hess dedicated his neonatology textbook to him, and the New York medical profession, along with Hess, celebrated his work at a banquet in 1939. Couney died in 1950, 7 years after his incubator show on Coney Island closed. Hospitals were by then welcoming premature babies and caring for them in incubators on a routine basis (Baker, 1996; Reedy, 2003).

References

Abbasi, J. (2017). Barry Marshall, MD: *H pylori* 35 years later. *JAMA, 317*(14), 1400–1402.

Ackerknecht, E. (1946). Incubator and taboo. *Journal of the History of Medicine, 144*.

Altman, L. (2005, October 11). Nobel came after years of battling the system. *New York Times*.

Baker, J. P. (1996). *The machine in the nursery, incubator technology and the origins of newborn intensive care*. Baltimore, MD: The Johns Hopkins University Press.

Burke, J. (1985). *The day the universe changed*. Boston: Little Brown and Company.

Campbell, C. (1986). *Anatomy of a fierce academic feud*. Available at https://www.nytimes.com/1986/11/09/education/anatomy-of-a-fierce-academic-feud.html

Douglas, E. (2001, February 16). Darwin's natural heir. *The Guardian*. Available at https://www.theguardian.com/science/2001/feb/17/books.guardianreview57

Editor. (1898). The danger of making a public show of incubators for babies. *The Lancet*, 390–391.

Liebling, A. (1939, June 3) Patron of the Preemies. *The New Yorker*, pp. 20–24.

Needleman, H. (1998). Clair Patterson and Robert Kehoe: Two views of lead toxicity. *Environmental Research, 78*(2), 71–78.

Patterson, C. (1965). Contaminated and natural Lead environments of man. *Archives of Environmental Health: An International Journal, 11*(3), 344–360.

Prusiner, S. (2014). *Madness and memory*. New Haven, CT: Yale University Press.

Reedy, E. A. (2003). From weakling to fighter: Changing the image of premature infants. *Nursing History Review*, 109–127.

Sapolsky, R. (2017). *Behave: The biology of humans at our best and worst*. New York: Penguin Pres.

Silverman, W. A. (1979). Incubator-Baby Side shows. *Pediatrics*, 127–141.

Specter, M. (2001, July 23). Rethinking the brain. *The New Yorker*, 42–53.

Tanenbaum, J. (2005). Delayed gratification: why it took everybody so long to acknowledge that bacteria cause ulcers. *Journal of Young Investigators*, February. Available via https://www.jyi.org/2005-february/2005/2/9/delayed-gratification-why-it-took-everybody-so-long-to-acknowledge-that-bacteria-cause-ulcers

University of California Museum of Paleontology website. (n.d.). Alfred Wegener (1880-1930). Available at http://www.ucmp.berkeley.edu/history/wegener.html

Wilson, E. (1974). *Sociobiology: A new synthesis*. Cambridge MA: Belknap Press.

Part II
Manipulation and Use of Social Influence in Science: The Financing, Design, and Dissemination of Research Studies and Results

Chapter 6
Sham Dealing and Sham Peer Review in Academic Publishing: Perspectives from a Case Study in a Mexican University

Florencia Peña Saint-Martin

Introduction

The changes in the Mexican universities and higher education institutions (HEIs) in their internal dynamics have been many and diverse, due to the impact of the structural adjustment policies imposed since the early 1980s (Ibarra, 2002). HEIs are now organized as private enterprises providing educational services and are forced to qualify as "productive" to get extra financial resources. In the logic of private enterprises' accountability, their outcomes are now evaluated by measuring their efficiency and "productivity." Some of the criteria used to assess this productivity are the number of students enrolled—particularly graduate ones—students' performance measured by the percentage getting their degrees on time, the percentage of full-time professors with a PhD, and the number of professors' publications (Peña & Fernández, 2016).

This new logic has promoted internal competition which has impacted the relationships of the members of the academic communities within and between different types of employees in complex and recursive ways. It has affected managers, administrative staff, professors, part-time teachers, and both undergraduate and graduate students. In addition, from 1984 on using the same productivity logic, membership in the National System of Researchers (*Sistema Nacional de Investigadores*, SNI) has almost become a requirement for full-time professors. This is a program of the National Council for Science and Technology (*Consejo Nacional de Ciencia y Tecnología*, CONACyT) to which only professors who can claim "high research productivity" can belong. Hence, membership not only provides symbolic capital for professors, it also has an important impact on the prestige

F. Peña Saint-Martin (✉)
Graduate Program of Physical Antrhopology, National School of Anthropology and History, Mexico City, Mexico

D. M. Allen, J. W. Howell (eds.), *Groupthink in Science*,
https://doi.org/10.1007/978-3-030-36822-7_6

of their HEI and the programs they work for. Being a member of the SNI also increases professors' revenues during a time in which basic salaries have stagnated (Ibarra & Rondero, 2008). "High productivity" is measured primarily through publications (especially in international journals), tutoring graduate students (mainly PhDs), and leading research groups (preferably international ones). The SNI clearly lays out its rules and its criteria for evaluating professors[1] (http://www.conacyt.mx/index.php/el-conacyt/convocatorias-y-resultados-conacyt/convocatorias-sistema-nacional-de-investigadores-sni/marco-legal-sni/reglamento-sni/841-reglamento2013-1/file, October 18 de 2017).

> The National System of Researchers was created by Presidential Agreement and published in the *Official Gazette of the Federation* on July 26, 1984, to recognize the work of people dedicated to produce scientific knowledge and technology. Recognition is granted through peer evaluation and consists of granting the appointment of a national researcher. This distinction symbolizes the quality and prestige of scientific contributions. In parallel to the appointment, economic stimuli are awarded, the amount of which varies with the assigned level.
>
> The purpose of the SNI is to promote and strengthen, through evaluation, the quality of scientific and technological research and the innovation that occurs in the country. The System contributes to the formation and consolidation of researchers with scientific and technological knowledge of the highest level as a fundamental element to increase culture, productivity, competitiveness and social welfare (CONACYT, http://www.conacyt.gob.mx/index.php/el-conacyt/sistema-nacional-de-investigadores, November 18, 2017, personal translation).

The impact of the SNI has been contradictory (Pérez Castro, 2009). On the one hand, it has increased the number of professors with tenure who have a PhD in almost all public HEIs (Didou & Gérard, 2010). This degree is virtually an indispensable requirement for being part of the system. Probably, this has helped professors become better at teaching and training, develop new scientific skills, and improve their tutoring of graduate theses and dissertations. It may also have increased their productivity (Ch & Barros, 2012) in terms of publishing more high-quality papers, as this too is an indispensable requirement of the system. Virtually, all the HEI launched their own programs to incentivize their professors' productivity. They try to motivate their academic staff with economic bonuses based on their productivity, which is evaluated using their own indicators (Heras, 2005).

However, this courting of "productivity" has also caused problems due to internal competition at universities. Alliances between professors have been formed in which they join efforts to meet certain ends. They reorganize their work in ways that allow them to more easily obtain the necessary requirements for becoming a member of the SNI and for obtaining bonuses. Some of these alliances worked out well. They achieved substantive contributions to academic activities and functioned harmoniously. Unfortunately, others transformed into teams that began to exclude and

[1] http://www.conacyt.mx/index.php/el-conacyt/convocatorias-y-resultados-conacyt/convocatorias-sistema-nacional-de-investigadores-sni/marco-legal-sni/reglamento-sni/841-reglamento2013-1/file, 18 October 2017.

paralyze colleagues and other academic groups that represented competition for them. In trying to benefit themselves and access positions of power, they developed informal, questionable ways to shun colleagues (Porter, 2012, 2016). So, what Brian Martin calls *suppression of dissent* (http://www.bmartin.cc/dissent/intro/definitions.html, November 21, 2017) has been used to eliminate what they perceive as "threats," leading to the elimination of any competition. In some HEIs, hidden and silent wars have been started by these aggressive groups. However, such groups try to make their behaviors appear to be legitimate and in accordance with the university's rules, often by sham dealing (Osborne, 2009). These dynamics have disrupted the personal relationships of the academic communities in not a few HEIs in Mexico. Porter (2012) has pointed out that there are what might be termed academic gangsters making the university's internal life difficult. Therefore, these policies sometimes damage the productivity they supposedly promote.

Both strategies (suppression of dissent and mobbing) are commonly used to carry out the removal of such perceived threats. Mobbing is perhaps the most difficult to bear for those who are targets. It is an assault using formal or informal power on the person or persons who "touch" the interests of individuals or groups.

> Suppression of dissent: action taken in an attempt to stop or penalize a person who makes a public statement or does something that is seen as a threat to a powerful interest group, such as a government, corporation or profession. Typical actions include ostracism, harassment, censorship, forced job transfer, reprimands and dismissal. Suppression is action against dissent that does not involve physical violence (Martin, https://www.uow.edu.au/~bmartin/dissent/intro/definitions.html, November 21, 2017).

If these actions are perpetrated by a group recurrently and in a prolonged time frame—which, unfortunately happens often—they are transformed into mobbing, which is:

> … a form of violence in which aggression toward a target chosen by an organized group is given primarily through hostile and dishonest communication. Messages are directed primarily to the context surrounding the target (directors, subordinates and peers), through: 1. attitudes that try to prevent the target to expressed, 2. promote their isolation, achieving collective rejection towards him/she, 3. promote his or hers discredit by minimizing their contributions and exaggerating or inventing errors, defects and faults, 4. promote the discredit of their work, using the same mechanisms, 5. compromise their health by assessing them hazardous tasks. Mobbing is distinguished from other forms of violence because it is perpetrated by an organized group and the communicational attacks are recurrent and systematic, as well as prolonged in time (https://congresomobbing.wordpress.com/2010/07/13/i-congreso-iberoamericano-sobre-acoso-laboral-e-institucional/, 14 November 2017, personal translation).

Suppression of dissent and mobbing are frankly abusive to certain individuals within educational institutions. As already pointed out, those who become a menace to the interests of persons or groups with formal or informal power are undermined. These forms of verbal and nonverbal aggression use communication as the "weapon." They are framed in the context of individual or group personal relationships and academic dynamics, and they are justified and portrayed as legitimate and even necessary.

Graduate Programs at HEI

Another variable to consider in these new dynamics is the requirement for Mexican institutions to have graduate programs of "high quality." This demand forces HEI to have programs that are attractive enough to lead young people to enroll in them. It is also a requirement that students get their degrees on time and with high-quality theses and dissertations. The CONACyT promotes this situation by creating a program to provide scholarships to students, benefits for professors, and extra resources for graduate programs to encourage this "high quality." The program has had different names; it is now called National Program of Graduate Studies of High Quality (*Programa Nacional de Posgrados de Calidad*, PNPC; http://www.conacyt.gob.mx/index.php/becas-y-posgrados/programa-nacional-de-posgrados-de-calidad, October 25, 2017). This set of processes has been established in the graduate programs of virtually all national public and even private universities.

However, since tutoring master's and PhD students is necessary to qualify for SNI membership, internal struggles for getting graduate students are also often generated. This has, once again, led not uncommonly to some professors shunning others, a process that is sometimes even directed at their students. On the other hand, the neoliberal public policies that have been enforced have allowed many young people enrolling in graduate programs to have a scholarship that becomes their source of income, thus sparing them from facing unemployment or holding precarious jobs.

Another effect of this dynamic has been that new young graduates may not be able to find a job as researchers or professors—positions that can lead to tenure. In not a few cases, despite their high academic qualifications, they end up becoming part of the administrative staff of universities. Because of their lack of expertise due to a lack of training as such, their performance in these jobs is subpar. Many of them become highly frustrated because they are engaged in activities that are not in line with their high professional qualifications. Therefore, it is not uncommon for them to develop envy and other negative feelings toward the professors within their same HEI. The latter have tenure and are usually receiving a salary for performing research, teaching, and outreach activities within the discipline they had studied. This scenario creates tension between administrators with this profile and professors that sometimes ends up in activities designed by the former to get revenge on the latter. Another important group of these graduates end up as part-time teachers with a low salary, no possibility for tenure, and none of the fringe and other benefits afforded to the professors. This too often generates negativity and a desire for revenge.

In this context, professionals with master's and PhD working as administrators and part-time teachers often end up discrediting the work of tenured academic staff. It is not uncommon to hear them say that students do not get their degrees on time because "there is a lack of proper supervision," thusly blaming the professors. They may also complain that the professors "do nothing" because they have assistants who are the ones who do the actual teaching. Part-time teachers, in particular, see themselves as the ones who carry the load with teaching, tutoring, organizing field-work, etc.—while professors take the credit. This scenario has not been conducive to a good working environment within HEIs. When the administrators with high professional profiles impugn the academic activities of the professors, clearly this creates a dynamic that is not conducive to the high academic efficiency that the HEIs need. This paper will provide an example of how this combination of factors can lead to institutionalized abuse against professors. This has negatively affected the very academic activities of the HEI that are being used as indicators of efficiency.

Key Concepts for the Analysis of the Case

> [Violence is] the intentional use of physical force or power, threatened or actual, against oneself, another person, or against a group or community, that either results in or has a high likelihood of resulting in injury, death, psychological harm, maldevelopment, or deprivation. (http://www.who.int/violenceprevention/approach/definition/en/, November 21, 2017)

Diana Scialpi (2005) was a pioneer bringing to light the phenomenon she called "institutional violence." It can take the form of "soft" violence (Bourdieu, 2000) taking place during collective interaction in a hidden or little visible, but nonetheless harmful, way.

> We can define the *political-bureaucratic violence* as a variant of political violence, perpetrated by political officials of the Public Administration and by high-ranking officers (senior staff and/or with executive functions) that have a social responsibility, legal and administrative employees of the State (Scialpi, 2002).

Sham Dealing Investigating *mobbing* using grounded theory and through interviews, Deborah Osborne came up with the concept she called *sham dealing*, and concluded that it is a form of aggression masquerading as legitimate and honestly performed action. She says that:

> Sham dealing is unfair dealing whilst a pretense of fair and genuine dealing is maintained. Sham dealing types of managerial actions are experienced as an additional form of bullying in workplaces and within the larger arena of the formal claims process (Osborne, 2009:16–17, http://www.bmartin.cc/pubs/09-4apcei/4apcei-Osborne.pdf, November 14, 2017)

> This type of simulated actions has the appearance of a legitimate treatment, but it is not (Osborne, 2009:16–17).

Sham Peer Review In line with Osborne, but independently, authors such as Twedt (2003), Chalifoux (2005), and Huntoon (2009) came up with the related idea of "sham peer review." They analyzed situations in which "facts" were manipulated in order to "fit the crime committed." The goal was to attain a predetermined outcome. Again, the "actions have the appearance of genuine dealing but are characterized by a deceptive misuse of legitimate process" (sham dealing, Osborne, 2009:1). He identifies several procedures which are illustrative of this process:

1. *Ambush tactic and secret investigations*. The targeted doctor is called to what he believes to be an informal and friendly meeting. Upon arrival, it becomes clear that the meeting has been set up to include many authorities from within the institution and that it is not going to be cordial. Everybody except him knows what it is really going on. They begin by questioning the doctor about concerns which they know he is not going to be able to address properly. This plot has been designed in advance with the intent of finding him guilty of some problematic behavior and making him the subject of sanctions including suspension.
2. *Depriving targets of records needed to defend themselves*.
3. *Guilty until proven innocent* (if he can).
4. *Numerator-without-denominator tactic*. That means that the accusation of wrongdoing does not take into consideration the number of similar cases that have happened elsewhere, nor the number of times the same doctor has acted correctly. This bias is used to promote and justify sanctions.
5. *Trumped-up and/or false charges*. "In sham peer review, where the hospital controls the entire process and acts as judge, jury, and executioner, the truth or falsity of charges makes no difference, and the truth and the facts do not matter because the outcome is predetermined, and the process is rigged" (p. 65).
6. *Peer Commissions findings biased because they are influenced by the biased analyses of previous reviews*.

Twedt (2003) argues that most of these reprisals are for whistleblowing and are the cost of the doctor's courage in denouncing irregularities in order to protect the public interest. Doctors that warn of unsafe conditions for their patients or work poorly done by a colleague are put in the spotlight by hospital administrators or by the management. Instead of receiving recognition and support for trying to improve services, they are disciplined or fired for being "disruptive" or accused of violating the confidentiality of their patients. Often, the hospital flips the accusation and the doctors are the ones who end up being marked for having employed bad practices. They may even be threatened with an internal investigation into their performance which may result in the inclusion of their names in the National Practitioners Data Bank in the list of doctors who have had complaints leveled against them. This may mean that finding work in another hospital can become nearly impossible (Twedt, 2003).

As will be seen, both administrative sham dealing and sham peer review also occur in HEIs.

A Case Background From 2006 to 2012, a female professor at an HEI had coordinated or co-coordinated 14 books. For 12 of these, she had requested and obtained the endorsement of her institution for being a co-editor, even though the HEI had not provided any financial support. The authorizations had involved three different administrations.

To give her the institutional endorsement, the chair of the Department of Publications had requested:

1. A printed copy and a CD with the versions of the chapters of the book, the introduction, the information in the legal page, and the index of authors.
2. A letter of the coordinator or coordinators of the book stating that the chapters had the necessary quality and format to be published.
3. Assurance that they had been peer reviewed by at least by two researchers and that the authors had worked with the suggestions given by them.
4. The actual peer reviews.

Once the chair checked this administrative and academic information, the authorization for the institution to appear as coeditor was given in a letter stating:

> In response to your request dated on XXX, asking for authorization to include our institution as coeditor of the book titled XXX, I let you know that after reviewing the academic and administrative documentation you have submitted, your request has been approved. Chair.

This mechanism, in addition to ensuring high academic rigor for the book, gave a vote of confidence to the professors of the institution who served as academic coordinators for it. Many of them had a history of publications, teaching, organizing events, etc. on the topics addressed in the coordinated books. Implicitly, it was also recognized that they had honestly and knowledgeably chosen the ideal peer reviewers from among the scientific community. The policies of higher education described above are meant to insure that its publications are a valid indicator of the quality of universities themselves, as well as that of its professors, students, and graduate programs. Logically, it is important to encourage them.

Institutional Abuse In this same HEI in 2012, a woman with a master's degree in one of the disciplines offered by the same institution was appointed to be the chair of the Department of Publications. She met the previously described profile of a staff member who had academic training but, because of the job restrictions in the country, ended up doing administrative activities or which she had no previous experience. She exhibited emotional negativity toward professors. As will be shown, the dynamics of the department from which this new official took the charge qualify as administrative abuse. In fact, it caused many more problems in addition to the one that will be analyzed here. This abuse not only affected the number of publications of the involved professors but also the prestige and the academic goals of the institution by having an impact on the performance indicators of professors, students, educational programs, and the institution itself.

In this case, a professor started the process of publishing a book. As she had many times before, she intended to increase the prestige of the institution she worked for by adding it as a co-publisher. The book involved was a result of a Conference held in the institution in 2011. Due to the large number of participants, the event had been very successful. By the end, there were 39 panels that included 215 authors and 170 papers from different institutions. Participants came from 13 countries and 15 states within Mexico. In addition, this first experience laid the foundation for similar events every 2 years. The conferences were scheduled to take place in Argentina (2013), Brazil (2015), Colombia (2017), and Cuba (2019).

The professor's experience led her to becoming the president of the Conference. She called the participants to submit their texts as book chapters for the publication of a book which was to be distributed at the next Conference in Argentina. Therefore, the support of the institution for this publication would promote its reputation internationally. In addition, it was important that the HEI appear as co-editor of the book because it resulted from an event that it promoted and housed.

The Facts To this end, while she was abroad on sabbatical leave in February 2012, she sent an e-mail to the chair of the Department of Publications letting her know that the work was in progress. She never received any reply. She received no precise instructions on how to proceed, notifications of any new mechanisms for publishing, nor any new agreements on the procedures that should be followed in the process.

The work was completed at the beginning of 2013 using the guidelines she had used in coordinating previous books. At the time the request for an institutional endorsement was made, the problems arose. The chair of the Department began to present obstacles to authorizing the institution to be co-publisher, even though the publication did not entail any economic cost. It was not until then that the chair sent information to the professor—through third parties—that there was a Publications Commission that had devised new publication procedures that were now going to be enforced. She had never been notified about this before, despite her having been the coordinator or co-coordinator of many previous books. As mentioned, this information had not been sent to her in response to her initial e-mail to the chair about the book.

The chair insisted that, in order to get the authorization to include the institution as a co-publisher, she had to submit the material to the Commission and start the publishing procedure all over again—including re-sending the chapters for peer review. This was demanded even though the book was ready after months of work and needed to be published by the next Conference to be held soon in Buenos Aires, Argentina.

As another example of abuse, the chair never sought out the professor for a personal conversation or called her into her office. Conclusions and instructions were always sent through third parties, and the professor was never informed about how her case was going to be followed up. For instance, the professor was ignored when the case was discussed by the Committee of Publications and was, therefore, unable to defend her reasoning; nor could she question negative decisions by the Committee concerning her requests. This treatment of her was in direct contradiction of the rules written the *General Conditions of Work* from the institution, which clearly state that any decisions concerning the interests of professors must be furnished to them in writing.

The honesty of this professor was also questioned in a highly offensive manner through a suggestion that she had sought out "friends" as peer reviewers, instead of choosing the best ones for the topic in which she was an expert. The chair also questioned whether she had followed up on the recommendations for changes that were offered by the peer reviewers. In the end, despite the intervention of the two other authorities of this HEI, the chair of Department of Publications, in a letter addressed to one of these authorities, refused to allow the HEI to be co-publisher. A copy of this decision was not even given to the professor who had been directly involved as an editor of the book. Because the professor did not get an official notice addressed to her, this action was also a violation of her rights.

The professor sent an official letter to the director of the institution addressing this issue, pointing out that:

1. The letter with the negative resolution of the Commission of Publications was not addressed to her, and she did not even receive a copy.
2. She had not been informed about nor called to a meeting in which her request was going to be dealt with.
3. The letter denying the authorization for the institutions to be a co-publisher was not signed by the Commission of Publications, but by the chair of the Department of Publications, and it did not even attach the statement of facts produced in the meeting.
4. A year later, she had not been given the official new procedures for publishing a book or for asking for other types of authorizations.

Therefore, she requested a copy of the documentation of this case. The Commission responded to the director—again, without a copy for the full-time professor. The Commission had twelve members but their letter only had seven signatures, without printed names to identify them. Their response included:

1. The date of the meeting in which the case was dealt with.
2. Statements that the peer reviews of the chapters:
   (a) Lacked an academic institution as endorsee.
   (b) There was no academic institution requesting them.
   (c) They did not have the proper format needed to draw conclusions on the matter.
   (d) They were, for the most part, printed on recycled paper, which made them illegible.
3. A statement that the dossier of the book lacked an index that tied each chapter to the relevant peer reviews.
4. That because of the above, the Commission decided to return the book, reiterating that the proper procedures must be followed.

The director did finally send the professor a letter with several attachments which elucidated:

1. The organization and functioning of the Commission of Publications.
2. The guidelines from the Department of Publications for the delivery of manuscripts.
3. The guidelines for publications.
4. Manuals for publications.
5. A copy of the statement of facts of the Technical Council in which the Technical Guidelines were approved.

Should not all of these documents and information been given to her as soon as she told the Department of Publications about the book in the first place? The only logical conclusion is that sham dealing was involved.

Final Thoughts

Needless to say, due to this long and tortuous process, the institution for which the professor worked did not appear as co-publisher of the book. This was despite the fact that, 2 years before, the Conference from which the book originated had been held there. The chair of the Department of Publications never owned up to her "mistakes," such as never replying to the email from the professor asking her for the information about the new publishing procedures. The dynamics of this case makes it possible to hypothesize that from the very beginning the chair had decided not to grant the institutional endorsement, and then set in motion a process consistent with the description of sham dealing and sham peer review.

From the moment that the professor sent a letter to the director of the HEI, she was re-victimized. She was mistreated by the authorities from whom she requested support (Corsi, 1995).

Of the tactics mentioned by Huntoon (2009), the following were used in this case:

- *Not giving the target of aggression the documentation and information necessary to defend herself.* This happened in several ways: the chair of the Department of Publications did not give the professor the procedures in response to her first e-mail. Once the case was proceeding, the chair did not tell her the dates on which the Commission of Publications was going to discuss her request or the decisions of the Commission of Publications.
- *Making prefabricated false charges.* Having been put in a position of defenselessness, it was only by the professor's insistence on a copy of the decisions made during the meeting that she was informed about the criteria that were being used to deny her request. However, of the list of "mistakes" and lack of proper documentation listed by the Commission, all of them were "repairable." Because the issues were being falsely described as unsolvable and the professor was not informed about them, and because the professor was denied the right to attend the meeting in which her case was discussed, it seems highly likely that sham dealing was behind this case. She clearly was never given the opportunity to explain anything or defend her activities and opinions. It is possible to conclude that the chair of the Department of Publications created a strategy designed to deny her request from the very beginning due to some prejudice against her.
- *Applying the criterion of "numerator without denominator."* The professor in question had published 12 previous books with institutional endorsement. This time, she had submitted the documents that were asked of her before for previous approvals for her work to the same office and in perfect order. So why was everything so messy this time? It is possible that the chair of the Department of

Publications had made certain that the files that were sent to the Commission to analyze would lead to a negative decision on the request?

- *Parallel communications which are outside of the formal channels for such discussion.* The chair talked with the members of the Commission and gave them her own view of all the irregularities that the full-time professor allegedly committed. However, at the same time, she prevented a direct relationship between the Commission and the professor regarding her request.
- *Peer validations prejudiced by the previous biased reviews.*
- Considering all this, it is possible to hypothesize that the chair had spoken with the members of the Commission in ways meant to bias them against a favorable opinion. No member of the Commission questioned why the professor was absent during discussions of her request nor bothered to make sure that she would receive their findings on time.

As already stated, this case was not the only one that showed similar dynamics working against publications by professors in this university. Hence, unfortunately, the chair was allowed to establish what amounts to institutional abuse toward professors as an internal policy. She belonged to the previously described group of highly trained academics in administrative jobs who are prone to exercising animosity by preventing a professor's work from being published. However, at the same time, she was damaging the institution's reputation by negatively affecting the indicators used by the academic community at large to evaluate the institution, its graduate programs, and its student's and professor's productivity. Unbelievable!

Note Peña, F. (2016). Maltrato institucional o de cómo los administrativos en las instituciones de educación superior pueden convertirse en un obstáculo para el trabajo académico. Estudios de caso. In: F. Peña y K. Fernández (editors), *Mobbing en la Academia Mexicana*, Ediciones Eón, Red del Programa para el Desarrollo Profesional Docente, Secretaría de Educación Pública: "Salud, Condiciones de Vida y Políticas Sociales" y Escuela Nacional de Antropología e Historia, Mexico City.

References

Bourdieu, P. (2000). *La dominación masculina.* Barcelona, Spain: Editorial Anagrama.

Ch, R., & Barros, T. (2012, November). El CONACYT: de carro completo a institución Ferrari. *Nexos.* http://www.nexos.com.mx/?p=15069, October 13, 2017.

Chalifoux, R. (2005). So what is a sham peer review? *MedGenMed, 7*(4). Published online November 15, 2005. http://www.ncbi.nlm.nih.gov/pmc/articles/PMC1681729/, December 2, 2017.

Corsi, J. (1995). *Violencia masculina en la pareja. Una aproximación al diagnóstico y a los modelos de intervención.* Buenos Aires, Argentina: Editorial Paidós.

Didou, S., & Gérard, E. (2010). *El Sistema Nacional de Investigadores, veinticinco años después.* México: ANUIES.

Heras, L. (2005). La política de educación superior en México: los programas de estímulos a profesores e investigadores. *Revista Venezolana de Educación*. [Online] volume 9, number 29, pp. 207–215. http://www.scielo.org.ve/scielo.php?script=sci_arttext&pid=S1316-49102005000200009&lng=es&nrm=iso, November 6, 2017.

Huntoon, L. R. (2009). Tactics characteristic of sham peer review. *Journal of American Physicians and Surgeons, 14*(3), 64–66. http://www.jpands.org/vol14no3/huntoon.pdf, October 25, 2017.

Ibarra, E. (2002). La 'nueva universidad' en México:Transformaciones recientes yperspectivas. *Revista Mexicana de Investigación Educativa, 7*(14), 75–105.

Ibarra, E. & Rondero, N. (2008). Regulación del trabajo académico y deshomologación salarial: balance general de sus ejes problemáticos. In T. Bertussi & G. González (coordinators), *Anuario educativo mexicano: visión retrospectiva 2005*, Universidad Pedagógica Nacional, Miguel Ángel Porrúa & H. Congreso de la Unión, Mexico City, pp. 569–601.

Osborne, D. (2009). Pathways into bullying. *4th Asia Pacific Conference on Educational Integrity, 28–30 September*. University of Wollongong, Wollongong, NSW, pp. 1–61. http://ro.uow.edu.au/apcei/09/papers/18/, July 25, 2014.

Peña, F., & Fernández, K. (2016). Neoliberalismo, democracia y mobbing: ¿Qué sabemos sobre su dinámica en las instituciones de educación superior? In F. P. K. Fernández (Ed.), *Mobbing en la Academia Mexicana* (pp. 15–39). México: Ediciones y Gráficos Eón, Red PRODEP "Salud, Condiciones de Vida y Políticas Sociales y Escuela Nacional de Antropología e Historia".

Pérez Castro, J. (2009). "El efecto Frankenstein: Las políticas educativas mexicanas y su impacto en la profesión académica", *Espiral. Estudios Sobre Estado y Sociedad, Número, 46*, 61–93.

Porter, L. (2012, April 30). La universidad secuestrada: el gánster academic. Laboratorio de Análisis Institucional del Sistema Universitario Mexicana.http://laisumedu.org/semanario, May 15, de 2017.

Porter, L. (2016). La salvación de la universidad. In F. Peñay & K. Fernández (Eds.), *Mobbing en la academia mexicana* (pp. 45–58). México: Ediciones y Gráficos Eón, Red PRODEP "Salud, Condiciones de Vida y Políticas Sociales y Escuela Nacional de Antropología e Historia".

Scialpi, D. (2002). La violencia laboral en la administración pública argentina. *Revista Venezolana de Gerencia, 7*(18): 196–219.

Scialpi, D. (2005). Violencia laboral y desamparo institucional aprendido, *Revista Jurisprudencia Argentina*, número especial: Mobbing: el acoso psicológico en el ámbito laboral 27 de abril. http://acosomoral.org/pdf/R%5B1%5D.J.A.%20Abril%202005.%20MOBBING%20%28Scialpi%29.pdf, November 3, 2017.

Twedt, S. (2003). Cost of courage. *Pittsburgh Post-Gazette*. http://www.post-gazette.com/pg/03299/234499.stm, December 12, 2017.

Chapter 7
Research Grants and Agenda Shaping

Brian Martin

Introduction

In 1969, Clyde Manwell was appointed the second professor of zoology at the University of Adelaide. He came with an outstanding research record. In 1971, he and his wife, Ann Baker, wrote a letter to the newspaper criticizing aspects of the government's fruit fly spraying program, triggering commentary in state parliament. The senior professor of zoology wrote to the Vice Chancellor, leading to an investigation that could have resulted in Manwell's dismissal. The saga, which lasted 4 years before resolution in Manwell's favor, involved media coverage, court cases, and student protest (Baker, 1986).

Manwell later wrote about his experience with Australia's leading competitive research grants scheme at the time. Prior to the complaint and publicity, Manwell had received a grant. Afterward, despite a publication record in the top 2% in his field, his grant was terminated without explanation (a rare occurrence), and his subsequent applications were unsuccessful, at a time when most applications in his field were funded. The implication was that the complaint against Manwell, or his challenge to pesticide orthodoxy, influenced grant assessors or panel members against his applications (Manwell, 1979).

Manwell's case can be considered a manifestation of altruism leading to unfairness: research grant panels are likely to award money to those who are most like themselves, including their ideas. Manwell had challenged conventional views and, therefore, was henceforth considered unworthy of support: he had become an "other" rather than one of "us."

Let's take a step back and look at the purpose of research grants. Researchers need time and resources to carry out their studies. Most commonly, they receive this via an appointment at a university or research institution, which provides a salary,

B. Martin (✉)
Humanities and Social Inquiry, University of Wollongong, Wollongong, NSW, Australia
e-mail: bmartin@uow.edu.au

D. M. Allen, J. W. Howell (eds.), *Groupthink in Science*,
https://doi.org/10.1007/978-3-030-36822-7_7

computing and library facilities, and sometimes a laboratory and support staff. In addition, for extra support, they can apply for research grants.

Grants come in all amounts and from various sources. They can be for $1000 or $10 million. They can be provided by a researcher's employer or can be "external," offered by some other organization. Two common types are competitive schemes, in which a panel chooses between numerous applications based on merit, and tied schemes, in which an organization provides funds for projects directly related to its interests. In a typical national competitive scheme, researchers from a wide range of disciplines can apply; applications are judged by experts, rankings are made and grants awarded to the highest-ranking applicants. In a typical tied scheme, a grant is given to a chosen researcher on a specified topic, for example, to carry out studies for the army or a breast cancer charity. There are all sorts of variants of these two types of schemes. Many tied schemes have some level of competition and some competitive schemes have thematic priorities.

Grant applications range from brief to lengthy and from simple to elaborate. Typically, they must follow a template that includes an exposition of the research proposed to be undertaken, a budget, and a listing of the applicant's achievements. For some schemes, writing an application is a major operation, taking weeks of effort (Graves, Barnett, & Clarke, 2011). For external competitive grants, applications may be vetted by superiors and administrative staff to ensure compliance with various requirements as well as to improve the quality of the application.

In principle, the grant system sounds sensible. Money to support research should go to those who undertake the most meritorious projects. However, there are various shortcomings, ranging from bias against individuals and projects to systemic problems due to the grant system itself.

Agenda Setting

There are a few other documented examples like Manwell's (e.g., Horrobin, 1974, 1996; Martin, 1986), though these are hardly enough to make a strong case that there is extensive bias in awarding grants. The methodological obstacles to investigating bias in grant systems are considerable. Deliberations are usually confidential, and committee members rarely speak out about disputes and problems. More fundamentally, if there is bias among expert assessors and panel members, it may be unconscious, so independent means are required to make judgments about the fairness of grant allocations. The challenge is that competitive grants are awarded based on the opinions of experts in the field, so claims about bias usually involve questioning expert judgment on the basis of some other experts or criteria.

Some critics of grant systems argue that there is a systemic bias against innovative projects (Nicholson & Ioannidis, 2012). Based simply on probabilities, a radical or unorthodox proposal is likely to be read by assessors who are closer to the mainstream than the converse. Whether or not there is any such bias in grant committees, many applicants feel that it is better to play safe, so beliefs about bias against unorthodox research can be self-fulfilling.

Over the years, I've had many discussions with colleagues about grant applications, theirs and my own. For many academics, applying for a grant is a strategic enterprise, with the topic, methods, and goals chosen to maximize the chance of success. Close attention is given to the members of grant panels, especially their areas of interest. If a particular panel member is likely to take carriage of your proposal, then you may be able to improve your odds by making the application appealing to that individual. When, as occurred periodically, a panel member came for a visit to the university to give a talk about grants committee operations and expectations, many academics would attend, seeking insights into how to tailor their applications to win approval. The implication is that many applicants subordinate what they really want to do and think is important to what they think will win favor with grant bodies.

Systematic slanting in topics funded is most obvious in tied grants, typically offered by corporations or government departments. For example, the military funds a wide range of research, thus having an influence over priorities in fields including oceanography, psychology, and computer science. As well as influencing priorities within fields, grant funding can influence the relative emphasis between fields. Military funds give more priority to nuclear physics than to ecology or law.

Researchers who are not reliant on grants have a greater opportunity to explore areas that serve the public interest, or just their own personal interests. However, the influence of grant systems affects them as well. This is because funding priorities influence the questions seen as important in a field. So, for example, if the computational challenges relating to encryption are given plenty of funding, they move higher on the priority list for other researchers too, and influence editors and even the setting up of journals.

Competitive grant schemes seem on the surface to be less tied to special interests. Competitive schemes typically draw on the expertise of top researchers, and these are the very researchers most likely to have succeeded based on their interest in areas that are well funded and are central to the field. So it is plausible that competitive schemes are inherently biased against dissident or unorthodox views and against research that addresses unfashionable topics. More generally, competitive schemes suffer the same shortcomings as any system reliant on peer review (Bartlett, 2011; Bornmann, 2011; Horrobin, 1990).

There are a number of studies of grant systems and the operations of grant bodies (Lamont, 2009; Mow, 2010; Thorngate, Dawes, & Foddy, 2009; Wessely, 1998). Undoubtedly, nearly all members of such bodies attempt to be fair, awarding grants according to the stated criteria. Also undoubtedly, there are cases involving insider bias, in which panel members award grants to each other, collaborators, or allies. This need not be conscious bias, and it is far more insidious when it is unconscious. (On the social psychology of panel peer review, see Olbrecht & Bornmann, 2010.)

Another aspect of grant systems is the enormous effort they entail. Part of this effort occurs in the central administration of the system and in peer assessments. Another and usually larger part is the effort required of applicants and their employers. If, for example, writing an application for a competitive scheme requires an effort similar to writing a paper for publication, and the success rate for applications is 20%, then the publication of five papers is sacrificed to the system itself, and this might be a nontrivial percentage of the additional papers published due to the successful grants, especially considering that grant recipients commonly attribute their outputs to the grant even when these outputs might have occurred anyway.

It is worth noting that for many researchers, especially in fields not requiring laboratories, their main requirements are time, computers, and library facilities. Additional funding is seldom crucial in the humanities. Yet even in such fields, applying for grants has become a necessary ritual for scholars seeking advancement because obtaining a grant is prestigious, for both the scholar and the institution. Grant successes become surrogates for research excellence even though in practical terms grants are inputs to research, not outputs. Institutions can provide incentives to those obtaining lucrative grants, including teaching relief, promotion, and leadership roles. Star researchers are sometimes lured to other institutions by the promise of a research-only position, support staff, travel funding, and other advantages. There is no similar glorification of star teachers.

The grant system can inadvertently lead to cementing of the status and success of successful applicants. Obtaining a grant can create more opportunities for research, thus helping develop a track record that in turn enables further grant successes. Thus, at the beginning, a slight superiority, or good luck, can compound over time into entrenched advantage. Those most likely to benefit this way are scholars who position themselves at the cutting edge of mainstream or fashionable topics.

Alternatives

The systemic biases in the usual sorts of grant schemes are easier to see when a comparison is made to alternatives. One option is ample funding for researchers as part of their appointments, so no grant applications are required. This would eliminate the excessive overheads of grant administration and grant writing. However, it might be argued that this would not provide sufficient incentive to make efficient use of resources, because poor performers would receive as much support as good ones.

A modification of this method is to provide research support based on productivity: the more papers a scientist produced, or the greater the number of citations received, the more internal and/or external funding is provided (Roy, 1984). This approach rewards those who achieve by conventional criteria. Special support might be provided to those at the beginning of their research careers, or who are making a major shift in research directions, to enable the building of a record of outcomes. However, this model of funding has no simple way of encouraging innovative, unorthodox projects, because typically it is harder to publish findings for such research. Furthermore, projects with a long gestation would not attract long-term funding: instead, the quest for funding might encourage short-term superficial projects with quick publication turnarounds.

Another model for funding is to introduce an element of randomness (Fang & Casadevall, 2016; Gillies, 2014). Applications might be received in the usual way.

Any application above a specified minimum of quality would be put in a pool, and successful applications chosen by lot. One advantage of such a scheme would be to enable researchers to pursue what they really want to do, including being as creative as they wish, because every application, assuming it satisfies the minimum criteria, would have an equal chance.

A modification of this model involves a combination of peer review and randomness. For example, each application would be peer reviewed and given a score. The score (perhaps a number from 1 to 10) would determine the number of lottery tickets assigned to the application. A top-quality application would have a better chance of being funded, but even applications seen as inferior by peers would have a chance.

Introducing a grant lottery would make formal what is already happening in many grant schemes that nominally operate entirely according to merit (Bornmann & Daniel, 2009; Cole, Cole, & Simon, 1981; Graves et al., 2011). Peer review introduces an element of luck, as the fate of an application depends sensitively on the choice of peer reviewers. For superlative applications and very poor ones, this may make no difference, but for a large number of good applications, the difference between success and failure may come down to tiny score differences, which means that luck plays an important role (Frank, 2016). The illusion that outcomes are based only on merit has some undesirable effects: unsuccessful applicants may become unnecessarily demoralized, and successful ones may falsely believe they are greatly superior to their less fortunate colleagues. When a random element is formally introduced to the selection process, it is easier to rationalize failure as bad luck and harder to claim success as impeccable evidence of superiority.

It is worth noting that despite billions of dollars of research funding being allocated in competitive research schemes, there is relatively little research into how effective they are in achieving their goals (Demicheli & Di Pietrantonj, 2007). For example, it would be possible to specify several models for funding, introduce them in well-defined fields, and measure outcomes years down the track. For example, it is possible to imagine the usual competitive scheme being compared to grants being awarded based on previous publications. Another possibility, involving some deception, would be to award some portion of grants to applications that did not gain peer support and then to compare outputs years later to those that did. The lack of empirical tests of the effectiveness of grant schemes suggests that they may be serving purposes other than improving research performance.

Conclusion

Research grant schemes are ostensibly intended to improve the quality and quantity of research. Schemes are subject to bias against particular individuals or types of projects, as shown by a few documented cases. However, this sort of bias is less important than the general effects of grant schemes and the increasing priority put on obtaining external research funding.

The creation and expansion of grant schemes may be related to their role as disciplining procedures, to subordinate researchers to outside agendas. This is most obvious for grants tied to particular areas. Most of these sorts of grants are provided by corporations and government agencies, thereby providing pressure to investigate topics and use methods amenable to the funders. Funding of this sort offers an incentive to report findings that do not challenge the agendas of the funders. In what is called the "funding effect," research results favor funder agendas far more than results of independently funded research (Krimsky, 2012). One explanation for this is that researchers realize, often unconsciously, that coming up with results unwelcome to the funder will mean that prospects for future funding are reduced.

Another effect of tied grants is that research areas for which there is less funding are less likely to be investigated. Groups that have little money, such as social justice activists, have little capacity to set research agendas.

The funding effect plays relatively little role in competitive grant schemes, in which decisions are typically made by scholars in relevant fields. These schemes can nevertheless provide a disciplining effect. Scholars, when seeking grants, are likely to slant their proposals to what they believe their peers will think is worthwhile in terms of topics and methods, thereby providing a subtle discouragement of unorthodox approaches. The disciplining effect of competitive schemes thus serves to orient research toward mainstream agendas, thereby serving the more prominent and influential figures in the field. Meanwhile, to the degree that these figures are seeking tied funding, mainstream agendas become oriented to the interests of governments and large corporations.

The increasing prestige of obtaining grant money is strange, at least on the surface, considering that grants are inputs rather than research outputs. If scholars were left to their own devices, they might be tempted to carry out investigations that go in a multitude of directions, including those that challenge elite agendas. This does occur to a certain extent, but is constrained to the extent that appointments, promotions, and honors go to those most successful in obtaining grants. Although researchers see themselves as autonomous, the grant process can contribute to maintaining the "ideological discipline" that they developed during their research training (Schmidt, 2000).

Acknowledgments The author thanks David Allen, Steven Bartlett, and Lutz Bornmann for useful feedback.

References

Baker, C. M. A. (1986). The fruit fly papers. In B. Martin, C. M. A. Baker, C. Manwell, & C. Pugh (Eds.), *Intellectual suppression: Australian case histories, analysis and responses* (pp. 87–113). Sydney, Australia: Angus & Robertson.

Bartlett, S. J. (2011). The psychology of abuse in publishing: Peer review and editorial bias. In S. J. Bartlett, *Normality does not equal mental health: The need to look elsewhere for standards of good psychological health* (pp. 137–160). Santa Barbara, CA: Praeger.

Bornmann, L. (2011). Scientific peer review. *Annual Review of Information Science and Technology, 45*, 199–245.
Bornmann, L., & Daniel, H.-D. (2009). The luck of the referee draw: The effect of exchanging reviews. *Learned Publishing, 22*, 117–125.
Cole, S., Cole, J. R., & Simon, G. A. (1981). Chance and consensus in peer review. *Science, 214*(20 November), 881–886.
Demicheli, V., & Di Pietrantonj, C. (2007). Peer review for improving the quality of grant applications. *Cochrane Database of Systematic Reviews*, (2), MR000003. https://doi.org/10.1002/14651858.MR00003.pub2
Fang, F. C., & Casadevall, A. (2016). Research funding: The case for a modified lottery. *MBio, 7*(2), e00422–e00416.
Frank, R. H. (2016). *Success and luck: Good fortune and the myth of meritocracy*. Princeton, NJ: Princeton University Press.
Gillies, D. (2014). Selecting applications for funding: Why random choice is better than peer review, *RT. A Journal on Research Policy & Evaluation, 2*, 1–14.
Graves, N., Barnett, A. G., & Clarke, P. (2011). Funding grant proposals for scientific research: Retrospective analysis of scores by members of grant review panel. *BMJ, 343*, d4797. https://doi.org/10.1136/bmj.d4797
Horrobin, D. F. (1974). Referees and research administrators: Barriers to scientific advance? *British Medical Journal, 27*(April), 216–218.
Horrobin, D. F. (1990). The philosophical basis of peer review and the suppression of innovation. *Journal of the American Medical Association, 263*(10), 1438–1441.
Horrobin, D. F. (1996). Peer review of grant applications: A harbinger for mediocrity in clinical research? *Lancet, 347*(9 November), 1293–1295.
Krimsky, S. (2012). Do financial conflicts of interest bias research? An inquiry into the "funding effect" hypothesis. *Science, Technology & Human Values, 38*(4), 566–587.
Lamont, M. (2009). *How professors think: Inside the curious world of academic judgment*. Cambridge, MA: Harvard University Press.
Manwell, C. (1979). Peer review: A case history from the Australian Research Grants Committee. *Search, 10*(3), 81–86.
Martin, B. (1986). Bias in awarding research grants. *British Medical Journal, 293*(30 August), 550–552.
Mow, K. E. (2010). *Inside the black box: Research grant funding and peer review in Australian research councils*. Saarbrücken, Germany: Lambert Academic Publishing.
Nicholson, J. M., & Ioannidis, J. P. A. (2012). Conform and be funded. *Nature, 492*(6 December), 34–36.
Olbrecht, M., & Bornmann, L. (2010). Panel peer review of grant applications: What do we know from research in social psychology on judgment and decision-making in groups? *Research Evaluation, 19*(4), 293–304.
Roy, R. (1984). Alternatives to review by peers: A contribution to the theory of scientific choice. *Minerva, 22*(Autumn-Winter), 316–328.
Schmidt, J. (2000). *Disciplined minds: A critical look at salaried professionals and the soul-battering system that shapes their lives*. Lanham, MD: Rowman & Littlefield.
Thorngate, W., Dawes, R. M., & Foddy, M. (2009). *Judging merit*. New York: Psychology Press.
Wessely, S. (1998). Peer review of grant applications: What do we know? *Lancet, 352*(25 July), 301–305.

Chapter 8
The Role of Communicating the Beliefs of the Clinician – Using the Placebo Effect in Clinical Practice

Paul Harris

There exists between the two primary persons involved in a therapeutic relationship many avenues of communication through which they exchange their thoughts, ideas, theories, beliefs, notions, and concepts. Over the years, there has been a shift in the use of these channels of communication by most physicians, healers, health-care practitioners, or doctors. This shift is complex in its nature, but can be summarized as moving away from interpersonal communication, away from hands-on touching the patient, away from getting to know the patient as a person, and away from communicating knowledge and understanding and compassion for the patient on the one hand and moving toward more reliance on lab data extracted from tests, probes, specimens, or evaluations of parts of the patient's corporeal self. As part of this shift, there is evidenced an increased reliance on tests that are purported to be more "objective" measures of the patient and which are based on reductionist ideals that have stripped away much of the humanistic aspects of the relationship between the doctor and the patient. Additional force is provided by industries involved in the development of and the funding of research designed to support this notion that this more "scientific" approach is always better. What might be at work is a groupthink surrendering by health-care professionals in general. The following will look at how the placebo effect has been used to these effects.

Attempts have been made to sterilize the relationship between the doctor and the patient, to arrive at a condition where the relationship does not enter the health-care equation as either a positive or a negative. As health care is seen more and more as a business, this dehumanization of the relationship between the doctor and the patient becomes a necessity, so that doctors and patients can be interchanged anywhere along the line of the health-care machine. Wrapped up in this evolutionary

P. Harris (✉)
Southern College of Optometry, Memphis, TN, USA

D. M. Allen, J. W. Howell (eds.), *Groupthink in Science*,
https://doi.org/10.1007/978-3-030-36822-7_8

change and this dehumanization of health care is a scapegoat of sorts called "placebo," thought to be a contaminant to be expunged from the doctor–patient relationship.

The placebo effect is a natural outcome of a normal therapeutic relationship between all health-care providers and their patients which cannot be eliminated or controlled, and all health-care providers should be learning to harness it to effect positive outcomes. The myth the application of the scientific method to the study of health care, the double-masked placebo-controlled study, will be unmasked for what it is.

Definitions

Placebo has come to mean many different things to many different people. "Placebo" is Latin for the phrase *I shall please*. The placebo becomes the embodiment of one persons' desire to please the other. The placebo effect is that which happens that can be attributed to the act of having been given a placebo. "The placebo must be differentiated from the placebo effect, which may or may not occur and which may be favorable or unfavorable. The placebo effect is defined as the changes produced by placebos" (Benson & Epstein, 1975).

Benson and Epstein state that, "A placebo is an active substance or preparation given to satisfy the patient's symbolic need for drug therapy and used in controlled studies to determine the efficacy of medicinal substances. Also, it is a procedure with no intrinsic therapeutic value" (Benson & Epstein, 1975). Thus, the placebo is seen as only working at a subconscious level to fulfill a *symbolic need* and that the caregiver is responding only at this level. This one-sided view does not recognize the role of the caregiver and the contribution of the ritual giving the placebo satisfies. They state that the only legitimate use placebos are as part of controlled studies, and that any studies which do not include a placebo arm are not valid. This simplifies the rules of thinking in the health-care professions by greatly narrowing studies that are to be taken seriously.

They also included the adjective "active" before the word "substance." The degree to which a substance is "active" or not emerges from one's perspective and understanding. In some situations, one person's "active" might be another person's "inactive" (Price, Finniss, & Benedetti, 2008). We might say that the potential for "action" is in the eye of the beholder and emerges from notions, ideas, concepts, and beliefs about the treatment in question.

Benson and Epstein continue with, "A placebo is any therapeutic procedure which is given deliberately to have an effect, or unknowingly has an effect on a patient, symptom, syndrome, or disease, but which is objectively without *specific* activity for the condition being treated" (Benson & Epstein, 1975). The broadening of the definition to any "therapeutic procedure" is significant.

Is there objective truth, which can be determined? Or is this a myth emboldening groupthink to stop searching or looking for true understanding? A cornerstone of the scientific method is that there exist objective data and that objective observations are possible and are the ideal conditions under which all research would be conducted. However, seeing, recognizing, and understanding emerge from the underlying frames of reference and requisite underlying knowledge base to allow such recognition and understanding. For example, until the insight about a twisted chain emerged, all those studying DNA were taking stabs in the dark at understanding.

Thomas Kuhn states, "If two people stand at the same place and gaze in the same direction, we must, under pain of solipsism, conclude that they receive closely similar stimuli. But people do not see stimuli; our knowledge of them is highly theoretical and abstract. Instead they have sensations, and we are under no compulsion to suppose that the sensations of our two viewers are the same." And, "... very different stimuli can produce the same sensations; and, finally, that the route from stimulus to sensation is in part conditioned by education. Individuals raised in different societies behave on some occasions as though they saw different things" (Kuhn, 1970). Thus, much of what is seen, even with the aid of measuring devices, is dependent on the knowledge and observational abilities of the observer. Kuhn states that basis for holding to one theory or another may better be based on belief, rather than on anything that can be proven. He states, "...that what each takes to be facts depends in part on the theory he espouses" (Kuhn, 1977). Here then is how groupthink may assert itself, unknowingly through unrecognized loopholes in logic where caregivers falsely believe they are driven by objective truth, when absolutes are nearly impossible to guarantee.

Beecher states, "A placebo is something, which is intended to act through a psychological mechanism. It is an aid to therapeutic suggestion, but the effect, which it produces, may be either psychological or physical" (Beecher, 1955). This is very open, being just about anything that the caregiver chooses to use to embody his or her intentions to help the patient get well and is very clear that the placebo works through or triggers a psychological mechanism. The placebo is seen as an aid to therapeutics.

Jean Comaroff is a sociologist whose work has looked at many of the dynamics of the doctor–patient relationship. "'Placebo' refers to that aspect of any treatment which is effective through symbolic rather than instrumental means. In this view, the placebo is, 'an active ingredient in practically every prescription.' Indeed, anything offered with therapeutic intent *may* be a placebo" (Comaroff, 1976). Therefore, every prescription given by every caregiver contains, as an integral element, a symbol, a potential to trigger a placebo response by the recipient. Taking this to be true, then two things emerge: (1) one can never fully separate out the effect of a specific treatment from the placebo effect and (2) the goal of knowing absolutely what a treatment effect is devoid of the placebo effect is unattainable. This then becomes a straw man argument for promoting the dumbing down of caregivers allowing the emergence of groupthink, spoiling innovation and true understanding.

Pearson states, "Placebo effects may also be viewed as a subset of a larger group of mind–brain–body effects such as the psycho-immunological effects of religious beliefs and devotional practices, and the effects of cultural and social economic systems on the prevalence and severity of specific diseases" (Pearson, 2002). Her work is part of an effort to identify the role that placebos play in everyday clinical practice and is part of the work of the National Center for Complementary and Alternative Medicine. This broadens the concept of a placebo to a special subset of much broader systems and gives potential mechanisms for the actions on a person.

Hart states that the word *placebo* entered the English language by a mistranslation of the 116th Psalm. "In the medieval Catholic liturgy, this verse opened the Vespers for the Dead; because professional mourners were sometimes hired to sing vespers, 'to sing placebos' came to be a derogatory phrase describing a servile flatterer" (Hart, 1999).

The Negative Connotations of Placebo

Benson and Epstein state, "Disdain for the placebo effect is the prevalent attitude in medicine today. The disdain for the placebo effect became prominent in medicine with the introduction of controlled drug investigations in the 1950's. The placebo effect is considered merely as a variable to be controlled and hence is ignored" (Benson & Epstein, 1975). Here, we see the strong influence on medical practice that the drug companies need to "test" their new products has created.

Comaroff states, "The more the doctor viewed medical practice as a scientific exercise, the more disparaging he was about placebo therapy" (Hart, 1999). To be more scientific means that one must disparage placebos and their use, and this is driven by self-image and the projection of that image to others. It is unclean to suggest that any aspect of modern scientific care might involve something intangible and unquantifiable, such as placebos and their effects.

Others condemn outright the use of placebos because it involves knowingly deceiving the patient. Comaroff states, "Doctors definitions tend to suggest that the placebo is an inert preparation, or form of therapy, which has little or no specific medical effect, but is given 'to humor rather than cure.' But definitions of this type *always* imply that the practitioner knowingly exploits such techniques to gratify the patient" (Beecher, 1955).

Bok states, "Clearly the prescription of placebos is intentionally deceptive only when the physician himself knows they are without specific effect but keeps the patient in the dark" (Bok, 1974). He continues, "As for the diagnostic and therapeutic use of placebos, we must start with the presumption that it is undesirable" (Bok, 1974). He gives no support for this statement, just that it should not be done. He goes further calling for the eradication of placebos. "Experiments involving humans are now subjected to increasingly careful safeguards for the people at risk, but it will be a long time before the practice of deceiving experimental subjects with respect to placebos is eradicated" (Bok, 1974).

Placebos Take a Licking but Keep on Ticking

Even though on an official basis the medical community disdains the use of placebos and is trying to get it out of the way so they can prove the efficacy of the therapeutic agents they use, placebos are there front and center.

Jean Comaroff interviewed physicians in the United Kingdom where they made explicit much of the thought which underlies the giving of placebos in clinical practice. Transcripts of these interviews provide tremendous insight into doctor–patient relationships. The following makes explicit the degree to which physicians, if given time to reflect will admit that they tend to overprescribe and when they do, often overprescribe a placebo (Comaroff, 1976).

> Dr. A., "I would say that I prescribe in 95 per cent of my consultations. That sounds high; it is high! Not all of these prescriptions are warranted in medical terms. You see, out here in Wales at least, when people go to the doctor, they expect a prescription. Even if you gave them a bottle of aspirins on prescription, it would have a high therapeutic value. You can't always call this a placebo, but I'd say that the placebo effect was about 50 per cent. It is very important that everybody gets a prescription. I very rarely prescribe a placebo though. Most of the things I give have a therapeutic effect of some kind. But for some of them it's the placebo effect rather than the therapeutic effect that is more important."

So, we must recognize that placebos are being prescribed regardless of the attitudes held by some. Kermen et al. showed that based on 412 responses to a questionnaire sent to 970 members of the American Academy of Family Physicians (43% response rate), 56% of respondents said they had used a placebo in clinical practice, 61% said they used placebos rather than offering no treatment at all, and only 8% questioned the ethics of using placebos (Kermen, Hickner, Brody, & Hasham, 2010).

Carroll states, "Too many studies have found objective improvements in health from placebo to support the notion that the placebo effect is entirely psychological" (Carroll, 2015). Tavel states, "The placebo effect also plays an important role for almost all conventional medical caregivers" (Tavel, 2014). He continues, "It is especially effective in relieving pain, anxiety, fatigue, insomnia, and depression but can go further to enhance the effectiveness of medical treatments with acknowledged physical benefits." So, there are specific conditions where the interactions between the doctor and patient, and the rituals the doctor and healthcare staff go through can and do have an effect in the way the patient reacts to their treatment.

Price et al. state, "Placebo factors have neurobiological underpinnings and actual effects on the brain and body" (Price et al., 2008). They continue, "The focus has shifted from the 'inert' content of the placebo agent to the concept of a stimulation of an active therapy within a psychosocial context."

Effect Size

How big is the placebo effect? Beecher combined the results of 15 studies involving 1082 subjects. Across these studies, he found that the placebos had an effect of 35.2% SD 2.2, which at the time was quite significant. Wong, using brain imaging, found that, "75% of the apparent efficacy of antidepressant medicine may actually be attributable to the placebo effect" (Wong, 2002). Wolf and Pinsky in studying the differences between a drug that was thought to be effective treating anxiety and tension versus a placebo found that the symptoms were made better in about 30% of the 31 subjects with the placebo alone (Wolf & Pinsky, 1954).

Placebo effects vary from 30% to 35% at the low to 75% in the examples given so far. In the normal course of many medical conditions, when a doctor does nothing, one-third get better, one-third get worse, and one-third stay about the same. Numbers close to or just above this one-third level of effectivity are often touted or extolled when a new study comes out, when in fact they are very close to baseline placebo effect levels as well as being close to expected outcomes of taking no action at all. Hrobjartsson and Gøtzsche state that the placebo effect "...cannot be distinguished from the natural course of the disease, regression to the mean (Price et al., 2008), and the effects of other factors" (Hrobjartsson & Gøtzsche, 2001).

Vedantam also looked at a series of studies over time and included many studies funded by drug companies, looking at studies where sugar pills of one sort another were used as the placebo. He showed that St. John's Wort cured 24% of the depressed people who received it. In the same studies, the cohort treated with Zoloft only attained a 25% cure rate, while those who got the placebo sugar pills had a 32% cure rate (Vedantam, 2002).

In a study which compared the effectiveness of a placebo versus anesthetic effects during dental procedures, the major factor turned out to be the suggestion of effectiveness by the caregiver at the time of the shot. Five hundred subjects were randomly given either an active anesthetic or a placebo. Randomly, within each group, some were told that what was being given to them would reduce their discomfort from the procedure and others were told nothing. Those who got the placebo with the verbal reassurance got more relief from pain than those getting the actual anesthetic with no reassurance at all (Gawande, 2002; Gracely, Dubner, Deeter, & Wolskee, 1985).

Freedman states that many placebo-controlled trials are not published (Freedman, Glass, & Weijer, 1996). The studies are done, and many are done well, but the results may not have been flattering to the new drug or treatment, so no one takes the time to prepare a report of findings and the results are not published. It is also known that subjects in clinical trials spend time guessing which condition they are in; because they are often told of the potential side effects of medications, which they may be given, they often figure out which arm of the trial they are in and doctors who are blinded to what they are giving also try to guess during the study period (Ney, Collins, & Spensor, 1986).

Placebo effects vary across cultures. In cases of ulcer treatment, in the United States, placebos were 36% effective in reducing discomfort, which matched the world average at the time of reporting. At the same time, rates for the effectiveness of placebo were 59% in Germany and only 7% in Denmark, The Netherlands, and Brazil (Moerman, 2002).

Why might this be? According to Amaral and Sabbatini, "The general idea is that the placebo effect appears as an involuntary conditioned reflex of the patient's body. In human beings, there exists, besides the first system of signals, a second one, language, that increases the possibilities of conditioning. For human beings, words can function as stimuli, so real and effective that they can mobilize us just like a concrete stimulus. Because words are symbols, abstractions, the conditioned stimulus can be generalizable. The placebo effect is an organic effect that occurs in patients due to Pavlovian conditioning on the level of abstract and symbolic stimuli. What counts is the reality present in the brain, not the pharmacological one. The nervous system expectation in relation to the effects of a drug can annul, revert or enlarge the pharmacological reactions to this drug" (Amaral & Sabbatini, 1999). This begins to get at the nature of why the effects are so variable from person to person as well as within the same person when going through different types of protocols, either experimental or clinical.

A patient who expects a drug to work shows comparable levels of dopamine released in their brain after an injection of either the real drug or a placebo (de la Fuente-Fernández et al., 2001). Expectation of symptom improvement is associated with increased endogenous striatal dopamine release in Parkinson's disease and increased endogenous opioid transmission in placebo analgesia. Expectation of symptom improvement is driven by frontal cortical areas, particularly the dorsolateral prefrontal, orbitofrontal, and anterior cingulate cortices (Lidstone & Stoessi, 2007; Reid, 2002). This leads to the observation that medication and placebo response rates in clinical trials are highly correlated (Walach, Sadaghiani, Dehm, & Bierman, 2005).

Placebo response rates in clinical trials are always a mix of true and false placebo effects. True placebo effects are being redefined based on the *meaning* of an intervention for a patient. These effects have been called *meaning effects*. A false placebo is a nonplacebo factor that appears to cause an improvement of a disease (Moerman & Jonas, 2002; Walach et al., 2005). The *meaning effect* can be seen as emerging within the individual and induced by complex interactions between the individual as he constructs meaning out of his medical situation, the medical system trying to intervene, physiological and psychological changes brought on by these interventions, inferences made by the person all resulting in an altered mental state and feeling of wellness (Walach et al., 2005).

Patterns of Discovery

There are three phases that occur, almost like clockwork when a new discovery is made. In the first phase, the world reacts positively because it is new, and it is great. The feeling in the air is often that a magic bullet has been found, and of course, there are no side effects. The inevitable second phase can be characterized as: the honeymoon is over. There are many reasons for this, including things like: for the first time the "new" gets compared to the best previous and it does not actually work much better; there is less support of all the communication between the caregiver and the subject/patient as it moves to a clinical tool, so there are fewer opportunities for all the positive meaning effects to emerge; and lastly the number of people getting the treatment increases, sometimes by orders of magnitudes, and this leads to the emergence of and recognition of side effects. Finally comes the sobering evaluation that takes place when what emerges is the realization that the new is actually not better than existing or even pure placebo effects. Some phases in these cycles can last a long time and groupthink might even cause an extended hold in place in the early parts of the cycle, when actual facts exist which should have allowed the professions to move on and recognize that the new thing actually should be discarded or improved more before full adoption takes place.

As an example, in a study of surgery vs. arthroscopic knee surgery, where incisions were made and simulations of all the routine sounds and commands that would occur versus actual surgery, follow-up at the 2-year point was quite revealing; 35% of the patients said that they felt less pain and were better able to get around, whether they were operated or not (Horowitz, 2002).

Few academics in medicine talk to their charges about displaying sympathy for the patient and its role, leaving those new to health caregiving with a lack of knowledge and examples that this should actually be done (Talbot, 2000). Lastly, factoring in for spontaneous remission or statistical regression to the mean effects means one must include a nontreatment and nonplacebo group in all studies, thereby increasing the costs of any study. This is the only way to know the relative roles of the treatment, the placebo or meaning effect, and the normal course of the condition being studied (Jaksic, Aukst-Margetic, & Jakovljevic, 2013).

Publication Bias

A thought experiment: If publishers or editors of journals favor research with positive effects shown for new treatments, we must recognize that a bias is in place which will distort everyone's view of the evidence base. If a treatment arm includes meaning effects which would enhance true placebo effects, this could make that new treatment look more effective than it really is. Conversely, a very effective meaning effect could take place in one area of a study more than in another leading to the masking of some real effect (Walach et al., 2005). "When placebo effects are large, it can be difficult to demonstrate drug effects in clinical trials" (Whalley, Hyland, & Kirsch, 2008). Unintended bias may also be revealed only by looking from the 30,000-foot view. "Studies reporting large effects of placebo are published in prestigious journals, whereas studies with no effects would be dismissed as 'failed experiments', and are published less often, later, in less prestigious journal and more often as abstracts" (Hrobjartsson, Kaptchuk, & Miller, 2011).

One last confounding aspect of experimental design is the role of informed consent, which may influence the outcome of some arms of an experiment differentially and thus either favor or reduce artificially the placebo or meaning effect, simply by the way the information is given (Hrobjartsson, Kaptchuk, & Miller, 2011). Tell the person in the experiment that they might experience this or that symptom, and this acts as a seed or trigger for the person actually attending to a possible symptom and experiencing and reporting it, when if it had not been mentioned it would never have been experienced or reported by the person.

Washout phase to weed out placebo responders Many randomized controlled trials are preceded by a so-called washout phase in which all participants take an inert pill and anyone who reacts favorably to it is eliminated. The result is that 30–40% of the subjects may be removed from the group. However, the fact that they reacted to the inert pill may have little impact on predicting their response to the actual clinical protocols about to be tested. Thus, the pool of subjects no longer is representative of the population at large but is skewed by the attempt to remove placebo responders (Talbot, 2000).

Doctor–Patient Relationship

Few of us can clearly articulate how we come to hold our beliefs. We are not sure how much is from our scientific background or from reading journals or keeping up to date with the latest and greatest. In fact, we may be deluding ourselves with a belief that we are on much firmer ground than can be proven. What we do know is that, "The physician's belief in the intrinsic worth of his medicine has always rivaled that of the patient" (Kuhn, 1977). And those beliefs are transmitted from the doctor to the patient in the subtlest ways at times.

Comaroff states, "Placebo therapy is an important element in an established ritual sequence, used by doctors to cope with problems of clinical uncertainty and of patient management" (Comaroff, 1976). As a matter of course, doctors faced with either the choice of having to explain something to a patient or family member when the explanation is either lengthy or complex for some condition or which might not have a clear-cut treatment protocol, or to give a prescription for something simple, might elect to give something instead. This keeps the doctor in control and saves lots of time. "Placebo therapy may be comprehended as a repertoire of techniques which enable the general practitioner to deal with complex and uncertain situations in a manner which conserves his time and energy" (Comaroff, 1976).

Time with doctors has been decreasing over the ages. In 1943, the average visit to the doctor lasted 26 minutes; this decreased to 17 minutes in 1985 and is about 13–16 minutes at the time of this writing in the United States. Less time with the patient translates into less opportunity to build the communication and trust necessary to effectively use the placebo effect for the benefit of the patient. Additionally, in certain clinic settings, patients rarely get to see the same doctor from visit to visit. They become a patient of the practice, not of a particular doctor. This undermines the kind of solid relationship that builds trust and a sense that your doctor understands your story (Talbot, 2000).

For Best Outcomes – Use All the Tools

To produce the best outcome with those patients we serve, we should consciously and progressively combine, like how one grades dose escalation of component parts, those nonspecific effects of the patient–practitioner relationship (Kaptchuk et al., 2008). Talbot states, "The physician who can marshal a placebo response with her words and manner probably comes closest to what many of us would think of as the profession's ideal – the kind of doctor who seems wholly committed to our welfare, not the insurance company's; who knows when and how to give us hope, who listens closely but doesn't feel constrained from delivering advice; who knows us because she has taken the time to know us" (Talbot, 2000).

The following sample equation is offered below to help improve the quality of care delivered:

$$\begin{aligned}&\text{Patient's Response} = \text{Stimulus}\left(\text{the actual care / treatment plan}\right)\\&*\text{Attitude} * \text{Appraisal} * \text{Comfort level with caregiver} * \text{Alignment}\\&\text{of belief systems of patient and caregiver in the domain being}\\&\text{worked in} * \text{"Bedside manner"}, *\text{etc.}\end{aligned}$$

The result is the patient's response. Everything to the right of the equal sign is what goes into producing the patient's response. Between each element is an "*", which might be thought of as a multiplier. If that factor is neutral, then it could be thought of as holding the value of 1.0. Anything multiplied by 1.0 remains the same. A modifier, which is strongly in play, is greater than 1.0 and increases the effect of the care. A modifier, which is negatively affecting things, is less than 1.0 and it decreases all the good being done in other areas. We can think of all these factors being in play and needing to be balanced, with the result causing the patient's response to their treatment to be much more than just a direct result of actual treatment.

Specifically, these factors include:

- Attitude: The mind-set one brings to the overall situation, the evaluation of things before the interactions have begun.

- Appraisal: A continuing evaluation of how things are going throughout the interaction with the caregiver. This can be thought of as modifying the attitude over time.
- Comfort level with caregiver: Affinity might be an apt description here, the higher the degree of comfort with the person and their office and their staff, etc., the more likely the patient/subject will benefit from the care.
- Alignment of belief systems of patient and caregiver in the domain being worked in: The more closely aligned they are together the greater the likelihood that increased benefits will be derived is seen.
- Bedside manner: The mannerisms and communication style used is something under the direct control, most of the times, of the caregiver and should be matched to the needs of the patient/subject as much as possible to improve outcomes.

In looking at things this way, the actual placebo does not appear, and the stimulus is just one of the parameters to be tweaked.

Lastly, are some clinical guidelines for improving effectiveness, not just in health care, but most likely in any interaction between people.

Clinical Guidelines for Improved Effectiveness

- Characteristics of optimal patient–practitioner relationship (Brody & Miller, 2011):
  - Warm, friendly manner
  - Active listening
  - Thoughtful silence while pondering a treatment plan
  - Communication of confidence
  - Communication of positive expectations
- Positive therapeutic effects can be produced by suggestions, past effects of active treatments, and cues that signal that an active medication of treatment has been given.
- Psychological mediators of these effects include expectations, desires, and emotions that target prospective symptom changes.
- Take time with your patient.
- Tell the patient in a caring manner the expected benefits of all treatments before administering them (Kuhn, 1970).
- Use open administration of drugs or treatments rather than hidden ones.
- Be aware of the context relative to the patient – adapt language and explanations to allow them to understand.
- Help your patient expect to feel good (or less bad).
- Help them to expect to perform better by explicitly stating your expectations in terms relevant to them in their lives.

Developments in research on placebos suggest that the time has come to translate the science of placebo effect into clinical and medical research and practice. The health-care provider or caregiver following these guidelines should be inoculated against groupthink and the negatives which come with surrendering one's values and judgment.

References

Amaral, J., & Sabbatini, R. (1999). Placebo effect: The power of the sugar pill. *Brain & Mind*, Published on the web, July 25, Center for Biomedical Informatics. www.epub.org.br/cm/n09/mente/placebo1_i.htm

Beecher, H. (1955). The powerful placebo. *JAMA, 159*, 1602–1606.

Benson, H., & Epstein, M. (1975). The placebo effect – A neglected asset in the care of patients. *JAMA, 232*(12), 1225–1227.

Bok, S. (1974). The ethics of giving placebos. *Scientific American, 231*(5), 17–23.

Brody, H., & Miller, F. G. (2011). Lessons from recent placebo research about the placebo effect – From art to science. *JAMA, 306*(23), 2612–2613.

Carroll, R. (2015). The placebo effect. The Skeptics Dictionary, on the web at www.skepdic.com

Comaroff, J. (1976). A bitter pill to swallow: Placebo therapy in general practice. *The Sociological Review, 24*(1), 79–86.

de la Fuente-Fernández, R., Ruth, T. J., Sossi, V., Schulzer, M., Calne, D. B., & Stoessl, A. J. (2001). Expectation and dopamine release: Mechanism of the placebo effect in Parkinson's disease. *Science, 293*, 1164–1166.

Freedman, B., Glass, K. C., & Weijer, C. (1996). Placebo orthodoxy in clinical research II: Ethical, legal, and regulatory myths. *The Journal of Law, Medicine & Ethics, 24*, 252–259.

Gawande, A. (2002). *A surgeon's notes on an imperfect science* (pp. 115–129). New York: Henry Holt & Co..

Gracely, R., Dubner, R., Deeter, W., & Wolskee, P. (1985). Clinician's expectations influence placebo analgesia. *The Lancet, 1*, 43.

Hart, C. (1999). The mysterious placebo effect. *Modern Drug Discovery, 2*(4), 30–40.

Horowitz, J. (2002). What the knees really need. Time, July 22.

Hrobjartsson, A., & Gøtzsche, P. (2001). Is the placebo powerless? – An analysis of clinical trials comparing placebo with no treatment. *New England Journal of Medicine, 344*(21), 1594–1602.

Hrobjartsson, A., Kaptchuk, T. J., & Miller, F. G. (2011). Placebo effect studies are susceptible to response bias and to other types of biases. *Journal of Clinical Epidemiology, 64*(11), 1223–1229.

Jaksic, N., Aukst-Margetic, B., & Jakovljevic, M. (2013). Does personality play a relevant role in the placebo effect? *Psychiatria Danubina, 25*(1), 17–23.

Kaptchuk, T. J., Kelley, J. M., Conboy, L. A., Davis, R. B., Kerr, C. E., Jacobson, E. E., et al. (2008). Components of placebo effect: Randomized controlled trial in patients with irritable bowel syndrome. *BMJ, 336*(7651), 999–1003.

Kermen, R., Hickner, J., Brody, H., & Hasham, I. (2010). Family physicians believe the placebo effect is therapeutic but often use real drugs as placebos. *Family Medicine, 42*(9), 636–642.

Kuhn, T. (1970). *The structure of scientific revolutions* (2nd ed. pp. 192–193, 195). Chicago: The University of Chicago Press.

Kuhn, T. (1977). *The essential tension* (p. 338). Chicago: The University of Chicago Press.

Lidstone, S. C., & Stoessi, A. J. (2007). Understanding the placebo effect: Contribution from neuroimaging. *Molecular Imaging and Biology, 9*, 176–185.

Moerman, D. E. (2002). *Meaning, medicine, and the placebo effect.* Dearborn: ResearchGate, University of Michigan. https://doi.org/10.1017/CBO9780511810855

Moerman, D. E., & Jonas, W. B. (2002). Deconstructing the placebo effect and finding the meaning response. *Annals of Internal Medicine, 136*, 471–476.

Ney, P. G., Collins, C., & Spensor, C. (1986). Double blind: Double talk or are there ways better to do better research? *Medical Hypotheses, 21*, 119–126.

Pearson, N. (2002). National Center for Complementary and Alternative Medicine, Project concept review – The placebo effect in clinical practice, Ph.D. (NCCAM, NIH) 301-594-0519.

Price, D. D., Finniss, D. G., & Benedetti, F. (2008). A comprehensive review of the placebo effect: Recent advances and current thought. *Annual Review of Psychology, 59*, 565–590.

Reid, B. (2002). The nocebo effect: placebo's evil twin. *The Washington Post*, April 30, Page HE01

Talbot, M., (2000). The placebo prescription. *The New York Times Magazine*, 9 Jan 2000.

Tavel, M. E. (2014). The placebo effect: The good, the bad, and the ugly. *The American Journal of Medicine, 127*(6), 484–488.

Vedantam, S. (2002). Against depression, a sugar pill is hard to beat. *The brain in the news*, May 15 (pp. 1–2).

Walach, H., Sadaghiani, C., Dehm, C., & Bierman, D. (2005). The therapeutic effect of clinical trials: Understanding placebo response rates in clinical trials – A secondary analysis. *BMC Medical Research Methodology, 5*(26), 1–12.

Whalley, B., Hyland, M. E., & Kirsch, I. (2008). Consistency of the placebo effect. *Journal of Psychosomatic Research, 64*, 537–541.

Wolf, S., & Pinsky, R. H. (1954). Effects of placebo administration and occurrence of toxic reactions. *Journal of the American Medical Association, 155*(4), 339–341.

Wong, K. (2002). Brain imaging study reveals placebo's effect. *Scientific American*, News in Brief On-line, January 2.

Chapter 9
Bias and Groupthink in Science's Peer-Review System

David B. Resnik and Elise M. Smith

Introduction

Peer review is a key part of the scientific enterprise. Most journals use peer review to evaluate articles submitted for publication; funding agencies use peer review to assess research proposals; and scholarly conference committees use peer review to evaluate abstracts and conference proceedings. Peer review serves mainly as a gatekeeping mechanism to ensure that published or funded research meets appropriate disciplinary or interdisciplinary norms including standards of rigor, reproducibility, validity, objectivity, novelty, and integrity.

The peer-review process involves subject-matter experts, and this lends a certain prestige and credibility to those scientific works that are positively reviewed. Peer review also serves to improve the quality of articles and research proposals and educate junior scholars about methodological standards (Resnik & Elmore, 2016). However, peer review is not perfect (Smith, 2006). Various socials scientists have opened the black box of scientific inquiry – including peer review – to reveal social norms held by peer-reviewers which can create bias (Latour & Woolgar, 1979). Specific studies have identified bias regarding academic rank, gender, race, nationality, and institutional affiliation that can undermine the impartiality and integrity of the peer-review system (Lee, Sugimoto, Zhang, & Cronin, 2012; Resnik & Elmore, 2016).

Bias may also be the result of groupthink – which exists when the psychological drive for consensus is so strong that any divergence from that consensus is ignored or rejected. This is not to say that a degree of consensus or agreement is not

D. B. Resnik (✉) · E. M. Smith
National Institute of Environmental Health Sciences, National Institutes of Health, Research, Triangle Park, NC, USA
e-mail: resnikd@niehs.nih.gov

D. M. Allen, J. W. Howell (eds.), *Groupthink in Science*,
https://doi.org/10.1007/978-3-030-36822-7_9

beneficial. Understandably, the public expects scientific findings which are endorsed by a large group of specialists to be sound and credible. Also, in undertaking research, there should be some agreement among scientists respecting working assumptions, certain hypotheses, and methodology, notwithstanding some uncertainty or divergence of opinion. For example, health-care providers must agree on standards of practice to apply the results of biomedical research. If there was no "common ground" or consensus, medical practice would be chaotic, unpredictable, and possibly unsafe. However, groupthink may be problematic if a complacent trust between members is created and individual critical reflection in scientific decision-making is no longer accepted or promoted.

This chapter describes scientific peer review, discusses some of the evidence for bias, examines the impact of biases related to groupthink, and considers some options for reforming the system to reduce the impact of bias.

Science's Peer-Review System

In the seventeenth century, the editors of *Philosophical Transactions of the Royal Society of London* instituted the first known instance of peer review to address the concerns of some of the members of the Royal Society that their journal was publishing highly speculative, rambling articles and works of fiction. However, peer review did not become standard practice in scientific publishing until the nineteenth century (Shamoo & Resnik, 2015). In the twentieth century, government agencies began using peer review to determine the allocation of funds for scientific projects. Peer review is now also used to make decisions concerning tenure and promotion in academic institutions and to award scientific prizes (Shamoo & Resnik, 2015).

Journal editors usually conduct an initial review of a manuscript submitted for publication to determine whether it fits the aims and scope of the journal and meets some minimum standards of quality. If a paper is deemed suitable for peer review, the editors invite researchers with expertise in its subject-matter to review it. Some journals allow authors to recommend potential reviewers or request that certain individuals not serve as reviewers. Most journals seek input from two reviewers, but some may ask for more, especially when reviewers disagree (Resnik & Elmore, 2016). Reviewer reports usually include some comments intended for the authors or editors, an evaluation of the manuscript based on journal criteria (e.g., originality, significance, statistical soundness, strength of the argument, quality of writing), and an overall recommendation (e.g., accept the manuscript as is, accept with revisions (minor or major), revise and resubmit, or reject). Editors usually follow the reviewers' recommendations given their expertise, but in instances when they disagree with the reviewers, editors may not (Shamoo & Resnik, 2015). Editors are responsible for conducting their own assessment of the manuscript and determining whether the reviewer reports are fair and competent (Resnik & Elmore, 2016).

The most common form of peer review in scientific publishing is the single blind: reviewers are informed of the authors' identities and affiliations but not vice versa.

Blinding reduces the unwanted effects created by power dynamics. For example, a junior scholar may hesitate to reject a paper because of significant methodological flaws if she was aware that a prestigious author knew her identity. The reviewer might be worried about being ostracized from her field of research because of her difference of opinion with an esteemed member in high standing in said group. Generally speaking, the purpose of single blinding is to encourage reviewers to make candid comments without fear of reprisal from disgruntled authors (Shamoo & Resnik, 2015). Informing the reviewers of the authors' identities allows them to disclose any conflicts of interest and consider relevant institutional factors into account during review. For example, if the reviewers know that the manuscript comes from a non-English-speaking country, they may decide to take this into account when evaluating the written presentation (Shamoo & Resnik, 2015).

An increasing number of journals have switched to a double-blind system in which neither party is told the other's identity or affiliation. The purpose of double blinding is to reduce bias related to gender, institutional affiliation, or nationality (see discussion below). However, studies have shown that nearly half the time reviewers can correctly identify the first author on the manuscript (Baggs, Broome, Dougherty, Freda, & Kearney, 2008; Justice, Cho, Winker, Berlin, & Rennie, 1998). Identification of authors may be more likely to occur in highly specialized fields where most researchers know each other's work through writing style, subject of research, and research cited (Resnik & Elmore, 2016). Laboratories usually are aware of their competition since research is often shared at conferences and through professional collaboration.

Some journals have gone to an open system in which authors and reviewers are told each other's identities and affiliations (Resnik & Elmore, 2016). The purpose of open review is to deter unethical behavior from reviewers, such as breach of confidentiality or theft of ideas (Resnik & Elmore, 2016). Open review may also allow for both authors and reviewers to be named on the paper which adds a degree of accountability as well as recognition for the peer review. Researchers who find peer-reviewers work particularly important may choose to name peer-reviewers openly by name in acknowledgments. However, scientists may prefer to not participate in an open review system because they fear reprisal (Ho et al., 2013).

Although anonymity may promote candid review, one might argue that secrecy in science is counterproductive and may ultimately reduce the quality of peer review. A recent trend is where researchers promote full transparency and expediency by using postpublication open peer review (Hunter, 2012). In journals, such as F1000 *Research,* authors send a publication to the journal which conducts a very basic an in-house review. The article is then put online without delay. Peer-reviewers then post reviews online and articles are often reviewed if requested. This public "review" period and ensuing debate allows researchers to cite manuscripts that have not yet completed peer review.

Researchers have argued that publishing work that will be later revised and republished could reduce quality control and may augment the incidence of unsound science or of misconduct (Teixeira da Silva & Dobránszki, 2015). It may be argued that although traditional peer review has flaws, it is better than publishing research without oversight. However, the goal of postpublication peer review is often to allow more continuous peer review, not less (Lauer, Krumholz, & Topol, 2015). When manuscripts may change, journals do openly mention when a paper is not yet peer reviewed.

Interestingly, the culture and integration of postpublication peer review are similar to prepublication archiving which originated in physics but has been adopted by many disciplines in the biomedical sciences. In prepublication archiving, researchers put a copy of their paper in an online repository, such as arXiv.org or bioRxiv.org, which is often cited with a specific digital object identifier (DOI) during or before any formal peer-review process in another journal. A considerable upside to this model is that identification of the provider or source of an idea occurs before any peer-review process. This helps to stop individuals from stealing ideas during the peer-review process. Some have even mentioned that open models are part of the "Open Science future" (Pulverer, 2016).

Numerous studies have examined how these different approaches impact the quality, consistency, and effectiveness of peer review, but thus far, the evidence has been inconclusive (Armstrong, 1997; Lee et al., 2012). For example, two small studies conducted by McNutt, Evans, Fletcher, and Fletcher (1990) and Fisher, Friedman, and Strauss (1994) found that blinding reviewers improves the quality of review, but larger studies conducted by van Rooyen, Godlee, Evans, Smith, and Black (1998), Justice et al. (1998), and Godlee, Gale, and Martyn (1998) found that blinding does not have this effect. While a study by Walsh, Rooney, Appleby, and Wilkinson (2000) concluded that openness improves the quality and courtesy of reviewer reports, other studies found no evidence that openness improves peer review (Godlee et al., 1998; Justice et al., 1998; van Rooyen et al., 1998, 1999, 2010). More research, therefore, is needed on the extent to which different approaches to peer review impact quality, consistency, and effectiveness.

Peer review by funding agencies varies considerably, depending on the method used. Some agencies convene in-person panels, while others may handle the review process remotely via secure websites or email, or by some combination of in-person and remote (Shamoo & Resnik, 2015). The National Institutes of Health (NIH), for example, uses study sections composed of experts to review research grants. The study section will usually meet in-person to review grant proposals and materials will be distributed in advance. A proposal will normally be assigned a primary and a secondary reviewer. These reviewers will present the proposal to the group and provide an assessment. The entire group will also evaluate the proposal and score it based on specific review criteria, including scientific significance, methodology, qualifications of the principal investigator, institutional resources, adequacy of the budget, preliminary research, and potential impact of the study (Shamoo & Resnik, 2015). The NIH requires reviewers to declare conflicts of interest (COIs) and prohibits individuals from reviewing proposals submitted by colleagues from their institution, or from recent collaborators, former students, or advisors. The final funding decision is made by NIH leadership, based on recommendations from the study section.

Bias in Peer Review

Although the peer-review system is designed to provide an "impartial" quality assessment, evidence indicates that various biases can impact decisions related to publication and funding (Lee et al., 2012; Shamoo & Resnik, 2015). One well-documented type of bias is the tendency for journals to publish positive or confirmatory results rather than negative ones. Initial studies of this phenomena conducted by Mahoney (1977), Easterbrook, Berlin, Gopalan, and Matthews (1991), and Stern and Simes (1997) found that clinical trials reporting positive results were more likely to be published than those reporting negative results, and subsequent research confirmed these findings (Lee et al., 2012). A systematic review and meta-analysis of studies of publication bias conducted by Dwan et al. (2013) found similar results. While there is a substantial evidence of a bias in favor of publishing positive results, it is unclear whether this bias is due to decisions made by reviewers, editors, or authors. It may be the case that most of the bias results from authors' decisions not to publish negative results rather than reviewer or editor preferences for positive results (Olson et al., 2002).

Numerous studies have shown that gender bias impacts the funding of grant proposals (Shen, 2013; Wenneras & Wold, 1997). Bornmann, Mutza, and Daniela (2007) conducted a meta-analysis of 21 studies of grant peer review conducted between 1979 and 2004 and found that men were 7% more likely than women to receive funding, although there was considerable variability in the impact of gender. The authors note that a variety of causal factors may contribute to this discrepancy, including fewer women on peer-review panels or in leadership positions. Waisbren et al. (2008) found that differences in grant funding success between male and female applicants disappeared when they controlled for academic rank, suggesting that gender biases in grant peer review may be a function of differences in career paths between men and women. Two studies of gender bias in NIH grant review by Kaatz and coauthors suggest that an awareness of an applicant's gender may function as a subconscious (implicit) influence on decision-making. These studies found that reviewers consistently gave female applicants lower scores than male applicants, even when they used similar words and phrases to describe their proposals (Kaatz et al., 2015, 2016).

Gender bias is more difficult to study in journal peer review than in grant review because most journals do not disclose the names of reviewers. However, Helmer, Schottdorf, Neef, and Battaglia (2017) obtained gender data from Frontiers journals, which include the names of the reviewers and associate editors alongside the article accepted for publication. They analyzed data from 126,000 authors, 43,000 reviewers, and 9000 editors for 41,000 articles published in 142 journals from the natural and social sciences, medicine, engineering, and the humanities and found that women are underrepresented in the peer-review process and that there is a strong same-gender preference (e.g., men editors give higher ranking to men authors; women give higher ranking to women). Grod et al. (2008) also found that acceptance rates for papers with female first authors increased significantly after

Trends in Ecology and Evolution adopted a double-blind review format. However, other studies have shown little to no bias regarding gender. For instance, a study in biosciences (989 responses) found that the gender of the first author had no significant effect on the reviewer's recommendations or acceptation rate (Borsuk et al., 2009). Other studies have found no significant difference in acceptance rates between male and female first-authored papers (Lane & Linden, 2009; Tregenza, 2002).

Despite efforts to encourage women to pursue careers in science, important gender disparities remain in science on a global scale and in most countries including the United States and Canada (Larivière et al., 2013). Overall, many different factors impact gender discrepancies in science, including culture, education, workplace environment, childbearing and rearing responsibilities, labor distribution within teams, and career decisions (Ceci & Williams, 2011). Although reviewers' implicit biases in peer review can play a role in the underrepresentation of women in science, it is but one among many confounding factors.

Like gender, race and ethnicity also appear to influence the peer-review process. Ginther and colleagues published several studies of racial and ethnic bias in the grant peer-review process in the United States. Their first study found that black applicants were 10% less likely than white applicants to receive funding for R01 grants when other relevant factors, such as education, training, previous awards, and publication record, were controlled for (Ginther et al., 2011). Another study found that biases against black applicants for NIH R01 grants decreased when one included medical school affiliation: blacks from medical schools were only 7.8% less likely to receive funding than whites (Ginther, Haak, Schaffer, & Kington, 2012). A third found that white women were no less likely than white men to receive funding, but that Asian and black women were less likely to receive funding, when controlling for relevant factors (Ginther, Kahn, & Schaffer, 2016). However, Jang et al. (2013) conducted a bibliometric analysis comparing research productivity of black and white applicants and found that the NIH peer-review process is not biased against black applicants. Racial and ethnic differences in funding disappear when one controls for research productivity (Jang et al., 2013).

There is also evidence of bias in peer review related to nationality and institutional affiliation (Lee et al., 2012). Ross et al. (2006) studied abstracts accepted at the American Heart Association's Scientific Sessions before and after it instituted double-blind review and found that blinding the reviewers to the authors' names reduced biases related to nationality and institutional affiliation. More specifically, Ross et al. (2006) showed that when the affiliations of researchers were made public, papers with US institutions were accepted 7.4% more often than during blinded review; papers with non-US institutions were accepted 0.9% less than during blinded review. A study of abstract acceptance by Timmer, Hilsden, and Sutherland (2001) also found evidence of bias related to nationality, and a study by Ernst and Kienbacher (1991) found that reviewers were more likely to accept articles submitted by authors who have the same nationality as that of the journal. Murray et al. (2016) found that funding success and the award amount were significantly lower for smaller institutions submitting grant applications to Canada's Natural Sciences and Engineering Research Council Discovery Grant program. However, Garfunkel, Ulshen, Hamrick, and Lawson (1994) found that institutional ranking in terms of NIH funding in the United States did not impact reviewers' recommendations or the acceptance rate for major papers submitted to a biomedical journal, although it did impact recommendations and acceptance rates for brief reports.

Groupthink and Bias in Science

We will now turn our attention to bias related to groupthink, which we will define as a situation in which the psychological drive for group consensus is so strong that dissent is hidden, rejected, or dissuaded.[1] The social psychologist Irving Janis (1972) coined the term "groupthink" to describe decision-making processes that have led to foreign-policy fiascos, such as the US' failed invasion of Cuba's Bay of Pigs in April 1961. American intelligence officials and military leaders wrongly assumed that the 1400 Cuban exiles who took part in the invasion would be able to instigate a successful venture to oust Castro, but they were vastly outnumbered by the Cuban army and surrendered within 24 hours (Janis, 1982). Janis observed that groupthink led to this ill-fated military venture by causing decision-makers to not examine evidence critically and consider alternative course of action. Janis' work built upon earlier studies of cohesiveness and conformity in group decision-making (Janis, 1972, 1982).

In scientific research, groupthink may lead researchers to reject innovative or controversial ideas, hypotheses or methodologies that challenge the status quo. Philosophers, historians, and sociologists have observed that scientists often resist new ideas, despite their reputation for open-mindedness (Barber, 1961; Kuhn, 1962). The great quantum physicist Maxwell Planck has been quoted as saying: "A new scientific truth does not triumph by convincing its opponents and making them see the light, but rather because its opponents eventually die, and a new generation grows up that is familiar with it" (Planck, 1962: 33–34).

In his seminal work on the history of science, *The Structure of Scientific Revolutions*, Kuhn described the role of conformity and close-mindedness in scientific advancement. According to Kuhn (1962), science progresses though different stages. In the first stage, known as normal science, scientists conduct their research within a paradigm that defines the field. A paradigm is a way of doing science that includes basic assumptions, beliefs, principles, theories, methods, and epistemic values that establish how one solves problems within the normal science tradition; normal science involves consensus within a scientific community. For example, Newtonian physics was a normal science tradition that established ways of solving problems related to motion and electromagnetic radiation (Kuhn, 1962). During the

[1] Our definition is loosely inspired by Irvin's definition (1972) but has been modified so as to apply to the context of science and peer review.

normal science stage, scientists attempt to apply the paradigm to problems they can solve and they resist certain theories, methods, and ideas that challenge the paradigm. At this stage, scientists tend to think outside the theoretical limits of the paradigm limiting novel ideas. However, as problems emerge that cannot be solved within the paradigm, scientists start to consider new ideas, theories, and methods that form the basis of a new and emerging paradigm. A scientific revolution occurs when the new paradigm replaces the old. For example, during the early twentieth century, Newtonian physics succumbed to quantum mechanics and relativity theory (Kuhn, 1962). A paradigm shift is not a purely rational process driven by logical argumentation and empirical evidence; rather, it involves a change in perception or a willingness to see the world in a different way (Kuhn, 1962). After the revolution, a new paradigm takes hold and the process repeats itself.

Some philosophers have argued that a certain amount of closed-mindedness, known as epistemological conservatism, is justified in scientific research. The rationale for this epistemological stance is that change in a network of beliefs should be based on substantial empirical evidence. Since changes in beliefs can consume a considerable amount of time and effort and our cognitive resources are limited, we should not change our beliefs, especially ones that play a central role in our worldview, without compelling evidence (Lycan, 1988; Quine, 1961; Resnik, 1994; Sklar, 1975). For example, because Einstein's general theory of relativity contradicted the fundamental principle of Newtonian physics that space and time are immutable, it took extraordinary proof – that is, that observation of the sun's gravity bending light from a star during a solar eclipse in 1919 – to confirm the theory (Buchen, 2009). While it seems clear that a certain amount of conservatism makes sense in research, scientists should be careful to avoid dogmatism. Although scientists should practice a degree a skepticism pertaining to hypotheses and theories that challenge the status quo, they should be open to new ideas and avoid dogmatism (Resnik, 1994).

Groupthink and Bias in Peer Review

Issues surrounding groupthink that we find in scientific norms may permeate the process of peer review, which may result in the rejection of innovative or controversial manuscripts and research proposals. It is plausible to hypothesize that lack of social diversity could contribute to groupthink in peer review. As noted earlier, Helmer et al. (2017) found that women are underrepresented in the population of peer-reviewers for Frontiers journals. Since racial and ethnic minorities are underrepresented in science (Committee on Science, Engineering, and Public Policy, 2010; Nelson, 2007), it is likely that they are also underrepresented in the reviewer population. It is possible that there is also a lack of diversity with respect to nationality and institutional affiliation in the reviewer population, although we know of no published research on this topic.

If we suppose that there is a lack of social diversity in the population of peer-reviewers, it is conceivable that this type of bias could impact the review process and that increasing reviewer diversity would decrease groupthink (Longino, 1990). However, it is important to recognize that this argument assumes that diversity with respect to social factors translates into increased willingness to accept ideas that challenge the status quo, and that lack of such diversity has the opposite effect, neither of which might be the case. Social diversity may also not lead to diversity with respect to opinions, beliefs, and epistemological norms (i.e., intellectual diversity) (Card, 2005). For example, a socially diverse group of researchers could still fall prey to groupthink because they lack intellectual diversity and favor the status quo or want to preserve their chances for peer recognition. Also, a socially homogenous group of researchers might not fall prey to groupthink because they are intellectually diverse and are open to new and controversial ideas.

Clearly, more research is needed on the relationship between social diversity and peer review. Some argue, based on standpoint theory, that marginalized groups may have a different or perhaps an even better view of social phenomena, given their position at the margins of society (Harding, 2004). Although some aspects of standpoint theory remain contentious as it methodologically and systematically questions the position of power it may be an effective tool to question the status quo.

There are different ways that groupthink could occur in the peer-review process. Because of the difficulty in finding peer-reviewers, editors may resort to using the same network of individuals repeatedly. Groupthink within this limited network may set in and reduce the diversity of reviews. The hyperspecialization of certain fields may also narrow the choice of qualified reviewers significantly and thus reduce their diversification. Moreover, with time, editors may become overly trusting toward certain peers, especially those with similar scientific stances. Editors may come to blindly trust individuals of high academic standing which may reduce the proper evaluation of the review.

Another type of groupthink involves the occurrence of dogmatism in the peer-review process itself; that is, a predisposition to reject innovative or controversial theories, hypotheses, or methods. Shamoo and Resnik (2015) have observed that a certain amount of dogmatism may be unavoidable in peer review because reviewers are chosen for their expertise, and experts are usually established researchers with theoretical and methodological commitments (or biases) that can compromise their open-mindedness. An anthropological perspective of peer review has shown that even when trying to promote fairness, peer-reviewers usually think that research that is similar to their own (in terms of methods, topics, results) is of a higher standard – making criteria for excellence somewhat subjective (Lamont, 2009). In this case, the status quo will most likely be maintained and novelty discouraged; in effect, past "truths" would be left unchallenged.

The presence of multidisciplinary panels on review boards often helps to reduce groupthink and bias. However, in journal peer review, there is no open multidisciplinary debate. To reduce or counteract closed-mindedness, editors could select reviewers who are not established researchers, but this strategy could potentially undermine the quality of peer review.

While there is anecdotal evidence (i.e., complaints from scientists) that intellectual dogmatism impacts peer review (Chubin & Hackett, 1990), it is difficult to obtain systematic data that supports this hypothesis (Lee et al., 2012). A study by Resnik, Gutierrez-Ford, and Peddada (2008) found that 50.5% of 283 scientists responding to a survey conducted at a government biomedical research institution claimed that they had experienced bias in the peer-review process. However, this study did not define bias and gathered data on scientists' perceptions of bias, not on bias itself.

An interesting study conducted by Resch, Ernst, and Garrow (2000) randomly assigned 398 reviewers to receive papers on conventional or nonconventional treatments for obesity. The papers were virtually the same with respect to research methodology and design; the main difference related to the type of intervention. One hundred and forty-one reviewers responded to the review request. Sixty-seven percent of the reviewers who received papers on the effectiveness of conventional treatment recommended publication as opposed to 57% of those who received paper on the effectiveness of nonconventional treatment. This difference was statistically significant, suggesting that reviewers are biased in favor of conventional therapies (Resch et al., 2000). While the study by Resch et al. presents some useful data related to bias in peer review, it is limited to certain types of bias in clinical research and may not generalize to other fields. Also, it does not address some of the deeper issues that underlie the bias, such as dogmatic allegiance to various theories, methods, ideas, and so on.

Research conducted by Campanario (2009) spans various fields of science and provides evidence for dogmatism in science. Campanario collected data on the peer-review process for 16 papers from the fields of medicine, biochemistry, chemistry, and physics; while these papers did eventually earn Nobel Prizes for the authors, they were severely panned during the peer-review process or were rejected. He obtained evidence concerning the review of these papers from the authors' autobiographies, personal accounts, Nobel lectures, and other written reports. For example, Arne Tiselius won the Nobel Prize in Chemistry in 1948 for his work on electrophoreses and adsorption, but the editors at *Biochemical Journal* where he initially sent his key paper rejected it because it focused too much on physical science. David Lee, Douglas Osheroff, and Robert Richardson received the Nobel Prize in Physics in 1996 for their discovery of superfluid helium, but *Physical Review Letters* initially rejected their work because the reviewers did not believe that the physical system they described was possible. They succeeded in overturning this decision by convincing the editors that their discovery would work. Murray Gell-Mann receive the Nobel Prize in Physics in 1953 for his work on the phenomenon of "strangeness" in particle physics, but the editors of *Physical Review* objected to use of the word "strangeness" and he had to change his terminology to "new unstable particles" (p. 553). Thomas Cech won the Nobel Prize in Chemistry in 1989 for discovering that some ribonucleic acid (RNA) molecules can act as enzymes, but the reviewers for his paper submitted to *Nature* strongly objected to his decision to characterize the properties he observed as "enzyme-like" or as a type of "catalysis" (p. 553). Most biochemists at that time believed that RNA cannot act as an enzyme.

In the discussion section at the end of his paper, Campanario offers dogmatism as a possible explanation for the encounters that these Nobel Prize winners had with scientific peer review: "A possible explanation for peer resistance to scientific discovery lies in the fact that new theories or discoveries often clash with orthodox viewpoints held by the referees (p. 558)." He also suggests that difficulties that some Nobel Prize winners have had with peer review may also be due to delayed recognition: some discoveries are so far ahead of their time that it takes other researchers years, perhaps even decades, to appreciate them (Campanario, 2009; Garfield, 1989; Stent, 1972). Of course, delayed recognition may simply be another form of dogmatism insofar as scientists fail to recognize research because it contradicts the status quo. In his conclusion, Campanario also observes: "Peer review has been shown to be plagued with many imperfections…there is a real risk that evidence contrary to the established views can be suppressed or disregarded (Campanario, 2009: 559)."

While Companario's research provides compelling evidence of dogmatism in scientific peer review, the sample for his study is highly selective, and the experiences these Nobel Prize winners had with peer review may not reflect other researchers' experiences. Nobel Prize winners are usually chosen for their highly innovative and influential contributions to science, and the dogmatism encountered by some Nobel Prize winners may not be as prevalent throughout science. However, it does seem reasonable to assume that non-Nobel Prize winning scientists may also encounter strong resistance to innovative research they submit to journals.

Conclusion

Although peer review is essential to the evaluation of scientific research, it is susceptible to various biases, some of which may result from or contribute to groupthink. To counteract groupthink in peer review, scientists should take steps to enhance the diversity of reviewers with regard to gender, race, nationality, institutional affiliation, and other social factors that could impact reviewer judgments. Intellectual diversity should also be promoted (e.g., including individuals using different methods and expertise) as well as funding and publication of innovative or controversial research that challenges the status quo. Editors and funding agency leaders should also stress open-mindedness in the review of research and seek to publish and fund innovative and controversial research that meets appropriate standards of rigor, reproducibility, objectivity, and integrity. To overcome confirmatory biases, editors should be open to publishing research that reports negative results if it meets appropriate scientific standards.

Journal editors and funding agency leaders should collect data on peer review, so that they can better understand how to control and/or mitigate biases that may impact the process. Journal editors and funding agency leaders should conduct their own, independent assessment of reviewer reports so that they can determine whether these reports are biased. Journals should also consider experimenting with procedures, such as double-blind review, which may minimize the impact of biases. Reviewers, editors, and funding agency leaders should try to address their own biases so that manuscripts and research applications can receive a fair hearing. Additional meta-research on the factors related to groupthink in science will help researchers, editors, and funding agency leaders understand how to promote neutrality and integrity in peer review.

Acknowledgments This research was supported, in part, by the National Institute of Environmental Health Sciences (NIEHS), National Institutes of Health (NIH), and the Fonds de Recherche du Québec en Santé (FRQS). This paper does not represent the views of the NIEHS, NIH, the FRQS, or any governmental organization.

References

Armstrong, J. S. (1997). Peer review for journals: Evidence on quality control, fairness, and innovation. *Science and Engineering Ethics, 3*(1), 63–84.

Baggs, J. G., Broome, M. E., Dougherty, M. C., Freda, M. C., & Kearney, M. H. (2008). Blinding in peer review: The preferences of reviewers for nursing journals. *Journal of Advances in Nursing, 64*(2), 131–138.

Barber, B. (1961). Resistance by scientists to scientific discovery. *Science, 134*(3479), 596–602.

Bornmann, L., Mutza, R., & Daniela, H. D. (2007). Gender differences in grant peer review: A meta-analysis. *Journal of Informetrics, 1*(3), 226–238.

Borsuk, R. M., Aarssen, L. W., Budden, A. E., Koricheva, J., Leimu, R., Tregenza, T., et al. (2009). To name or not to name: The effect of changing author gender on peer review. *Bioscience, 59*(11), 985–989.

Buchen, L. (2009). May 29, 1919: A major eclipse, relatively speaking. Wired, May 29, 2009. Available at: https://www.wired.com/2009/05/dayintech_0529/. Accessed 17 Apr 2017.

Campanario, J. M. (2009). Rejecting and resisting Nobel class discoveries: Accounts by Nobel Laureates. *Scientometrics, 81*(2), 549–565.

Card, R. F. (2005). Making sense of the diversity-based legal argument for affirmative action. *Public Affairs Quarterly, 19*(1), 11–24.

Ceci, S. J., & Williams, W. M. (2011). Understanding current causes of women's underrepresentation in science. *Proceedings of the National Academy of Sciences of the United States of America, 108*(8), 3157–3162.

Chubin, D., & Hackett, E. (1990). *Peerless science: Peer review and U.S. science policy*. Albany, NY: State University of New York Press.

Committee on Science, Engineering, and Public Policy. (2010). *Expanding underrepresented minority participation: America's science and technology talent at the crossroads*. Washington, DC: National Academies Press.

Dwan, K., Gamble, C., Williamson, P. R., Kirkham, J. J., & Reporting Bias Group. (2013). Systematic review of the empirical evidence of study publication bias and outcome reporting bias – An updated review. *PLoS One, 8*(7), e66844.

Easterbrook, P. J., Berlin, J. A., Gopalan, R., & Matthews, D. R. (1991). Publication bias in clinical research. *Lancet, 337*(8746), 867–872.

Ernst, E., & Kienbacher, T. (1991). Chauvinism. *Nature, 352*(6336), 560.

Fisher, M., Friedman, S. B., & Strauss, B. (1994). The effects of blinding on acceptance of research papers by peer review. *Journal of the American Medical Association, 272*(2), 143–146.

Garfield, E. (1989). Delayed recognition in scientific discovery: Citation frequency analyses aids the search for case histories. *Current Contents, 23*, 3–9.

Garfunkel, J. M., Ulshen, M. H., Hamrick, H. J., & Lawson, E. E. (1994). Effect of institutional prestige on reviewers' recommendations and editorial decisions. *Journal of the American Medical Association, 272*(2), 137–138.

Ginther, D. K., Haak, L. L., Schaffer, W. T., & Kington, R. (2012). Are race, ethnicity, and medical school affiliation associated with NIH R01 type 1 award probability for physician investigators? *Academic Medicine, 87*(11), 1516–1524.

Ginther, D. K., Kahn, S., & Schaffer, W. T. (2016). Gender, race/ethnicity, and national institutes of health r01 research awards: Is there evidence of a double bind for women of color? *Academic Medicine, 91*(8), 1098–1107.

Ginther, D. K., Schaffer, W., Schnel, J., Masimore, B., Liu, F., Haak, L. L., et al. (2011). Race, ethnicity, and NIH research awards. *Science, 333*(6045), 1015–1019.

Godlee, F., Gale, C. R., & Martyn, C. N. (1998). Effect on the quality of peer review of blinding reviewers and asking them to sign their reports: A randomized controlled trial. *Journal of the American Medical Association, 280*(3), 237–240.

Grod, O. N., Budden, A. E., Tregenza, T., Koricheva, J., Leimu, R., Aarssen, L. W., et al. (2008). Systematic variation in reviewer practice according to country and gender in the field of ecology and evolution. *PLoS One, 3*(9), e3202.

Harding, S. (2004). Asocially relevant philosophy of science? Resources from standpoint theory's controversiality. *Hypatia, 19*(1), 25–47.

Helmer, M., Schottdorf, M., Neef, A., & Battaglia, D. (2017). Gender bias in scholarly peer review. In: P. Rodgers (Ed.). *eLife, 6*, e21718.

Ho, R. C., Mak, K. K., Tao, R., Lu, Y., Day, J. R., & Pan, F. (2013). Views on the peer review system of biomedical journals: An online survey of academics from high-ranking universities. *BMC Medical Research Methodology, 13*, 74.

Hunter, J. (2012). Post-publication peer review: Opening up scientific conversation. *Frontiers in Computational Neuroscience, 6*, 63. (August 30).

Jang, J., Vannier, M. W., Wang, F., Deng, Y., Ou, F., Bennett, J., et al. (2013). A bibliometric analysis of academic publication and NIH funding. *Journal of Informetrics, 7*(2), 318–324.

Janis, I. L. (1972). *Victims of groupthink: A psychological study of foreign policy decisions and fiascoes* (2nd ed.). Boston: Houghton Mifflin Company.

Janis, I. L. (1982). *Groupthink: Psychological studies of policy decisions and fiascos*. Boston: Cengage Learning.

Justice, A. C., Cho, M. K., Winker, M. A., Berlin, J. A., & Rennie, D. (1998). Does masking author identity improve peer review quality? A randomized controlled trial. PEER investigators. *Journal of the American Medical Association, 280*(3), 240–242.

Kaatz, A., Lee, Y. G., Potvien, A., Magua, W., Filut, A., Bhattacharya, A., et al. (2016). Analysis of National Institutes of Health R01 application critiques, impact, and criteria scores: Does the sex of the principal investigator make a difference? *Academic Medicine, 91*(8), 1080–1088.

Kaatz, A., Magua, W., Zimmerman, D. R., & Carnes, M. (2015). A quantitative linguistic analysis of National Institutes of Health R01 application critiques from investigators at one institution. *Academic Medicine, 90*(1), 69–75.

Kuhn, T. S. (1962). *The structure of scientific revolutions*. Chicago: University of Chicago Press.

Lamont, M. (2009). *How professors think: Inside the curious world of academic judgment*. Cambridge, MA: Harvard University Press.

Lane, J. A., & Linden, D. J. (2009). Is there gender bias in the peer review process at Journal of Neurophysiology? *Journal of Neurophysiology, 101*(5), 2195–2196.

Larivière, V., Ni, C., Gingras, Y., Cronin, B., & Sugimoto, C. (2013). Global gender disparities in science. *Nature, 504*(7479), 211–213.

Latour, B., & Woolgar, S. (1979). *Laboratory life: The social construction of scientific facts*. London: Sage.

Lauer, M. S., Krumholz, H. M., & Topol, E. J. (2015). Time for a prepublication culture in clinical research? *Lancet, 386*(1012), 2447–2449.

Lee, C. J., Sugimoto, C. R., Zhang, G., & Cronin, B. (2012). Bias in peer review. *Journal of the American Society for Information Science and Technology, 64*(1), 2–17.
Longino, H. (1990). *Science as social knowledge*. Princeton, NJ: Princeton University Press.
Lycan, W. G. (1988). *Judgement and justification*. Cambridge, UK: Cambridge University Press.
Mahoney, M. J. (1977). Publication preferences: An experimental study of confirmatory bias in the peer review system. *Cognitive Therapy and Research, 1*(2), 161–175.
McNutt, R. A., Evans, A. T., Fletcher, R. H., & Fletcher, S. W. (1990). The effects of blinding on the quality of peer review. A randomized trial. *Journal of the American Medical Association, 263*(10), 1371–1376.
Murray, D. L., Morris, D., Lavoie, C., Leavitt, P. R., MacIsaac, H., Masson, M. E., et al. (2016). Bias in research grant evaluation has dire consequences for small universities. *PLoS One, 11*(6), e0155876.
Nelson, D. J. (2007). *A national analysis of minorities in science and engineering faculties at research universities*. Norman, OK: University of Oklahoma.
Olson, C. M., Rennie, D., Cook, D., Dickersin, K., Flanagin, A., Hogan, J. W., et al. (2002). Publication bias in editorial decision making. *Journal of the American Medical Association, 287*(21), 2825–2828.
Planck, M. (1962). Quoted in Kuhn, T. S. 1962). *The structure of scientific revolutions* (pp. 33–34). Chicago: University of Chicago Press.
Pulverer, B. (2016). Preparing for preprints. *EMBO Journal, 35*(24), 2617–2619.
Quine, W. V. (1961). *From a logical point of view*. New York: Harper and Rowe.
Resch, K. I., Ernst, E., & Garrow, J. (2000). A randomized controlled study of reviewer bias against an unconventional therapy. *Journal of the Royal Society of Medicine, 93*(4), 164–167.
Resnik, D. B. (1994). Methodological conservatism and social epistemology. *International Studies in the Philosophy of Science, 8*(3), 247–264.
Resnik, D. B., & Elmore, S. A. (2016). Ensuring the quality, fairness, and integrity of journal peer review: A possible role for editors. *Science and Engineering Ethics, 22*(1), 169–188.
Resnik, D. B., Gutierrez-Ford, C., & Peddada, S. (2008). Perceptions of ethical problems with scientific journal peer review: An exploratory study. *Science and Engineering Ethics, 14*(3), 305–310.
Ross, J. S., Gross, C. P., Desai, M. M., Hong, Y., Grant, A. O., Daniels, S. R., et al. (2006). Effect of blinded peer review on abstract acceptance. *Journal of the American Medical Association, 295*(14), 1675–1680.
Shamoo, A. E., & Resnik, D. B. (2015). *Responsible conduct of research* (3rd ed.). New York: Oxford University Press.
Shen, H. (2013). Mind the gender gap. *Nature, 495*(7439), 22–24.
Sklar, L. (1975). Methodological conservatism. *Philosophical Review, 84*(3), 374–400.
Smith, R. (2006). Peer review: A flawed process at the heart of science and journals. *Journal of the Royal Society of Medicine, 99*(4), 178–182.
Stent, G. S. (1972). Prematurity and uniqueness in scientific discovery. *Scientific American, 227*(6), 84–93.
Stern, J. M., & Simes, R. J. (1997). Publication bias: Evidence of delayed publication in a cohort study of clinical research projects. *British Medical Journal, 315*(7109), 640–645.
Teixeira da Silva, J. A., & Dobránszki, J. (2015). Problems with traditional science publishing and finding a wider niche for post-publication peer review. *Accountability in Research, 22*(1), 22–40.
Timmer, A., Hilsden, R. J., & Sutherland, L. R. (2001). Determinants of abstract acceptance for the Digestive Diseases Week--a cross sectional study. *BMC Medical Research Methodology, 1*, 13.
Tregenza, T. (2002). Gender bias in the refereeing process? *Trends in Ecology & Evolution, 17*(8), 349–350.
van Rooyen, S., Delamothe, T., & Evans, S. J. (2010). Effect on peer review of telling reviewers that their signed reviews might be posted on the web: Randomised controlled trial. *British Medical Journal, 341*, c5729.

van Rooyen, S., Godlee, F., Evans, S., Black, N., & Smith, R. (1999). Effect of open peer review on quality of reviews and on reviewers' recommendations: A randomised trial. *British Medical Journal, 318*(7175), 23–27.

van Rooyen, S., Godlee, F., Evans, S., Smith, R., & Black, N. (1998). Effect of blinding and unmasking on the quality of peer review: A randomized trial. *Journal of the American Medical Association, 280*(3), 234–237.

Waisbren, S. E., Bowles, H., Hasan, T., Zou, K. H., Emans, S. J., Goldberg, C., et al. (2008). Gender differences in research grant applications and funding outcomes for medical school faculty. *Journal of Women's Health (Larchmont), 17*(2), 207–214.

Walsh, E., Rooney, M., Appleby, L., & Wilkinson, G. (2000). Open peer review: A randomised controlled trial. *British Journal of Psychiatry, 176*, 47–51.

Wenneras, C., & Wold, A. (1997). Nepotism and sexism in peer-review. *Nature, 387*(6631), 341–343.

Chapter 10
Law Versus Science

Brian Martin

Introduction

Pieter Cohen, a professor of medicine at Harvard University, has carried out research into the effects of nutritional supplements, the sorts commonly consumed by bodybuilders. Cohen published his findings in scientific journals and also publicized them more widely. Following this, Jared Wheat, the owner of the supplement producer Hi-Tech Pharmaceuticals, sued Cohen for defamation (Robbins, 2017).

This might have seemed to be an obvious SLAPP – Strategic Lawsuit Against Public Participation – namely a legal action serving to restrain legitimate participation in matters of public interest. SLAPPs use various torts, most commonly defamation, to scare targets. In US courts, plaintiffs hardly ever win because of the First Amendment right to petition the government, for example, to write letters of complaint to politicians and public officials. However, the point of SLAPPs is seldom to win in court but rather to discourage participation in public matters (Pring & Canan, 1996; Sheldrick, 2014).

Because of the damaging effect of SLAPPs, many US states have passed anti-SLAPP laws. Massachusetts had such a law, so it seemed that Wheat's suit should have been dismissed. However, a judge overruled the state's anti-SLAPP law, saying it prevented the plaintiff from obtaining a trial by jury.

Cohen, backed by Harvard, had to defend in court. They won, but only in legal terms. Defending the case required a considerable amount of time, effort, and emotional energy. Wheat stated that he hoped his legal action would discourage other scientists from making "baseless allegations," and advised scientists to "think twice and do better research, knowing you can get sued if you do this" (quoted in Robbins, 2017). The legal action stimulated commentary by Cohen and others that referred to similar cases and reflected on the inappropriateness of using legal forums for dealing with scientific disagreements (Bagley, Carroll, & Cohen, 2017; Carroll, 2017; Katz & Redberg, 2017).

B. Martin (✉)
Humanities and Social Inquiry, University of Wollongong, Wollongong, NSW, Australia
e-mail: bmartin@uow.edu.au

D. M. Allen, J. W. Howell (eds.), *Groupthink in Science*,
https://doi.org/10.1007/978-3-030-36822-7_10

Wheat's case against Cohen is an example of how legal actions can influence the path of scientific research. Most commonly, they discourage research on specific topics or from particular perspectives.

In this chapter, I describe several ways that laws and legal actions can restrain scientific research. The next two sections describe relevant aspects of science and law. Then, I address the use of defamation actions against researchers, showing the role of domain shifting and illustrating the chilling effect of legal action. Next is a section on laws against euthanasia and how they indirectly discourage research in the area. After this is a discussion of intellectual property and how a legal regime set up to foster innovation can actually constrain it. Finally, I present a framework for analyzing responses to legal constraints on scientific research.

Legal interventions into scientific issues can be interpreted as attempts by self-interested groups to stymie or slant knowledge claims to their own advantage. In some cases, the interventions are from outsiders to the scientific enterprise, while in others, they are from insiders. Most scientists take the easy way out by avoiding research that might or has come under legal attack: for them, maintaining a strife-free career is more important than pursing principled action. Only occasionally do scientists unite against legal threats and constraints.

The Domains of Science and Law

To understand the effect of legal actions on research, it is useful to consider key features of science and law, especially the contrasts between them. Both science and law are enterprises that pursue truth in some sense. Science operates by processes of observation, experiment, theory development, and theory testing, aiming to develop and verify ways of explaining the world, both the natural and the social world. Scientists undertake research and publish it openly, so it is available for scrutiny, subject to critique and potentially the launching pad for further investigations. Decisions about what counts as a scientific fact or a valid theory are made through a sort of consensus process. There is no authority that pronounces the truth or falsity of a claim. Scientific knowledge emerges through collective processes of making claims and counterclaims until all or most researchers agree.

Law is a system of rules, based on statutes or precedents, that are applied to particular cases. Interpretations of the law are made by judges. Law can change, through legislation or reinterpretation. Judgments are published for all to read, but less to question than to understand and show relevance to future cases.

For some purposes, the formal differences between science and law are less important than the fact that they are different domains, each with its own set of procedures, practitioners, criteria, and aims. The aim of science is truth, whereas the aim of law is justice.

A legal action against a scientist, such as Wheat's suit against Cohen, involves movement from one domain to another, namely from science to law. It thus can serve to hinder the normal operation of science, with outcomes such as hindering particular researchers or discouraging certain types of research. Rather than research being assessed by peers according to scientific criteria, it is assessed by judges or juries according to entirely different sets of rules.

Another important factor in domain shifting is cost. Some research can be expensive in terms of salaries and equipment, but this cost is usually covered by funders – typically universities, governments, or corporations, not by individual scientists. Defending a legal action can be very expensive, involving tens or hundreds of thousands of dollars, and onerous for an individual and sometimes for an organization. There is also a significant cost in terms of time. Although lawyers run a case on behalf of a defendant, often the defendant spends many hours preparing documents. This represents an opportunity cost in research time foregone. Wheat's initial claim against Cohen was for $20 million. Although this might be considered an ambit claim or as a form of intimidation, even a judgment awarding $1 million in damages would be devastating for most individual defendants.

Constraints on Science

It needs to be said that science is never unfettered. Although truth is the guiding light for researchers, some truths are deemed undesirable. To take an extreme example, studying the effects of nuclear explosions on people and the environment could be done by dropping bombs on populations. Nazi doctors' experimentation on prisoners is considered a crime. Various treaties and laws, for example, on land mines and animal experimentation, constrain research. Some governments have attempted to control research on encryption and stem cells. Studies of vulnerable groups, such as children and prisoners, are limited by the requirements of institutional review boards and ethics committees.

Science is thus constrained in many ways, in part by legal restrictions. The search for truth needs to be undertaken in the context of other values. How then is it possible to assess whether a legal action is a legitimate expression of some public interest or a harmful restraint on the search for knowledge? Various factors can be considered, including widely endorsed principles, involvement by affected parties in deciding on rules affecting science, and examination of who benefits from legal actions. To take two contrasting examples, research to improve methods of torture is in conflict with human rights principles, whereas research on nutritional supplements has the potential to benefit consumers. Hence, legal restraints on torture research can be justified far more easily than legal restraints on supplements research.

In some cases, specific legal restrictions on research are clearly imposed in the service of vested interests. For example, in the United States, the influence of the National Rifle Association is sufficiently great that Congress in 1996 passed a law preventing federal funds for injury prevention at the Centers for Disease Control and Prevention from being used to promote gun control. The result is that gun violence is grossly understudied (Stark & Shah, 2017). However, when laws are used to inhibit research, often there are other rationales than straight-out censorship. All sorts of laws affect scientific research directly or indirectly, for example, laws on environmental protection, animal welfare, building codes, vehicle safety, minimum wage, employment contracts, pension funds, broadcasting, and monopolies. To illustrate the issues involved, three cases will be examined in more detail: defamation, euthanasia, and intellectual property.

Defamation

Defamation law is commonly seen as an attempt to balance two competing values: protection of reputation and protection of free speech. One person's speech can hurt another person's reputation. When someone feels their reputation has been harmed by another's speech, they can go to court seeking damages, and this very possibility serves to inhibit reputation-damaging speech. On the other hand, defamation suits can inhibit speech that serves the public interest, so the law provides defenses. For example, a defendant may be able to defeat a charge of defamation by demonstrating the truth of statements made. Other defenses include qualified privilege, for example, when a teacher gives grades that hurt a student's reputation, and parliamentary privilege, when an elected representative makes statements in parliament.

Publication of scientific papers, and reports of research, potentially can harm the reputation of individuals, including other scientists whose ideas or contributions are challenged. This sets the stage for invoking defamation law in ways that block or discourage research.

Alex de Blas was a student at the University of Tasmania. For her fourth year of undergraduate study, called the honors year, she wrote a thesis about pollution from the Mt Lyell mine in the state of Tasmania. The owners of the mine threatened de Blas and the university with an action for defamation, demanding that it not be published (Montgomery, 1994).

Hilary Koprowski was a pioneer in developing a vaccine for polio. In a mass test of his vaccine in the late 1950s, it was given to nearly a million people in what today is the Congo. Decades later, a few individuals proposed that this vaccination campaign may have inadvertently led to the emergence of the disease AIDS. Tom Curtis, a journalist for the *Houston Post,* learned about this theory, investigated further, and wrote a story in *Rolling Stone,* generating enormous interest (Curtis, 1992). Koprowski sued Curtis and *Rolling Stone* for defamation. The case was highly expensive, and eventually *Rolling Stone* settled, paying Koprowski $1 and issuing a "clarification." In the discovery phase of the proceedings, Curtis had to provide all his interview notes. He had planned a follow-up article, but this was cancelled. Furthermore, if he had wanted to do further interviews, he would have had to tell interviewees that anything they told him might be accessed in a future legal action. Koprowski's legal action thus had a severe chilling effect on further investigation of the polio-vaccine theory for the origin of AIDS (Martin, 2010).

Euthanasia Research

Research on euthanasia is severely restricted by the law, though not by direct legal action. In Nazi Germany in 1939, Hitler initiated a program of killing people with disabilities, euphemistically called euthanasia, thereby stigmatizing the term for decades to come. After World War II, interest in peaceful death for humanitarian reasons developed largely as a result of medical advances. Technologies such as defibrillators and feeding tubes mean that people who once would have died can be maintained alive, but often with greatly reduced quality of life. Some, suffering greatly from lack of autonomy, indignity, breathlessness, or intractable pain, sought an early death.

In most countries, the means for a violent death abound, including guns, high places, trains, and rope. On the other hand, means for peaceful death have been increasingly limited, with drugs that might provide fatal overdoses being restricted. This has led to a push for legalization of voluntary euthanasia. There are three main options for a peaceful death. The first, called active euthanasia, involves a doctor giving a patient a legal injection. The second, called physician-assisted suicide or physician-assisted dying, involves a doctor giving a patient a prescription for lethal drugs; the patient, if wishing to die, then takes the drugs. The third option, called self-deliverance or do-it-yourself euthanasia, involves a person obtaining lethal drugs or constructing an exit bag and then ending their life, without assistance.

In most countries, it is legal to commit suicide but illegal to help someone to end their life. Most of the writing in the area is about the ethics and legalities of euthanasia with little attention to research. It can be argued that the legal restraints on euthanasia have created a related restraint on research.

Even in places where euthanasia is illegal, it still occurs. For example, sympathetic doctors may covertly give patients access to lethal drugs or give patients lethal injections. To research this practice requires great care. Roger Magnusson (2002) carried out interviews with Australian doctors, documenting an underground euthanasia practice, and revealed that doctors sometimes botched their attempts to help patients die, usually because of lack of knowledge and training. This is one of the few interview-based studies of euthanasia practiced in places where it is illegal. Such research is restrained for two reasons: subjects of the research – doctors who assisted patients to die – are wary of revealing actions that could lead to deregistration or criminal prosecutions, and the research itself is generally unwelcome by governments and medical authorities that oppose legalization of euthanasia.

Russel Ogden, an academic at Kwantlen Polytechnic University in British Columbia, pursued research into assisted dying and do-it-yourself euthanasia. In the course of his studies, he observed several individuals ending their lives (e.g., Ogden, 2010). This sort of investigation, vital to learning how dying intended to be peaceful actually operates and can sometimes go wrong, was not welcomed in some quarters within his university. Ogden encountered obstacles to his research at several universities (Hager, 2015).

Advocates of everyone having the option of a peaceful death have looked for a "peaceful pill," a metaphor for any means by which individuals can reliably end their lives peacefully. The current preferred option is the drug pentobarbital, commonly called Nembutal. It is available at veterinary supply shops in some countries but highly restricted in many. For the "Nutech" group searching for a peaceful pill, one path would be to develop the capacity to synthesize Nembutal cheaply and easily (Côté, 2012). However, efforts along these lines have so far not succeeded, being limited by human and financial resources. Governments do not sponsor this sort of research, except perhaps for classified military and national security purposes.

Laws against euthanasia thus restrain scientific research in several ways. Investigations into the ways doctors and others (such as relatives) covertly end the lives of individuals to end their extreme suffering are rare, in large part due to criminal sanctions against helping others to die. Obstacles include obtaining project approval from research institutions and obtaining the trust of doctors to learn about their practices. A similar difficulty faces those, like Russel Ogden, who study do-it-yourself euthanasia. Finally, research into means for peaceful dying is restrained by stigma and resources.

Some would say that research into euthanasia is undesirable, especially if it helps justify euthanasia, discourages improvement in palliative care, and increases the number of people whose lives are ended prematurely. On the other hand, others believe research into euthanasia can contribute to improved quality of life, for example, by determining how deaths can be more peaceful, by better judging when euthanasia is warranted, and by investigating the potential for abuse.

Intellectual Property

The term "intellectual property" refers to a variety of laws, including copyright, patents, trademarks, and plant variety rights. Their common feature is putting legal restrictions on the use of ideas. For example, under current copyright law, as soon as a person writes some original words (such as the words in this chapter), they are copyrighted, and others cannot legally reproduce them for profit. Copyright can be assigned to others or sold. Copyright currently lasts for 70 years after the author's death.

The rationale for intellectual property is to stimulate the production of new ideas and devices. It operates by giving a temporary monopoly over the ideas and devices, to enable the creator to gain a benefit. The curious feature of intellectual property is that it legally restrains innovation in the name of stimulating innovation. Unlike material objects, ideas can be used by many people at the same time. Only one person can be wearing a pair of shoes at a time, whereas a poet can enjoy her poem while millions of others are reading it too.

To optimally stimulate the production of new ideas, the duration of protection needs to be adjusted to provide a balance between encouraging the creator (through restraining use by others) and enabling others to build on a creator's work. For example, novels usually have most of their sales within the first year of publication. Therefore, it can be argued that there is no need for copyright to extend beyond 1 year or perhaps a few years. Very few authors write more or better works by knowing that their copyright extends decades beyond their death. Excessive copyright terms, which keep being extended, restrain creativity by others. A classic example is Mickey Mouse, under copyright to the Disney Corporation. This copyright now does nothing to stimulate greater creativity by the original creator of Mickey Mouse, meanwhile preventing others from using Mickey Mouse for their own creations. Copyright with such a great duration thus serves to restrain innovation. It is a "monopoly privilege" enforced by law (Drahos, 1996).

Scientific research is partially protected from the restraints involved with intellectual property. Scientific papers are copyrighted in the usual way. Initially, the author holds copyright, but many journal publishers ask authors to assign them copyright for the purposes of sales, databases, and other uses. Other authors can quote from published papers as long as the quotes not too long, according to fair use provisions. This allows other authors to quote portions of a text for the purposes of exposition or criticism.

Courts have interpreted copyright of scientific papers as applying only to the expression, namely the words used, not to the ideas. Furthermore, scientific formulas cannot be copyrighted. Therefore scientists can use the ideas developed by other scientists immediately. The usual expectation is that the creator is cited, and indeed being cited by others is often what scholars most desire.

Patents provide another avenue for intellectual property to both encourage and restrain scientific and technological innovation. Patents provide protection for inventions for a limited time, which allows inventors to benefit from their creations, but can also restrain research and development. Sometimes companies buy patents covering inventions they never intend to use, as a means of suppressing competition with the technology that is currently the basis for their business. In other words, a rival technology is available, but it could threaten profits from current investments, so the rival technology is put on ice by purchasing patents covering it but not using them (Dunford, 1987). For example, General Electric obtained patents in order to slow down the introduction of fluorescent lights, in order to protect its sales of incandescent lights. In this case, a law designed to stimulate invention was used to suppress invention. Patent law is based on the presumption, sometimes false, that patent protection will be used to innovate rather than suppress innovation.

In the pharmaceutical industry, patents enable extraordinary profits, in conjunction with other techniques, especially marketing. Companies research new drugs, looking especially at ones that address chronic conditions such as arthritis, high cholesterol, and high blood pressure. These are especially profitable because drug use continues for months or years. When government regulators approve a suitable drug, massive marketing can establish it as a standard prescription. This marketing includes advertising, free samples for doctors, and free "educational trips" for doctors to seminars and conferences. Companies write papers about the drugs based on their in-house research and recruit academics to be ghost authors. Published in leading medical journals, such papers give credibility to claims about the drug, and the company's marketing machine uses the publications as publicity.

When a drug patent expires, sometimes a company can patent and introduce a new drug that is quite similar and market it as superior. This is one of the methods of evergreening, which basically means using tricks to unfairly extend patent protection.

Because the criteria for granting patents are so easy to satisfy, some companies obtain dozens of patents for various aspects of a product, thereby preventing competitors from marketing competing products. By means of such "patent thickets," innovation is hindered. Then, there are patent trolls: companies that obtain patents and, rather than using them, search for companies that have inadvertently violated them, aggressively seeking payment in compensation. Patent trolling in essence uses intellectual property as a tool of extortion rather than innovation.

Pharmaceutical prescription drugs have become a source of major corruption (Gøtzsche, 2013). In some cases, researchers fiddle results, for example, by looking for adverse effects for only a short period or excluding certain types of people from studies (Goldacre, 2012). Drugs are promoted despite evidence that they are killing people. Some companies have been fined billions of dollars, indicating the massive scale of the corruption involved.

Intellectual property law is part of what enables abuses in the pharmaceutical industry. However, more significant than corruption is the distorting effect on research of the massive profits enabled by patent protection. The counterpoint to investigation of drugs that can be patented is a lack of investigation of substances that cannot be patented and indeed of anything that cannot be patented. For example, in one study, exercise was found to be as effective as antidepressants in dealing with depression (Craft & Perna, 2004). However, exercise cannot be patented, so companies have little incentive to study its benefits. The result is that billions of dollars are invested in researching and promoting antidepressants, while nonpatentable options, including diet, mindfulness, and exercise, are underresearched. The same sort of distortion of research agendas occurs in other areas.

In the case of pharmaceutical drugs, the impact of law on scientific advance is indirect, unlike the use of defamation law. Patent law offers a set of incentives that, in the hands of a powerful industry, compliant governments, and a willing medical profession, encourage research in some areas and starve it in others.

Responses

When law operates to suppress or inhibit scientific research or findings, there are several possible responses. Three are described here: acquiescence, law reform, and resistance.

One option is to acquiesce by avoiding doing anything that might cause offence. In the case of defamation, this might mean not undertaking research that might trigger threats of legal action. Pieter Cohen, for example, could acquiesce by discontinuing his research into nutritional supplements. This option is basically capitulation to legal obstacles. Put starkly, this might seem unacceptable to anyone committed to free inquiry. Yet, it is actually quite common, representing the chilling effect of the possibility of being sued. Many scientists avoid topics that might lead to adverse actions against them (public denunciations, loss of funding, threats of dismissal) and instead choose topics where there is ample funding and the promise of a welcoming response from others in the field.

A second response is to push for reform of laws that serve to inhibit research. Defamation law reform is an example. Michael Curtis (1995), in an article stimulated by Hilary Koprowski's defamation suit against *Rolling Stone* and Tom Curtis, argues for heightened legal protection for scientific speech. Similarly, Kate Sutherland (2010), in a discussion of Canadian defamation law inspired by a legal action against the publisher of a book review, argues for defamation law reform. Many commentators have recommended changes in laws on intellectual property (Halbert, 1999; Shulman, 1999). However, despite critiques of legal regimes and calls for law reform, in practice this path is both uncertain and slow. Concerns about scientific advance are a low priority in defamation law reform, where the interests of mass media and internet corporations are more influential, and in reform of intellectual property law, where the influence of the corporate beneficiaries of current law (software companies, pharmaceutical manufacturers, Hollywood producers, genetic engineering companies) is overwhelming.

A third possible response is to challenge the legal action by exposing it and mobilizing support against it, in an attempt to make the action counterproductive for the plaintiff. This approach is based on a model of outrage management, also called the backfire model (Martin, 2007). When a powerful individual or group does something that others might see as unfair – for example, sexual harassment, police beatings, massacres of peaceful protest, and genocide – the perpetrator often uses one or more methods to reduce public outrage:

- Cover up the action
- Devalue the target
- Reinterpret what happened by lying, minimizing consequences, blaming others, and reframing
- Use official channels to give an appearance of justice
- Intimidate or reward people involved

The classic case involving defamation is called McLibel. In the late 1980s, members of an anarchist group called London Greenpeace (not related to Greenpeace International) produced a leaflet titled "What's wrong with McDonald's?" telling, among other things, about poor working conditions for McDonald's workers and the unhealthy nature of McDonald's food. McDonald's, notoriously litigious, infiltrated the small London Greenpeace group, collected information, and sued five activists for defamation. Two of them, Helen Steel and Dave Morris, defended in court, triggering the formation of a large-scale support network. After the longest case in British history, McDonald's won in court but its reputation was severely damaged: it was a public relations disaster. McDonald's defamation action backfired (Donson, 2000; Vidal, 1997).

McDonald's used all five methods to reduce outrage. It tried to hide its use of infiltrators, devalued the members of London Greenpeace, reframed its action as defending the reputation of McDonald's, and used official channels (a court action) to make its action seem legitimate. The legal action intimidated three of the London Greenpeace activists, who capitulated.

Steel, Morris, and their supporters countered each one of these methods. They reproduced hundreds of thousands of copies of the leaflet "What's wrong with McDonald's?" and publicized the defamation action. Steel and Morris behaved with restraint. As ordinary workers (a gardener and a postman), they were hard to devalue. McLibel campaigners framed the defamation action as censorship. Campaigning itself went outside the legal domain. Finally, Steel and Morris resisted the intimidation of the legal action and refused to accept a generous settlement payment.

In summary, to counter the usual methods used to reduce outrage, opponents can increase outrage in these ways:

- Expose the action
- Validate the targets
- Interpret the events as unjust (censorship in the case of McLibel)
- Avoid or discredit official channels; instead, mobilize support
- Resist intimidation and rewards

This provides a general approach to addressing many uses of the law that inhibit scientific research that serves the public interest. In relation to defamation, the idea is to make legal threats and actions backfire by giving more attention to whatever is targeted for censorship (Jansen & Martin, 2003, 2015). The same approach can be used to analyze the struggle between the music industry and individuals who download songs, a case involving intellectual property (Martin, Moore, & Salter, 2010).

In the 1990s, the government of South Africa, to deal with the large number of AIDS cases, sought to import a generic HIV/AIDS drug: compulsory licensing and parallel importation are permitted by international intellectual property agreements. Nevertheless, dozens of pharmaceutical companies sued the government, putting their profits above the health of South Africans with AIDS. To challenge this abuse of power, AIDS activists and public health groups publicized the pharmaceutical companies' legal action, put the focus on AIDS patients, reframed the issue from patent law to health being sacrificed to corporate greed, mobilized support, and mounted numerous protest actions. The opponents of the companies thus used all five methods of increasing outrage (Halbert, 2005: 87–111).

Conclusion

Three types of legal restraint on research were examined here. The first is the most obvious: defamation threats and actions against researchers that deter research on topics that would potentially benefit the community. There are relatively few cases like this. However, defamation law has a more significant influence on research via the chilling effect: researchers will shy away from some topics because of the risk of being sued.

In the case of defamation, a key factor in restraining research is domain shifting. Rather than respond to research findings by scientific criticism or presenting contrary findings – the usual method in science – defamation suits shift the engagement to the legal domain, where money and legal technicalities take priority over scientific claims.

Laws against voluntary euthanasia are not directed at research but nonetheless discourage research on euthanasia by making research more difficult to undertake and by restricting funding for it.

Intellectual property provides a different sort of effect on research, via incentives. Patents, in conjunction with marketing and government regulatory processes, allow pharmaceutical companies to make massive profits from blockbuster drugs, thereby providing an incentive to prioritize investigating drugs with this potential. The spinoff effect is that research into other ways of improving health, including via exercise, diet, and nonpatentable substances, receives less attention than it would otherwise.

The implication of these case studies is that studying the adverse effects of law on science requires going beyond the most obvious cases of suppression. It is important to recognize that some restraints on research can be justified, so it is necessary to carefully assess the justifications. It is also important to look for indirect effects of laws, which can be deeper and more pervasive than the relatively few cases that receive attention.

Acknowledgments The author thanks David Allen, Pieter Cohen, Debora Halbert, Anneleis Humphries, and Qinqing Xu for useful feedback on drafts.

References

Bagley, N., Carroll, A. E., & Cohen, P. A. (2017). Scientific trials—In the laboratories, not the courts. *JAMA Internal Medicine*, November 6. https://doi.org/10.1001/jamainternmed.2017.5730

Carroll, A. E. (2017). Why a lot of important research is not being done: Lawsuits have an intimidating effect on an already difficult enterprise. *New York Times*, December 4.

Côté, R. N. (2012). *In search of gentle death: The fight for your right to die with dignity*. Mt. Pleasant, SC: Corinthian Books.

Craft, L. L., & Perna, F. M. (2004). The benefits of exercise for the clinically depressed. *Primary Care Companion to the Journal of Clinical Psychiatry, 6*(3), 104–111.

Curtis, M. K. (1995). Monkey trials: Science, defamation, and the suppression of dissent. *William & Mary Bill of Rights Journal, 4*(2), 507–593.

Curtis, T. (1992). The origin of AIDS. *Rolling Stone* 626 (19 March), 54–61, 106, 108.

Drahos, P. (1996). *A philosophy of intellectual property*. Aldershot, UK: Dartmouth.

Donson, F. J. L. (2000). *Legal intimidation: A SLAPP in the face of democracy*. London, UK: Free Association Books.

Dunford, R. (1987). The suppression of technology as a strategy for controlling resource dependence. *Administrative Science Quarterly, 32*, 512–525.
Goldacre, B. (2012). *Bad pharma: How drug companies mislead doctors and harm patients.* London, UK: Fourth Estate.
Gøtzsche, P. C. (2013). *Deadly medicines and organised crime: How big pharma has corrupted healthcare.* London, UK: Radcliffe.
Hager, M. (2015). Confidentiality agreement handcuffs prominent assisted-suicide researcher. *The Globe and Mail*, January 6.
Halbert, D. J. (1999). *Intellectual property in the information age: The politics of expanding ownership rights.* Westport, CT: Quorum.
Halbert, D. J. (2005). *Resisting intellectual property.* London, UK: Routledge.
Jansen, S. C., & Martin, B. (2003). Making censorship backfire. *Counterpoise, 7*(3), 5–15.
Jansen, S. C., & Martin, B. (2015). The Streisand effect and censorship backfire. *International Journal of Communication, 9*, 656–671.
Katz, M. H., & Redberg, R. F. (2017). Science requires open discourse. *JAMA Internal Medicine*, November 6. https://doi.org/10.1001/jamainternmed.2017.5763
Magnusson, R. S. (2002). *Angels of death: Exploring the euthanasia underground. Melbourne.* Melbourne, VIC: University Press.
Martin, B. (2007). *Justice ignited: The dynamics of backfire.* Lanham, MD: Rowman & Littlefield.
Martin, B. (2010). How to attack a scientific theory and get away with it (usually): The attempt to destroy an origin-of-AIDS hypothesis. *Science as Culture, 19*(2), 215–239.
Martin, B., Moore, C., & Salter, C. (2010). Sharing music files: Tactics of a challenge to the industry. *First Monday, 15*(12).
Montgomery, B. (1994). Thesis claims "defame." *The Australian,* June 1, p. 21.
Ogden, R. D. (2010). Observation of two suicides by helium inhalation in a prefilled environment. *American Journal of Forensic Medicine and Pathology, 31*(2), 156–161.
Pring, G., & Canan, P. (1996). *SLAPPs: Getting sued for speaking out.* Philadelphia: Temple University Press.
Robbins, R. (2017). A supplement maker tried to silence this Harvard doctor — and put academic freedom on trial. *StatNews,* January 10.
Sheldrick, B. (2014). *Blocking public participation: The use of strategic litigation to silence political expression.* Waterloo, ON: Wilfred Laurier University Press.
Shulman, S. (1999). *Owning the future.* Boston: Houghton Mifflin.
Stark, D. E., & Shah, N. H. (2017). Funding and publication of research on gun violence and other leading causes of death. *Journal of the American Medical Association, 317*(1), 84–86.
Sutherland, K. (2010). Books reviews, the common law tort of defamation, and the suppression of scholarly debate. *German Law Journal, 11*(6), 656–670.
Vidal, J. (1997). *McLibel.* London, UK: Macmillan.

Chapter 11
Conjectures Masquerading as Facts

Andrew C. Papanicolaou

Introduction

Error, hyperbole, and fraud, variously motivated, have always been part and parcel of all human endeavors including science. But in science at least they are not inevitable; not to the degree that they could compromise the esteem it is held by the society that supports it. Had I thought otherwise, I would have no good reason for proceeding with this essay.

Seekers after knowledge are often motivated by wonder, a fact that Aristotle duly noted some centuries ago. Often, they are also motivated by the thirst for recognition and, occasionally, by greed for power—facts that Aristotle was too much of a gentleman to dignify with a comment. Undoubtedly, though, he must have known of the existence of those less than pure motives for the itinerant sophists were still frequenting the agoras of cities and the courts of affluent patricians and were by no means rare or unrepresentative exemplars of humanity. Nor, for that matter, are the scientists of today any less representative than the rest of the people when it comes to the propensity for sin and error. One expects, though, that they can recognize and correct them once they are pointed out to them more readily than the man on the street.

The expectation is reasonable and in most cases is not disappointed. It appears, though, that with the increasing industrialization of all academic endeavors; with the increasing emphasis on production and on attracting funding that gives universities more and more the appearance of businesses and the scientists more and more that of merchants; with the proliferation of professional journals that must attract research papers or perish; with the increasingly loud siren calls of travel around the world's resorts for the presentation of "new" scientific facts and theories by the same conferees two and three and five times in a single year; in short, with the

A. C. Papanicolaou (✉)
The University of Tennessee, College of Medicine, Knoxville, TN, USA

D. M. Allen, J. W. Howell (eds.), *Groupthink in Science*,
https://doi.org/10.1007/978-3-030-36822-7_11

visibly increasing temptations that assail the profession, the suspicion grows that pure motives among the scientists may now be in short supply and that the quality of their work may be slowly giving way to excessive quantity— the several peer-reviewed publications per year— that is needed for academic survival.

I cannot be sure that the appearance of gradual decay is true; that both the ethics and the competence of academics is not what once was or that the quality of their output is constantly degrading. Nor do I intend to investigate this interesting topic. Instead, in this essay, I wish to appose shortcomings that are evident in this field of endeavor, irrespective of whether they are more or less numerous and obvious than what they were at the time of Galileo or of Bohr or the time of my master's thesis advisor than they are today. As for my motive for recounting them, it is simply the belief that they can all be remedied once they are articulated and become known.

I will be commenting on four examples of such shortcomings, all borrowed from the area of cognitive neuroscience in which I can claim a modicum of competence. In the next section of this essay (section "Word Salads"), I will describe unreasonable errors due to either plain incompetence in the use of language or due to sloppy thinking, a distinction that, in practice, hardly matters. In the subsequent sections, I will describe rather insidious exaggerations of the truth. That is, affirmations that have repercussions beyond academia and may affect individuals and social institutions directly. They include claims regarding the nature of the human will and decision-making (section "Affirmations About the Will"), the ability of mind-reading in brain activation patterns recorded through the modern functional neuroimaging methods (section "Affirming the Reality of Thought-Reading"), and the ability to discern, again through functional neuroimaging, the consciousness level of comatose patients (section "Affirming the Discovery of Objective Brain Signs of the Level of Consciousness"). I consider these claims insidious particularly today, where the conviction in the authority of scientific pronouncements has, for large sectors of the general public, replaced the conviction in the authority of religious pronouncements.

Word Salads

It is a well-known fact that most terms regarding psychological functions of the nervous system used by systems neuroscientists, cognitive scientists, psychiatrists, and psychologists are borrowed from colloquial speech, sometimes with and at other times without modifications. The problem is that colloquial expressions are notoriously inconsistent. Consequently, a cursory look at the relevant professional literature will suffice to show that the inconsistency is carried over into the scientific nomenclature. Even the meaning of terms denoting such basic psychological realities as *feeling*, *sentiment*, *emotion*, *motive*, *mood*, *affect*, and even *sensation* and *perception* varies substantially from author to author. This creates the need for each of them to define anew the same terms before proceeding with the presentation of their theories, the rationale for the design of their experiments and the interpretation of their data.

Some investigators have, in fact, made their mark in their respective fields by introducing new technical terms that would delimit and define better the basic concepts and the corresponding terms. The effort is laudable, but the results are hardly worth the effort and the notoriety it bestowed on the innovators. I trust that few people will venture to suggest that Gazzaniga's (1992) and Ramachandran's and Blakeslee's (1998) renaming the infamous *homunculus* of old *General* and *Interpreter,* respectively, has advanced our conception of how patterns of brain signals become experiences one iota. Few also would think that renaming *habits* or *sensory-motor automatisms* as *non-declarative memories* or renaming *iconic* and *echoic memory* as *scratchpad* and *phonological loop* has enhanced our understanding of the mechanisms of immediate or short-term memory. Fewer still would be in a position to declare with a straight face that *attention* is (or is not) among the *Executive Functions*, given that both claims are made, often in the same publication, or to state in no uncertain terms whether or not what humanity for millennia has been calling *thinking* differs in anything substantial from the relatively new term *working memory.* Yet, most accept without complaint the proliferation of near-synonyms that enhance the already reining semantic anarchy and terminological disorder.

But besides vacuous verbal adjustments of the terminology, there are others that, far from being vacuous, aspire to correct the disorder by adopting terms from other disciplines where the terms do have definite meaning. I am referring here to the use of terms like *processing* as in *processing colors* or even *processing anger,* where the *processing* is meant to impart the rigor of engineering and information science to psychological descriptions. Unfortunately, however, what exactly these terms mean when applied to percepts or sentiments remains obscure since processing denotes many diverse events and activities. But the confusion is further exacerbated by the reverse procedure in which neuroscientists, psychologists and cognitive scientists indulge where technical terms like *necessary conditions* as in "*x is a necessary condition or necessary antecedent for y*" are substituted by non-committal expressions like "*x is involved in y*" or "*y is mediated by x*" One may take such substitutions of precise expressions by deliberately imprecise ones as implicit confessions of ignorance on the part of their users of the implied relation of x to y if it were not for the fact that the *involvement* sometimes is said to be *mild* and at other times *great,* which implies, instead, pretention to definite and more detailed knowledge of the said relation.

Then we have the real word salads where, once again, unquestioned conjectures and widely shared beliefs are spoken of as if they were definite facts: We all accept as fact that the various brain networks process, that is, convey and transform signals. Yet, much more often, we read that the brain processes *information* rather than *signals.* We all accept that the eyes are necessary for vision as is the visual cortex. Many also believe that the brain suffices for visual perception as it does for all psychological phenomena, so they feel free to declare that as a matter of fact the brain or parts of it perceive, decide, and sometimes inform us of what it or they perceive or decide and sometimes decide against telling us. Lest the readers of this essay suspect that I am falsely accusing colleagues of such absurdities, let me quote a passage from the source (that need not be specified) where I encountered them for the first time some years ago: a textbook among many that are meant to teach freshmen and sophomores the essentials of psychology:

> "..but the emotional reactions are controlled to a great extent by your right hemisphere. If you experienced something that upset or aroused you your right hemisphere would send out the neural commands that caused you to blush, smile, laugh or even "feel sick to your stomach." But your "emotional" hemisphere would also send a message across the corpus callosum to let your left "executive" hemisphere know what was happening in case you might need to respond to the situation with more than a blush or a smile…"

And, lest the readers think that such senseless word salads are only to be found in elementary textbooks written for presumed simple-minded undergraduates of a bygone era, I refer them to the more recent volume of Bennett and Hacker (2003) pointing to the same abuses of reason and of language employed by nearly all the prominent contemporary cognitive neuroscientists and "neurophilosophers."

The misdemeanors of members of the scientific community thus far recounted consist of affirmations that are false or confused but whose repercussions are hardly felt outside academia. There are others, however, that do have repercussions on that part of the general public which, to a considerable extent, has adopted science as its new religion. Examples of the latter will be presented in subsequent sections of this essay. All of them consist of conjectures that are treated by many scientists as facts. In the following sections, I will examine each of these affirmations in turn.

Affirmations About the Will

The proposition, "*each and every decision, much like any other human experience and action, is caused by a definite set of antecedent neuronal events in the brain,*" is not only the expression of a metaphysical belief but a perfectly legitimate scientific hypothesis, that is, an empirically falsifiable one. It follows then that if the neuronal causes of decisions were identified and if on their basis alone one could predict reliably what decision a person would make, it could be asserted that the decisions were determined by these neuronal events and the issue of freedom of the will would definitively have to be revised accordingly. Therefore, the fundamental question to be answered first is: has the aforementioned legitimate hypothesis been supported by empirical evidence? The answer provided by many neuroscientists is yes. But as it will become clear in the following paragraphs, this answer is entirely unjustified.

Two sets of studies, begun over 30 years ago, were conducted with the intention to test the hypothesis under consideration. The first set consisted of electrophysiological studies involving either surface event-related electroencephalographic recordings of normal subjects (e.g., Libet, 2003; Libet, Gleason, Wright, & Pearl, 1983; Matsuhashi & Hallett, 2008; Schneider, Houdayer, Bai, & Hallett, 2013) or single cell recordings from the brains of awake and cooperating patients (e.g., Fried,

Mukamel, & Kreiman, 2011) while the participants made simple decisions of button-pressing and also determining the time they became aware of deciding when to press the button. Similar tasks were performed in the second set of studies involving regional cerebral blood flow measurements using fMRI (e.g., Lau, Rogers, Ramnani, & Passingham, 2004).

In all cases, it was reported that decisions were invariably preceded by particular neuronal events (or, in the case of the fMRI studies, by local changes in blood flow rates that are interpreted as indices of neuronal activity). On the basis of these results, the conclusion was drawn that the neuronal causes of decisions were in fact identified. These conclusions, however, were from the very beginning challenged (see, e.g., Breitmeyer, 2002; Klemm, 2010; Pockett, Banks, & Gallagher, 2009; Roskies, 2006, 2010) on several grounds that will be summarized below, and new experiments cast doubt on the same conclusions (e.g., Miller & Schwarz, 2014; Miller, Shepherdson, & Trevena, 2011; Schurger, Mylopoulos, & Rosenthal, 2016). All the relevant arguments were recently revisited by Papanicolaou (2017a) re-evaluated by Kihlstrom (2017), by Kirsch and Hyland (2017) and by Breitmeyer (2017) and summarized by Papanicolaou (2017b). The following factors were found to render the conclusions plainly invalid.

First, none of the experiments were ecologically valid for two reasons:

(a) The decisions to be made were of no consequence (they all involved deciding when to press a button, as the subjects had agreed to do beforehand), although they were considered psychologically equivalent to consequential ones in which the action has significant repercussions (e.g., where the button-press would signify a vote or the placing of a signature on a document signifying a financial commitment).
(b) The decisions were only nominally "free," in that the subjects were already committed to "deciding" several times within each testing session.

Second, the subjects had to perform simultaneously several tasks and not only the decision task, namely:

(a) Choosing the time to make the movement.
(b) Identifying with (millisecond) precision when they so chose by perceiving the position of a dot moving around the face of a clock, or something analogous to it.
(c) Remembering the position of the dot at the end of the trial to report it; and
(d) Performing the movement and, in some cases, also identifying when the movement was performed.

Each of these cognitive and perceptual tasks obviously involves different perceptual and cognitive operations, all of which require focal yet necessarily divided attention. Now, in each of these tasks, according to the principle motivating all these studies that each experience has a neuronal cause, the neuronal antecedents found preceding each button-pressing decision could not be attributed to those decisions any more than to any of the other simultaneously proceeding tasks.

Third, when the subjects are instructed to "decide freely" when to press the button but without having to monitor the clock in order to time their decisions, the neuronal event that precedes the button-pressing disappears (Miller et al., 2011). This result shows plainly that the event in question must be a marker of one or more of the other simultaneously evolving psychological processes but definitely not a marker of the decisions.

Fourth, to what process the neuronal event that precedes the button-press corresponds is completely unspecifiable because its timing varies from a fraction of a second in the event-related studies, to 10 whole seconds in the context of the fMRI studies. Therefore, the different studies disclose different types of neuronal events and considering any of them as the cause of any of the simultaneously unfolding psychological processes is definitely arbitrary. Equally clear is that the event recorded electroencephalographically cannot be considered the cause of the decision to button-press because it disappears even when the same button-pressing decisions are made. Moreover, the events recorded from single cells and, more so than those recorded through fMRI, cannot be considered causes of the decision for the above named reasons and because individuals of a species that take whole seconds to implement simple decisions would likely disappear.

The failure of securing evidence of neuronal causes of seemingly "free" decisions certainly does not imply that no such causes exist. But it does demonstrate that the claims made that the presumed freedom of the human will has proven to be an illusion because science has discovered its neuronal causes are flatly wrong. Science has discovered no such thing. What has happened instead is that some scientists confuse their conjectures and metaphysical assumptions with empirical evidence—a confusion they often ascribe to zealots of other causes such as religious or political. Abstaining from doing so is important for the future of the science we practice and perhaps more important for what we teach the public that sustain our practices.

Affirming the Reality of Thought-Reading

In the words of some investigators (e.g. Owen, Schiff, & Laureys, 2009) "*...recent advances in imaging technologies and in particular the ability of fMRI to detect reliable neural responses in individual participants in real time are beginning to reveal patients' thoughts...*"(p.400). Assuming, as nearly every neuroscientist does, the principle of correspondence between experiences like thoughts and intentions and sets or patterns of brain signals to be valid, it appears perfectly reasonable to seek to identify such patterns with the modern functional neuroimaging methods. However, for reasons that will be offered shortly, it is not at all reasonable to claim that such patterns have been identified. And no one is "beginning to read" anyone's thoughts.

In the first place, we must distinguish between concepts and instances of concepts, that is, individual experiences (percepts, thoughts, hopes, and intentions). Concepts, by all accounts, are abstract entities constituted of features that are common to all the individual instances or tokens they represent. The concept "table" for instance consists of all the features that individual tables, or mental images of all tables one can conjure up, possess. Being abstract entities does not mean that they are exempt from the principle of correspondence. In fact, each is supposed to correspond to a distinct pattern of neuronal signals emanating from a particular assembly of functionally interrelated neurons—a mnemonic engram or circuit.

The cell assemblies of the different concepts are dormant when we do not think of the concept. They become reverberating circuits, thus forming a pattern of signals, once sensory input from a particular table (to continue with this example) activates them. This description is a summary of the most widely accepted current model of concept representation in the brain (see, e.g., Papanicolaou, 2017c). According to it, when we see and recognize a table, the subjective experience we have will correspond to the amalgamation of the input signals representing the specific object we happen to encounter, the signals emanating from the activated and the reverberating cell assembly or mnemonic circuit of the concept table and, needless to say, all the other signals corresponding to all other perceived or unconsciously processed sensations (e.g., of body position and motion) and all other fleeting thoughts—including our mood—that define the psychological present at the time of the encounter with the object "table." The latter group of signals corresponding to all biological and psychological functions account for the bulk of the global activation pattern immersed into which are the signals that correspond to the experience of the table (see Papanicolaou, 2017c for a detailed exposition of the process of extracting concept-specific activation patterns from global brain activation). Given that the precise conditions that define each moment of our experiential stream, or William James' famous stream of consciousness, are never the same, the particular experience of the particular table (or any other percept and any other individual thought) is unique and un-repeatable. Given also the basic principle of correspondence, the particular activation pattern of the particular experience of the table will also be unique and unrepeatable, if for no other reason, than for the fact that the pattern corresponding to the next experience of the same table will be produced by a slightly or not so slightly aged brain.

In view of the above facts, it is not clear how the activation pattern corresponding to the individual experience can ever be disentangled from the global activation pattern into which it is immersed. Certainly, to even begin discerning its outline inside the global pattern of signals, we first have to have a clear idea about the activation pattern corresponding to the *concept table*. The most expedient method used to visualize that pattern is to repeat the individual experience of the table many times, obtain the corresponding global patterns, and average them algebraically. By doing so, we would hope to thus extract the features of the global pattern that repeat reliably from the one experience to the next and correspond to the only set of pattern features that remain invariant across all instances of experiencing "table." This would be the pattern made of the *reverberating activity of the neuronal engram of the concept **table***. Needless to say, thus far, there is no evidence whatsoever that the activation pattern of any concept of concrete objects like a chair (let alone intentions, affects, and abstract thoughts) has been isolated and visualized.

Thus far, investigators have managed to derive, mostly using fMRI, patterns specific to broad concept categories such as "faces," "cats," and "man-made objects" (e.g., Carlson, Schrater, & He, 2003; Haxby et al., 2001; Kamitani & Tong, 2005) but always too broad and too few to establish a reasonable degree of specificity. But even those are so far unreliable (nonreproducible from study to study). Additionally, their specificity—that is, the degree to which they correspond to the particular intended concepts or some feature that is shared by those but other concepts as well—is uncomfortably low (for an extensive discussion, see Papanicolaou, 2017d). Whether or not at some future date the patterns of some specific concepts will be visualized sufficiently distinctly and reliably is an open question. But even if that question is answered in the affirmative, the possibility of isolating in individuals global activation patterns anything other than concept patterns (which is not the same as the patterns of individual thoughts) is extremely small. Nevertheless, rumors persist that at least percepts of objects are already discerned with the fMRI and intentions as well. In the following paragraphs, therefore, examples of these studies will be presented and interpreted.

A good example of such discernment is the study of Kay, Naselaris, Prenger, and Gallant (2008; see, also Cox & Savoy, 2003; Kamitani & Tong, 2005; Miyawaki et al., 2008). However, the relationship established in this and similar studies is one between stimuli and activation patterns in the visual cortex, but not between experiences and patterns. Conceivably, the same results could have been obtained by using as a subject a suitably equipped robot, a "zombie," or a comatose patient (so long as the patient's eyes were kept open and the visual input could reach the visual cortex), none of whom is said to have experiences. Nevertheless, it is possible that percepts and the neuronal code of pictures in the visual cortex involve similar activation patterns. If that proves to be the case, if the same pattern obtains when one thinks of a pencil as when one sees one, then one may claim that single "words" in the brain's book have been read and that individual contents of consciousness have been discerned in the flow of brain activity. But that the equivalent of such single "word" reading will eventually be expanded to reading of the entire stream of consciousness is a virtually impossible scenario for reasons that have already been suggested. At any event, as of now, nothing of the sort has transpired.

Affirming the Discovery of Objective Brain Signs of the Level of Consciousness

In recent years, analysis of the resting state of brain activity has resulted in the identification of "resting state networks," including the so-called default mode network or DMN, which obtain when people, though awake and vigilant, remain at rest with the eyes closed avoiding deliberate processing of environmental input or engaging in any specific cognitive activity. Under such resting conditions, the hemodynamic response (fluctuations of local blood flow rates) within certain brain areas and between them is correlated. Several sets of areas with correlated hemodynamic activity have been isolated and each is named a *resting state network*. Most of these networks are also activated during particular tasks and are named according to the function they apparently mediate: visual, motor, attentional, etc. (see Papanicolaou, 2017e for a review).

Of special interest is the DMN, which is interpreted by some investigators as the network that corresponds to the function of conscious awareness that is the prerequisite of having particular conscious experiences, such as intentions, thoughts, decisions, or sentiments. In normal subjects, the network is typically (but not always) found to consist of the following areas: the posterior cingulate cortex and the precuneus, the medial prefrontal cortex, and the inferior parietal lobule, bilaterally (see, e.g., Buckner, Andrews-Hanna, & Schacter, 2008 for a review). The integrity of this "consciousness network" is judged by (a) the strength of the correlation of the hemodynamic response of voxels within one constituent area or "hub" and among hubs and (b) the intensity of the hemodynamic responses in the hubs. Departures from normal values of correlation and/ or intensity are interpreted as signs of diminishing levels of consciousness.

Having such an objective measure of consciousness is obviously important. It has serious theoretical but also practical repercussions in the handling the unacceptably high rate of misdiagnosis, on the basis of behavioral signs, of the degree of compromised consciousness in intensive care wards (Schnakers et al., 2008). It is also important in deciding when to terminate assisted respiration and proceed with organ harvesting, in predicting restitution of consciousness, and other such urgent matters. Unfortunately, and for reasons that will be summarized below, hints or explicit affirmations to the contrary notwithstanding, the fact is that at present, no such visualization has been achieved.

What has been achieved instead are glimpses, more or less tenuous albeit promising, of some aspects or distinguishing features of neurophysiological events that might serve as markers of the still occult neuronal network or networks of consciousness. It is with these that we will deal in this section.

In one such study, the DMN and other resting networks were studied in a group of normal subjects during a normal consciousness state and during states of light and deep propofol-induced anesthesia associated with varying degrees of disruption of awareness (Boveroux et al., 2010). During the normal state of consciousness, the DMN consisted of the structures that define it most consistently, plus structures reported as parts of the DMN but less consistently so (such as the superior frontal sulci, the parahippocampal cortex, the lateral temporal areas, and, the brainstem and the thalamus) raising serious doubts about the nature of the network. On the other hand, during the state of induced unconsciousness, the degree of connectivity in all the above networks except the sensory ones was reduced, and a linear relation was found between the degree of network integrity (i.e., strength of correlations of the hemodynamic fluctuations of the constituent structures) and level of consciousness. Although gradual, these changes have been conveniently segregated into three discrete states (see, e.g., Monti, Laureys, & Owen, 2010): "coma," "vegetative state," also termed "unresponsive wakefulness syndrome," (Laureys et al., 2010) and "minimally conscious state." Additionally, there is a state characterized by perfectly normal consciousness yet nearly complete inability to communicate via any form of behavior requiring the voluntary musculature except vertical eye movements, called the *locked-in* syndrome. This state is often confused with the vegetative state, although it does not involve any known deviations from the normal state of consciousness.

The first attempts to establish relations between brain physiology and the various levels of aberrant consciousness (Levy et al., 1987; Rudolf et al., 1999; Schiff et al., 2002; Laureys et al., 1999) initially focused on the amount of brain activity, assessed through blood flow and glucose utilization measurements using positron emission tomography (PET). They found substantial reduction of that activity in the vegetative state as compared to the resting state of normal subjects. Similar reductions in global activity—close to half of the amount recorded during the normal state of awareness—are also observed in normal subjects during deep anesthesia (Alkire et al., 1999) and deep, slow-wave sleep (Maquet et al., 1997). But global reductions do not constitute a sufficiently sensitive and specific marker because some vegetative patients do not show substantial reductions in global activity, whereas some normal conscious volunteers do. Consequently, regional activity reductions were studied in search of a more accurate marker.

Such regional decreases in the activity of two DMN structures (the posterior cingulate and the left precuneus) among vegetative patients were found in a study by Kim, Kim, An, and Im (2010) through glucose utilization measurements. In a similar study, Laureys et al. (1999) addressed both the possibility that reduction in the activity of DMN structures and reduction in the degree of connectivity among them may identify deviations from the norm, specific to the vegetative state. They found that in the patients a subset of areas typically considered part of DMN showed reduced activity. In addition, they found that the posterior cingulate cortex, which almost invariably features as one of the main DMN component structures, was less "connected" with premotor and prefrontal areas. The utility of the connectivity measure was successfully exploited in subsequent studies to differentiate among normal resting conscious states and states varying in degree of aberration from normal consciousness. Boly et al. (2009) reported that in one patient in the vegetative state, the degree of connectivity between the posterior cingulate and precuneus with the thalamus was lower than that found in a control group of 41 normal subjects. Yet, the degree of connectivity among the cortical regions of DMN did not differ from that observed in normal individuals. These data suggest that a possible distinctive feature between activity patterns indicative of normal versus compromised consciousness is reduction of the functional connectivity in the cortex and the thalamus.

But a rather different suggestion emerges from a larger study of the same kind, by the same group of investigators (Vanhaudenhuyse et al., 2010). In that study, the existence of the normal DMN was duly identified and the expected integrity of that network among (fully conscious) patients in the "locked-in" state was verified, as was the anticipated negative relation between the degree of connectivity of DMN and the different levels of compromised consciousness. Yet this time, reduction in connectivity between the thalamus and the cortical components of DMN was not recognized as the distinctive feature differentiating conscious from nonconscious states. Rather, degree of connectivity of the precuneus was found to be the aspect of the DMN that differentiated normally conscious from minimally conscious and from unconscious individuals.

In spite of differences in findings, these studies have established that aspects of the DMN and other networks as well differ in conscious from unconscious groups of individuals. But because they differ in different ways (i.e., in amount of activity, in degree of connectivity, and in connectivity between different structures) from one study to the next, no one particular form of difference could be identified as the marker differentiating the subjective state of awareness and unawareness. Consequently, no neurophysiological scale for assessing level of consciousness or the prospects of regaining consciousness emerged from these studies. For the construction of such a scale, the pattern of structures that varies either in amount of activation, or in degree of connectivity, or in both must first be established, and established not on a group level but on the level of individual subjects and patients. Assessments of the current state of consciousness, as well as predictions of the likelihood of regaining consciousness, are only practically meaningful at the level of the individual patient, not at the level of the group.

It could, of course, be urged that the day for contemplating such inferences is drawing near because, as the next study to be described shows, we are in a position now to specify brain activity features with sufficient accuracy for a machine to differentiate and accurately classify activity patterns as belonging to conscious as opposed to nonconscious patients. In this study (Phillips et al., 2011), an attempt was made to classify objectively, by means of an automated algorithm, activity patterns obtained with metabolic PET measurements between fully conscious patients and presumably unconscious ones.

The attempt was successful. That is to say, all patients clinically diagnosed to be in the vegetative or wakeful unawareness state were classified as unconscious and most patients in the locked-in state were (correctly) classified as conscious. These results are clearly encouraging; yet, their clinical utility at present is not as clear. What has been demonstrated is that there are two kinds of activation patterns: the one common among patients in the vegetative state and the other common among fully conscious individuals. On that basis, we may assert that there is a pattern that characterizes most people who we know with certainty to be conscious. We may also assert that there is another type of pattern that is sufficiently distinct from the first and characterizes people whose consciousness is in doubt—the very doubt that motivated this sort of investigation in the first place. Therefore, although the first pattern may be said to possibly be the marker of the presence of a subjective state of consciousness because it happens to be found in most people who are certainly conscious, the second may only be said to characterize people in the vegetative state *but not all people that are unconscious* without begging the question.

It is certainly true that definite proof of the presence of conscious awareness on the basis of any brain activity pattern is impossible for the same reason that such proof is impossible on the basis of any physiological measurement, whether it be a peculiarity of the electroencephalographic (EEG) record or the outcome of some volumetric measurement or other of the structural MRI. And a definite proof will remain impossible even if the typical pattern indicative of the presence of conscious experience were already known, because an unknown number of potential deviations from that may result in loss or reduction of consciousness. But empirical science does not require definite proof nor can inductive inference attain it. It only requires sufficiently high likelihood that a particular statement, say, the statement "this patient is not conscious" or "is unlikely to regain consciousness," is true. And although what constitutes sufficiently high likelihood is always a matter of debate, most reasonable people will recognize when sufficient evidence has accumulated to warrant confidence in these predictions and assessments. But until the time comes that the relevant facts are established, it behooves us not to substitute for them our conjectures either unwittingly or deliberately for the purpose of self-aggrandizement or gratuitous aggrandizement of the discipline we serve.

References

Alkire, M. T., Pomrett, C. J., Haier, R. J., Gianzero, M. V., Chan, C. M., Jacobsen, B. P., et al. (1999). Functional brain imaging during anesthesia in humans: Effects of halothane on global and regional cerebral glucose metabolism. *Anesthesiology, 90*(3), 701–709.

Bennett, M., & Hackett, P. (2003). *Philosophical foundations of neuroscience*. Oxford, UK: Blackwell Publishing.

Boly, M., Tshibanda, L., Vanhaudenhuyse, A., Noirhomme, Q., Schnakers, C., Ledoux, D., et al. (2009). Functional connectivity in the default network during resting state is preserved in a vegetative but not in a brain dead patient. *Human Brain Mapping, 30*, 2393–2400.

Boveroux, P., Vanhaudenhuyse, A., Bruno, M., Noirhomme, Q., Lauwick, S., Luxen, A., et al. (2010). Breakdown of within- and between-network resting state functional magnetic resonance imaging connectivity during propofol-induced loss of consciousness. *Anesthesiology, 113*, 1038–1053.

Breitmeyer, B. G. (2002). In support of Pockett's critique of Libet's studies of the time course of consciousness. *Consciousness and Cognition, 11*, 280–283.

Breitmeyer, B. G. (2017). What's all the recent free will ado about? *Psychology of Consciousness Theory, Research, and Practice, 4*, 330–333.

Buckner, R. L., Andrews-Hanna, J. R., & Schacter, D. L. (2008). The brain's default network: Anatomy, function, and relevance to disease. *Annals of the New York Academy of Sciences, 1124*, 1–38.

Carlson, T. A., Schrater, P., & He, S. (2003). Patterns of activity in the categorical representations of objects. *Journal of Cognitive Neuroscience, 15*(5), 704–717.

Cox, D. D., & Savoy, R. L. (2003). Functional magnetic resonance imaging (fMRI) brain reading: Detecting and classifying distributed patterns of fMRI activity in human visual cortex. *NeuroImage, 19*, 261–270.

Fried, I., Mukamel, R., & Kreiman, G. (2011). Internally generated preactivation of single neurons in human medial frontal cortex predicts volition. *Neuron, 69*, 548–562.

Gazzaniga, M. S. (1992). *Nature's mind, the biological roots of thinking, emotions, sexuality, language, and intelligence*. New York: Basic Books.

Haxby, J. V., Gobbini, M. I., Furey, M. L., Ishai, A., Schouten, J. L., & Pietrini, P. (2001). Distributed and overlapping representations of faces and objects in ventral temporal cortex. *Science, 293*, 2425–2430.

Kamitani, Y., & Tong, F. (2005). Decoding the visual and subjective contents of the human brain. *Nature Neurosci, 8*, 679–685.

Kay, K. N., Naselaris, T., Prenger, R. J., & Gallant, J. L. (2008). Identifying natural images from human brain activity. *Nature, 452*, 352–355.

Kihlstrom, J. F. (2017). Time to lay the Libet experiment to rest: Commentary on Papanicolaou (2017). *Psychology of Consciousness Theory, Research, and Practice, 4*, 324–329.

Kim, Y. W., Kim, H. S., An, Y. S., & Im, S. H. (2010). Voxel-based statistical analysis of cerebral glucose metabolism in patients with permanent vegetative state after acquired brain injury. *Chinese Medical Journal (Engl), 123*, 2853–2857.

Kirsch, I., & Hyland, M. E. (2017). Methodological determinism and the free will hypothesis. *Psychology of Consciousness Theory, Research, and Practice, 4*, 321–323.

Klemm, W. R. (2010). Free will debates: Simple experiments are not so simple. *Advances in Cognitive Psychology, 6*, 47–65.

Lau, H. C., Rogers, R. D., Ramnani, N., & Passingham, R. E. (2004). Willed action and attention to the selection of action. *NeuroImage, 21*, 1407–1415.

Laureys, S., Celesia, G., Cohadon, F., Lavrijsen, J., Leon-Carrion, J., Sannita, W., et al. (2010). Unresponsive wakefulness syndrome: A new name for the vegetative state or apallic syndrome. *BMC Medicine, 8*, 68.

Laureys, S., Goldman, S., Phillips, C., Van Bogaert, P., Aerts, J., Luxen, A., et al. (1999). Impaired effective cortical connectivity in vegetative state: Preliminary investigation using PET. *NeuroImage, 9*, 377–382.

Levy, D. E., Sidtis, J. J., Rottenberg, D. A., Jarden, J. O., Strother, S. C., Dhawan, V., et al. (1987). Differences in cerebral blood flow and glucose utilization in vegetative versus locked-in patients. *Annals of Neurology, 22*, 673–682.

Libet, B. (2003). Timing of conscious experience: Reply to the 2002 commentaries on Libet's findings. *Consciousness and Cognition, 12*, 321–331.

Libet, B., Gleason, C. A., Wright, E. W., & Pearl, D. K. (1983). Time of conscious intention to act in relation to onset of cerebral activity (readiness-potential).The unconscious initiation of a freely voluntary act. *Brain: A Journal of Neurology, 106*, 623–642.

Maquet, P., Degueldre, C., Delfiore, G., Aerts, J., Peters, J., Luxen, A., et al. (1997). Functional neuroanatomy of human slow wave sleep. *The Journal of Neuroscience, 17*, 2807–2812.

Matsuhashi, M., & Hallett, M. (2008). The timing of the conscious intention to move. *The European Journal of Neuroscience, 28*, 2344–2351.

Miller, J., & Schwarz, W. (2014). Brain signals do not demonstrate unconscious decision making: An interpretation based on graded conscious awareness. *Consciousness and Cognition, 24*, 12–21.

Miller, J., Shepherdson, P., & Trevena, J. (2011). Effects of clock monitoring on electroencephalographic activity: Is unconscious movement initiation an artifact of the clock? *Psychological Science, 22*, 103–109.

Miyawaki, Y., Uchida, H., Yamashita, O., Sato, M., Morito, Y., Tanabe, H., et al. (2008). Visual image reconstruction from human brain activity using a combination of multiscale local image decoders. *Neuron, 60*, 915–929.

Monti, M., Laureys, S., & Owen, A. (2010). The vegetative state. *Clinical Reviews, 341*, 292–296.

Owen, A. M., Schiff, N. D., & Laureys, S. (2009). A new era of coma and consciousness science. *Progress in Brain Research, 177*, 399–411.

Papanicolaou, A. C. (2017a). The myth of the neuroscience of will. *Psychology of Consciousness: Theory, Research, and Practice, 4*, 310–320.

Papanicolaou, A. C. (2017b). The claim "the will is determined" is not based on evidence. *Psychology of Consciousness: Theory, Research, and Practice, 4*(3), 334–336.

Papanicolaou, A. C. (2017c). Overview of basic concepts. In A. C. Papanicolaou (Ed.), *The Oxford handbook of functional neuroimaging*. New York: Oxford University Press.

Papanicolaou, A. C. (2017d). Imaging the networks of consciousness. In A. C. Papanicolaou (Ed.), *The Oxford handbook of functional Neuroimaging*. New York: Oxford University Press.

Papanicolaou, A. C. (2017e). The default mode and other resting networks. In A. C. Papanicolaou (Ed.), *The Oxford handbook of functional neuroimaging*. New York: Oxford University Press.

Phillips, C. L., Bruno, M. A., Maquet, P., Boly, M., Noirhomme, Q., Schnakers, C., Vanhaudenhuyse, A., Bonjean, M., Hustinx, R., Moonen, G., Luxen, A., & Laureys, S. (2011). "Relevance vector machine" consciousness classifier applied to cerebral metabolism of vegetative and locked-in patients. *Neuroimage, 56*, 797–808.

Pockett, S., Banks, W. P., & Gallagher, S. (2009). *Does consciousness cause behavior?* Cambridge, MA: MIT Press.

Ramachandran, V. S., & Blakeslee, S. (1998). *Phantoms in the brain: Probing the mysteries of the human mind*. New York: William Morrow.

Roskies, A. L. (2006). Neuroscientific challenges to free will and responsibility. *Trends in Cognitive Sciences, 10*, 419–423.

Roskies, A. L. (2010). How does neuroscience affect our conception of volition? *Annual Review of Neuroscience, 33*, 109–130.

Rudolf, J., Ghaemi, M., Ghaemi, M., Haupt, W. F., Szelies, B., & Heiss, W. D. (1999). Cerebral glucose metabolism in acute and persistent vegetative state. *Journal of Neurosurgical Anesthesiology, 11*(1), 17–24.

Schiff, N., Ribary, U., Moreno, D., Beattie, B., Kronberg, E., Blasberg, R., et al. (2002). Residual cerebral activity and behavioural fragments can remain in the persistently vegetative brain. *Brain, 125*, 1210–1234.

Schnakers, C., Ledoux, D., Majerus, S., Damas, P., Damas, F., Lambermont, B., et al. (2008). Diagnostic and prognostic use of bispectral index in coma, vegetative state and related disorders. *Brain Injury, 22*(12), 926–931.

Schneider, L., Houdayer, E., Bai, O., & Hallett, M. (2013). What we think before a voluntary movement. *Journal of Cognitive Neuroscience, 25*, 822–829.

Schurger, A., Mylopoulos, M., & Rosenthal, D. (2016). Neural antecedents of spontaneous voluntary movements: A new perspective. *Trends in Cognitive Sciences, 20*, 77–79.

Vanhaudenhuyse, A., Noirhomme, Q., Tshibanda, L., Brun, O. M., Boveroux, P., Schnakers, C., et al. (2010). Default network connectivity reflects the level of consciousness in non-communicative brain-damaged patients. *Brain, 133*, 161–171.

Part III
Examples and Personal Experiences

Chapter 12
Key Opinion Leaders and the Control of Knowledge

Joel Lexchin

Why Are Key Opinion Leaders (KOLs) Necessary?

Since the end of World War II, there has been a divide in medical research leading to new medicines. At the risk of oversimplifying the situation, public funding goes into the generation of new basic science knowledge, for example, how neurochemicals function in the brain. Industry funding then takes this knowledge and uses it to develop medicines (Stevens et al., 2011). In 2012, pharmaceutical companies that were members of the Pharmaceutical Research and Manufacturers of America (PhRMA) spent over $48 billion USD on research and development (R&D) (Pharmaceutical Research and Manufacturers of America, 2013).

For the past couple of decades, the pharmaceutical industry has operated on a blockbuster model, relying on drugs that generate $1 billion, or more, in worldwide sales to provide the rate of return that shareholders have come to demand. Clinical trials that fail to demonstrate effectiveness or that raise significant safety concerns can dramatically affect the sale of products. Witness what happened following the July 2002 publication of the results of the Women's Health Initiative trial that found that the estrogen/progestin combination caused an increased risk of cardiovascular disease and breast cancer in postmenopausal women (Writing Group for the Women's Health Initiative Investigators, 2002). By June 2003, prescriptions for Prempro®, the most widely sold estrogen/progestin combination, had declined by 66% in the United States (US) (Hersh, Stefanick, & Stafford, 2004) and sales of estrogen replacement therapy were off by a third in Ontario (Austin, Mamdani, Tu, & Jaakkimainen, 2003). Now that the days of traditional blockbusters are seemingly over, they have been replaced by so-called niche busters, drugs that can be sold to small therapeutic markets that cost hundreds of thousands of dollars per year per

J. Lexchin (✉)
School of Health Policy and Management, Faculty of Health, York University, Toronto, ON, Canada
e-mail: jlexchin@yorku.ca

D. M. Allen, J. W. Howell (eds.), *Groupthink in Science*,
https://doi.org/10.1007/978-3-030-36822-7_12

patient. Although the economic model has moved on, the effects of negative studies on sales have not changed.

In order to avoid these scenarios and continue to expand revenue, companies have evolved from controlling the development of new drugs to also controlling the knowledge about those drugs, ensuring that theirs is the primary message that reaches doctors and patients (Gagnon, 2009). However, companies know that messages coming directly from them are likely to be viewed very skeptically. As a result, the concept of using "key opinion leaders" (KOLs) as an "independent" source of information has significantly expanded since the mid- to late-1990s (Millard, 2008). In the US, a 2007 survey found that 16% of physicians, or about 141,000, received payments for serving as a speaker or being part of a speakers' bureau (Campbell et al., 2007). More recently, in just 5 months of 2013, companies made what appear to be speaker payments of $400 or greater to 55,000 doctors (Sismondo, 2015).

Some KOLs are clinicians who are hired to give small-scale talks, but, for major programs, KOLs are typically well-known and highly respected leaders in their field who are especially effective at transmitting messages to their peers. Pharmaceutical companies hire KOLs to consult for them, to give lectures, to run continuing medical education sessions, to conduct clinical trials, and occasionally to make presentations on their behalf at regulatory meetings or hearings (Elliott, 2010). This chapter will focus on why people are willing to take on the role of a KOL, how they rationalize their position, how they are viewed by pharmaceutical companies and what the consequences are for how pharmaceutical knowledge is disseminated.

KOL Motivation

Some KOLs earn hundreds of thousands of dollars a year (Harris & Carey, 2008; Harris, 2008; Carey & Harris, 2008) and there are instances where their actions could lead to allegations that these people have been "bought." Two psychiatrists at a Texas state hospital resigned after being told that they would face disciplinary actions for accepting hundreds of thousands of dollars in speaking and consulting fees from AstraZeneca while also promoting one of its drugs to state officials (Silverman, 2015). In another case, Dr. Jack Gorman, a paid consultant to Forest Laboratories, wrote an extremely favorable article about escitalopram (Lexapro) (Gorman, Korotzer, & Su, 2002), a drug made by Forest, that was published in a special industry-funded supplement of *CNS Spectrums*, a neuropsychiatric journal that Gorman edited. Gorman stated at the time that the article was published that he was not paid personally to write it (Petersen, 2002). Typically, in the past, articles coming from industry-funded symposia, such as the one where Gorman first presented his paper, often had promotional attributes and were not peer-reviewed (Bero, Galbraith, & Rennie, 1992).

The suspicion that KOLs, like Gorman, are being bought is reinforced by a number of studies that have shown that authors who have a relationship with a company that produces a controversial product are more likely to express a positive attitude about the product, to downplay negative evidence about the drug and to adopt a promotional tone in their writing compared with authors who do not have a relationship. Examples where this has occurred involved calcium channel antagonists (Stelfox, Chua, O'Rourke, & Detsky, 1998), the oral hypoglycemic agent rosiglitazone (Wang, McCoy, Murad, & Montori, 2010), hormone replacement therapy (Fugh-Berman, McDonald, Bell, Bethards, & Sciali, 2011) and antidepressants (Cosgrove, Bursztajn, Erlich, Wheeler, & Shaughnessy, 2013). One way of interpreting these examples is that companies have effectively "bribed" authors, but the question remains whether authors were influenced as a result of their association with the companies or if their opinions preceded their involvement with the companies.

It is inevitable that some people can be bribed – in fact, some KOLs admit this reality. Sergio Sismondo, who teaches philosophy at Queens University in Canada, interviewed a series of KOLs and found at least six instances where physicians demanded speaking engagements in exchange for prescribing a company's product, or where sales representatives offered speaking engagements if doctors agreed to prescribe their products (Sismondo & Chloubova, 2013). In some cases, companies employed doctors as KOLs whose records included disciplinary actions related to problems with patient care or drug prescribing or who had received warning letters from the FDA over problems with how they conducted drug research (Aldhous, Giles, & Stenger, 2010). But rather than companies bribing doctors or doctors being swayed by the money being offered to them, the most likely scenario is that companies predominantly recruit people who already hold opinions favorable to their drugs.

Two examples serve to illustrate this process. Daniel Carlat, a psychiatrist in Massachusetts, described how a representative from Wyeth approached him to give talks about the antidepressant Effexor XR (venlafaxine). Carlat had already prescribed the drug to several patients, and it seemed to work as well as its competitors. He reasoned that if talked to primary-care doctors about Effexor, he would be doing nothing unethical. In his view, Effexor was a perfectly effective treatment option, with some data to suggest advantages over its competitors (Carlat, 2007). The second example is Dr. Peter Libby, chief of cardiovascular medicine at Harvard's Brigham and Women's Hospital. Libby gave talks for pharmaceutical companies because he felt that it was important for researchers to impart their knowledge to others (Kolata, 2008). Carlat and Libby were both speaking because of altruistic motives not primarily because of the benefits that they received from being KOLs.

What applies to Carlat and Libby applies to all of the 13 KOLs that Sismondo interviewed. They were uniformly quite emphatic that they believed in the products that they were promoting and that they believed that what they were doing helped to educate doctors. One who is quoted said, "If I don't believe the data, I won't do it. If I don't think the agent on label has a real role or a real niche, if it's not one I'm supportive of, then I don't do it. If I feel the drug company is pushing a sales pitch more than a proper therapeutic use, I won't do it" (Sismondo & Chloubova, 2013).

Although most KOLs are "true believers" in the drugs that they are promoting, they also readily acknowledge that there are other factors involved in their decision to work for drug companies. Some allow that the money that they are paid is the main reason for giving the talks and even when money is not the main motivating factor, they feel that they are entitled to the reimbursement to compensate them for the time that they spend when they could be seeing patients (Sismondo & Chloubova, 2013). In addition, they appreciate the various "perks" that come with the job such as the research funding that they receive, the increase in the number of publications that they author by means of ghost writing (Ghost writing is the practice whereby a pharmaceutical company directly or indirectly hires a "ghost" writer to write a journal article with a specific message and then finds a researcher or clinician who is willing to sign his or her name to the article. Typically, the ghost writer is either not acknowledge or is vaguely thanked for his or her help on the manuscript.), acquiring early knowledge about new drugs, being at the vanguard of their specialty and the psychological reward that comes from their egos being stroked (Elliott, 2010; Sismondo & Chloubova, 2013: Sah & Fugh-Berman, 2013). Eric Turner, a former reviewer for the FDA, at one point gave talks for Eli Lilly and described his experience. "The first thing they do is ferry you to a really nice hotel. And sometimes they pick you up in a limo, and you feel very important, and they have really, really good food" (Elliott, 2010).

KOLs and the Denial of Conflict of Interest

Beyond their sincere belief in the product that they are promoting and the education that they are delivering, KOLs deny that they can be influenced by any conflict of interest that their position creates. One KOL defended his integrity by saying that he was "not just a paid monkey reading slides," while another insisted that he "won't be a paid stooge for somebody" (Sismondo & Chloubova, 2013). A Florida rheumatologist echoed these comments: "It's not just like reading a script. I talk about it [the drug he is promoting] and answer questions" (LaMendola, 2009).

KOLs often claim that their talks are controlled by the FDA and therefore not biased because the drug companies have designed the contents of the slides to be consistent with what the FDA allows to appear on the label (Sismondo & Chloubova, 2013; LaMendola, 2009). Some justify what they are doing by pointing to other conflicts, criticizing the medical journals that editorialize against conflict of interest while accepting money for journal advertising or academics who speak out on conflict of interest but continue to take research money from industry (Sismondo & Chloubova, 2013). Others invoke benefits to doctors and patients from their talks; doctors are educated about the medications and, as a result, patients get better therapy (Sismondo & Chloubova, 2013). Even when KOLs recognize that there may be a bias in their talks, they are quick to defend themselves. "There is always the potential that somehow I'm getting in under the radar and then springing this very subtle and very pernicious sales message...I'm listening to myself every time I speak, and I have to ask myself the question: 'Is what I'm saying truthful?'" (Weber & Ornstein, 2010).

In taking the position that they will not be affected by conflict of interest, KOLs are echoing the stance taken by doctors in general when questioned about their relationships with industry. When internal medicine residents were asked if they thought that their prescribing would be influenced by pharmaceutical promotion, 61% answered no, but at the same time, only 16% thought that their colleagues would be similarly unaffected (Steinman, Shlipak, & McPhee, 2001). Forty-two percent of general practitioners in the Edinburgh area in Scotland felt that pharmaceutical industry involvement in continuing medical education created a conflict of interest, but 85% did not perceive their involvement with the industry as biasing their prescribing behavior (Rutledge, Crookes, McKinstry, & Maxwell, 2003). Only 7% of authors of clinical practice guidelines who had a relationship with pharmaceutical companies whose drugs were considered in the guidelines thought that their drug recommendations would be affected by that relationship (Choudhry, Stelfox, & Detsky, 2002).

These belief patterns are consistent with cognitive dissonance theory whereby the discomfort between what doctors do and what they believe has to be resolved. Based on an analysis of transcripts from focus groups, Chimonas and colleagues describe the ways in which doctors resolve the dissonance. "They avoided thinking about the conflict of interest, they disagreed that industry relationships affected physician behavior, they denied responsibility for the problem, they enumerated techniques for remaining impartial, and they reasoned that meetings with detailers were educational and benefited patients" (Chimonas, Brennan, & Rothman, 2007). KOLs exhibit all of these behavioral patterns. What is more, as KOLs deliver positive messages about a drug, they internalize these beliefs in order to resolve any residual psychological differences that may exist between doubts that they may have about the merits of the drug and the message that they are paid to deliver (Sah & Fugh-Berman, 2013).

Industry's Position on KOLs

One way of judging the importance that pharmaceutical companies place on KOLs is the fact that roughly one-third of the marketing budget for pharmaceutical companies is spent on KOLs (Millard, 2008; Elliott, 2010). This amounts to an average of about $38 million USD on each product as it moves from clinical testing to launch (PR Newswire, 2006). Companies are willing to spend this amount of money because of the return that they get. According to an internal Merck document, doctors who attended a lecture by a KOL on Vioxx (rofecoxib) wrote an additional $623.55 worth of prescriptions for the drug over a 12-month period compared with doctors who did not attend. "After factoring in the extra cost of hiring a doctor to speak, Merck calculated that the 'return on investment' of the doctor-led discussion group was 3.66 times the investment, versus 1.96 times for a meeting with a sales representative" (Hensley & Martinez, 2005). Whereas in 1998, in the United States, the number of talks by sales representatives and KOLs were about equal at just over

60,000 each annually, by 2004, there were almost twice as many talks by KOLs compared to sales representatives (Hensley & Martinez, 2005) – a reflection of the economic benefits of using KOLs instead of sales representatives.

Both outside observers and industry insiders acknowledge that the revenue that KOLs generate is why they are hired by drug companies. Eric Campbell, a Harvard Medical School professor, said, “The only reason the companies hire doctors is to increase sales. They call it education and the doctors call it education, but it’s about making money” (LaMendola, 2009). Steve Nissen, a cardiologist with the Cleveland Clinic, offered basically the same opinion. “If they can get one of them [a KOL] to favor their product, it will influence others. Why would they spend the money if it wasn’t effective?” (Fauber, 2009). Anton Ehrhardt, the senior medical director for the global medical affairs division of Millennium Pharmaceuticals, was quite open about the value of KOLs. “The ‘dirty little secret’ in this field…is that people working in pharma view the KOLs as sales agents” (Millard, 2008). According to Kimberly Elliott, a former drug company sales representative, her company “would routinely measure the return on our investment, by tracking prescriptions before and after their [KOLs’] presentations…If that speaker didn’t make the impact the company was looking for, then you wouldn’t invite them back” (Moynihan, 2008).

KOLs are not hired because of the number of prescriptions that they write as individuals but, in the words of one firm that specializes in managing KOLs for drug companies, because their talks, research, publications, positions in professional societies and other actions can influence the prescribing habits of thousands of doctors (Moynihan, 2008; Opinion Leader Development, 2014). These firms use sophisticated software to find KOLs through tracking a variety of metrics including publications, clinical trials, grants, academic credentials, prescribing patterns, and positions on guideline committees (Millard, 2008). Once a potential KOL is identified, then drug company marketing staff “evaluate their views and influence potential,” build relationships with them, and turn them into “product champions” (Moynihan, 2008). If KOLs do not have the impact that companies expect of them, they are not invited back by the company (Moynihan, 2008).

Increasingly, the process of training KOLs is outsourced to firms that run sessions to teach KOLs communication techniques. For example, one marketing firm’s website states that “[i]t’s vital that advocates are able to communicate and influence colleagues with clarity and conviction. To ensure speakers are at the top of their game, we have developed a communication skills programme for clinicians” (Sismondo, 2015). They are taught how to explain scientific concepts to audiences. In the process, KOLs become involved in the promotional plans for the product that they will be speaking about. There are confidential individual management plans developed for KOLs. One such plan included entries such as “so-and-so will meet with him on such-and-such a date with this expected result, and then we’ll invite him to do this” (Sismondo & Chloubova, 2013).

Controlling Knowledge

KOLs are provided with slide decks prepared by the pharmaceutical company and are expected to stick strictly to the message in those slides (Sismondo & Chloubova, 2013).

The reason for this rigid adherence to the script is twofold. First, companies do not want to run afoul of regulatory authorities by openly promoting off-label prescribing (i.e., prescribing for nonapproved indications) and second, companies have carefully prepared the message that they want doctors to hear – they do not want any extraneous information to interfere with that message. According Elliott, "I would give them all the information I wanted them to talk about, I would give them slides, they would go through specific training programs on what to say and what not to say so it would be beneficial for my company" (Miller, 2008).

The talks that KOLs give can be scientifically valid but also deceptive at the same time, for example, by touting the benefits of their company's drug but not mentioning that other drugs are equally or more efficacious. Alternatively, KOLs may be hired to give presentations or write articles emphasizing the negative aspects of individual drugs or drug classes without ever mentioning the product made by the company paying them. Dr. Adriane Fugh-Berman recounts how she was asked by a medical education company representing an unnamed pharmaceutical manufacturer to be the author of a review article about interactions between herbs and warfarin, an anticoagulant. The reason why the company wanted the article published was that it was planning on introducing a competitor to warfarin and viewed a piece critical of warfarin as a marketing tool. When Fugh-Berman received a draft of the article to edit or amend, she declined to participate, but later found out that virtually the same article was submitted to a journal under another author's name (Fugh-Berman, 2005). There are never any KOLs talking about the role of generics, that is, off-patent, drugs for the simple reason that there is no profit incentive for the brand-name companies to sponsor such talks.

Finally, KOLs are used in disease mongering, widening the boundaries of treatable illness, in order to expand markets for those who sell and deliver treatments. As GlaxoSmithKline was planning the introduction of its treatment for irritable bowel syndrome into the Australian market, its first step was to set up an Advisory Board, comprising one KOL from each Australian state. The Advisory Board's chief role would be to provide advice to GlaxoSmithKline on current opinion in gastroenterology and on "opportunities for shaping it" (Moynihan, Health, & Henry, 2002).

Just as KOLs need to maintain the illusion that they are independent to be able to justify continuing to give talks, likewise the pharmaceutical companies need to maintain the fiction that KOLs are independent sources of information. This supposed independence is the main reason that doctors trust KOLs more than sales representatives. If KOLs are shown not to be independent, then they lose their value to the companies. However, it is precisely when KOLs start to act independently and deviate from the messages that companies are cultivating, that their value to the company starts to be questioned. Daniel Carlat became increasingly uneasy about the benefits and harms of Effexor – an antidepressant that he was giving talks about. At the end of one event, he mentioned that data in support of Effexor were mainly short term, and that there was a possibility that other products were just as effective. Several days later, he received a visit from the district manager for the company who said, "My reps told me that you weren't as enthusiastic about our product at your last talk. I told them that even Dr. Carlat can't hit a home run every time. Have you been sick?" (Carlat, 2007).

Even more telling is what happened to John Norton after he wrote a series of case reports reflecting his experience with the side effect profile of a certain medication made by a company for which he often spoke. The picture he painted of that product was less favorable than that of a drug made by a competitor. Once those case reports became public, his invitations to speak dropped from four to six times per month to essentially none (Norton, 2000).

Conclusion

The point here is not the personal integrity of KOLs, but the fact that the information that they are given and trained to deliver has been shaped by the companies whose primary goal is to increase sales of their drugs. Data need to be interpreted and, for obvious reasons, companies are going to put the best spin on that data. Other views about the data are not being heard to anywhere near the same extent because no other stakeholder in the pharmaceutical world has resources to match those of the drug companies.

In 2004 alone, companies in the United States spent $57.5 billion on marketing to doctors and consumers (Gagnon & Lexchin, 2008). When one voice drowns out all the others and that voice predominantly sings the praises of drugs, then medicine suffers and patients fail to get the treatment that they are entitled to. KOLs are part of that marketing machine and cannot be viewed as impartial experts; they are hired to help sell the product. As Jerry Seinfeld once put it, "you're either helping me or selling me but they're not the same thing" (Seinfeld, 1993).

References

Aldhous, P., Giles, J., & Stenger, B. (2010). Pfizer's payments to censured doctors. *New Scientist, 206*(2758), 8.

Pharmaceutical Research and Manufacturers of America. (2013). *Biopharmaceutical research industry profile*. Washington, DC.

Austin, P. C., Mamdani, M. M., Tu, K., & Jaakkimainen, L. (2003). Prescriptions for estrogen replacement therapy in Ontario before and after publication of the Women's Health Initiative Study. *JAMA, 289*, 3241–3242.

Bero, L., Galbraith, A., & Rennie, D. (1992). The publication of sponsored symposiums in medical journals. *New England Journal of Medicine, 327*, 1135–1140.

Campbell, E., Gruen, R., Mountford, J., Miller, L., Cleary, P., & Blumenthal, D. (2007). A national survey of physician-industry relationships. *New England Journal of Medicine, 356*, 1742–1750.
Carey, B., Harris, G. (2008, July 12). Psychiatric group faces scrutiny over drug industry ties. *New York Times*.
Carlat, D. (2007, November 25). Dr. drug rep. *New York Times*.
Chimonas, S., Brennan, T., & Rothman, D. (2007). Physicians and drug representatives: Exploring the dynamics of the relationship. *Journal of General Internal Medicine, 22*, 184–190.
Choudhry, N., Stelfox, H., & Detsky, A. (2002). Relationships between authors of clinical practice guidelines and the pharmaceutical industry. *JAMA, 287*, 612–617.
Cosgrove, L., Bursztajn, H., Erlich, D., Wheeler, E., & Shaughnessy, A. (2013). Conflict of interest and the quality of recommendations in clinical guidelines. *Journal of Evaluation in Clinical Practice, 19*, 674–681.
Elliott, C. (2010 [cited 2015 April 13]). The secret lives of big pharma's 'thought leaders'. *The Chronicle of Higher Education*. Available from: http://chronicle.com/article/The-Secret-Lives-of-Big/124335/
Fauber, J. (2009, January 12). Drug firms wine, dine and pay up for doctors' speeches. *Milwaukee-Wisconsin Journal Sentinel*.
Fugh-Berman, A. (2005). The corporate coauthor. *Journal of General Internal Medicine, 20*, 546–548.
Fugh-Berman, A., McDonald, C., Bell, A., Bethards, E., & Sciali, A. (2011). Promotional tone in reviews of menopausal hormone therapy after the Women's Health Initiative: an analysis of published articles. *PLoS Medicine, 11*, e1000425.
Gagnon, M. (2009). *The nature of capital in the knowledge-based economy: The case of the global pharmaceutical industry*. Toronto, ON: York University.
Gagnon, M. A., & Lexchin, J. (2008). The cost of pushing pills: A new estimate of pharmaceutical promotion expenditures in the United States. *PLoS Medicine, 5*(1), e1.
Gorman, J., Korotzer, A., & Su, G. (2002). Efficacy comparison of escitalopram and citalopram in the treatment of major depressive disorder: pooled analysis of placebo-controlled trials. *CNS Spectrums, 7*(4 (suppl 1)), 40–44.
Harris G. (2008, October 4). Top psychiatrist didn't report drug makers' pay. *New York Times*.
Harris, G., Carey, B. (2008, June 8). Researchers fail to reveal full drug pay. *New York Times*.
Hensley, S., & Martinez, B. (2005, July 15). New treatment: To sell their drugs, companies increasingly rely on doctors – for $750 and up, physicians tell peers about products; talks called educational – Dr. Pitt's busy speaking tour. *Wall Street Journal*.
Hersh, A. L., Stefanick, M. L., & Stafford, R. S. (2004). National use of postmenopausal hormone therapy: Annual trends and response to recent evidence. *JAMA, 291*, 47–53.
Kolata, G. (2008, April 15). Citing ethics, some doctors are rejecting industry pay. *New York Times*.
LaMendola, R. (2009, September 19). Doctors' speeches on brand-name drugs can net thousands. *South Florida Sun-Sentinel*.
Millard, W. (2008). Dispatch from the pharmasphere: An industry's fault lines on display. *Annals of Emergency Medicine, 51*, 175–180.
Miller N. (2008, June 21). Paid doctors just drug spruikers, says insider. *Sydney Morning Herald.*
Moynihan, R. (2008). Key opinion leaders: Independent experts or drug representatives in disguise? *BMJ, 336*, 1402–1403.
Moynihan, R., Health, I., & Henry, D. (2002). Selling sickness: The pharmaceutical industry and disease mongering. *BMJ, 324*, 886–891.
Norton, J. (2000). Is academic medicine for sale? *New England Journal of Medicine, 343*, 508.
Opinion leader development: KOL (2014 [cited 2015 April 15]). Available from: http://www.kolonline.com/services-development.asp
Petersen, M. (2002, November 22). Madison Ave. has growing role in the business of drug research. *New York Times*.

PR Newswire. (2006). Pharma brands earmark $38 million for thought leaders: [cited 2015 April 14]. Available from: http://www.prnewswire.com/news-releases/pharma-brands-earmark-38-million-for-thought-leaders-53883072.html

Rutledge, P., Crookes, D., McKinstry, B., & Maxwell, S. (2003). Do doctors rely on pharmaceutical industry funding to attend conferences and do they perceive that this creates a bias in their drug selection? Results from a questionnaire survey. *Pharmacoepidemiology and Drug Safety, 12*, 663–667.

Sah, S., & Fugh-Berman, A. (2013). Physicians under the influence: Social psychology and industry marketing strategies. *Journal of Law, Medicine & Ethics, 41*, 665–672.

Seinfeld, J. (1993). *SeinLanguage*. New York: Bantam Books.

Silverman, E. (2015, April 21). Psychiatrists with ties to AstraZeneca resign from Texas state hospital. *Wall Street Journal*.

Sismondo, S. (2015). How to make opinion leaders and influence people. *CMAJ, 187*, 759–760.

Sismondo, S., & Chloubova, Z. (2013). "You're not just a paid monkey reading slides:" how key opinion leaders explain and justify their work. *BioSocieties, 11*, 199–219.

Steinman, M., Shlipak, M., & McPhee, S. (2001). Of principles and pens: Attitudes and practices of medicine housestaff toward pharmaceutical industry promotions. *American Journal of Medicine, 110*, 551–557.

Stelfox, H., Chua, G., O'Rourke, K., & Detsky, A. (1998). Conflict of interest in the debate over calcium-channel antagonists. *New England Journal of Medicine, 338*, 101–106.

Stevens, A., Jensen, J., Wyller, K., Kilgore, P., Chatterjee, S., & Rohrbaugh, M. (2011). The role of public-sector research in the discovery of drugs and vaccines. *New England Journal of Medicine, 364*, 535–541.

Wang, A., McCoy, C., Murad, M., & Montori, V. (2010). Association between industry affiliation and position on cardiovascular risk with rosiglitazone: Cross sectional systematic review. *BMJ, 340*, c1344.

Weber, T., Ornstein, C. (2010 [cited 2015 April 15]). Dollars for docs: who's on pharma's top-paid list? *ProPublica*. Available from: http://www.propublica.org/article/profiles-of-the-top-earners-in-dollar-for-docs

Writing Group for the Women's Health Initiative Investigators. (2002). Risks and benefits of estrogen plus progestin in health postmenopausal women: Principal results from the Women's Health Initiative randomized controlled trial. *JAMA, 288*, 321–333.

Chapter 13
Conflict Between Public Health Science and Markets: The Case of Tobacco Research – Illustrations from Tobacco and CO²

Augustine Brannigan

Introduction: Beyond Unconscious Bias to the Manufacture of Doubt

The idea of "groupthink" in science arises from concerns about how psychological conditions among researchers working in groups bias their conduct of objective research. In this chapter, we examine a different issue. What if ignorance is the outcome of institutional processes designed to suppress knowledge? The cases identified here involved the conscious creation of and exploitation of scientific ambiguity, confusion, doubt, and denial of important scientific facts. The objective was to countermand the control of commodities injurious to individuals and the environment. This occurred primarily in the area of public health science. In these cases, the evidence of injury suggested by scientific methods, including epidemiology and biomedical experiments, is said to have been deliberately obfuscated by producers and their industry experts.

These cases involve:

(a) Injuries to individuals using such consumer products as cigarettes, pharmaceuticals, and other healthcare products and implants resulting in preventable disease and death
(b) Diseases contracted by workers who are recklessly exposed to known toxic manufacturing materials such as asbestos, tetraethyl lead, barium, chromium, and radiation (to name a few) and
(c) Potentially catastrophic degradation of the biosphere including destruction of the atmosphere's protective ozone layer, the destruction of forests and lakes as a result of acid rain created by the sulfur emissions from industrial smoke

A. Brannigan (✉)
University of Calgary, Calgary, AB, Canada
e-mail: branniga@ucalgary.ca

D. M. Allen, J. W. Howell (eds.), *Groupthink in Science*,
https://doi.org/10.1007/978-3-030-36822-7_13

stacks, and atmospheric warming and worldwide coral decline due to CO^2 emissions from fossil fuel consumption

Two recent investigations of these diverse situations are found in David Michaels' (2008a, 2008b) *Doubt is their Product* and Oreskes and Conway's (2010) *Merchants of Doubt*. Where do these titles originate? In 1964, the US Surgeon General published a landmark report establishing patterns of epidemic levels of cancer, emphysema, and heart disease associated with cigarette use. In the face of undeniable evidence of long-term increases in disease, the strategy of the industry was characterized in a private memo sent in 1969 by a senior executive at Brown and Williamson Tobacco to other executives. It read as follows: "Doubt is our product since it is the best means of competing with the body of fact that exists in the mind of the general public. It is also the means of establishing that there is a controversy. If we are successful in establishing a controversy at the public level, then there is an opportunity to put across the real facts about smoking and health" (cited in Proctor, 2011, 289).

This logic originated in the defense of the tobacco industry, but *the manufacture of doubt* has become an effective strategy in other areas. For example, in 1992, Republican pollster and strategist, Frank Luntz advised political candidates who were critical of climate change to use scientific uncertainty as a political tactic. "Voters believe there is *no consensus* about global warming within the scientific community. Should the public come to believe that the scientific issues are settled, their views about global warming will change accordingly. Therefore, *you need to make the lack of scientific certainty a primary issue in the debate . . . The scientific debate is closing [against us] but not yet closed*" (emphasis in the original) (cited in Michaels, 2008b: 92). Through a series of case studies, Oreskes and Conway (2010), Michaels (2008a, 2008b) and Proctor (2011) trace how the merchants of dangerous products employ industry scientists and form alliances with university scientists who are friendly to industry to dispute the evidence of harm, that is, to contest, minimize, and deny harm and to delay regulations injurious to profits. The paradigm case is tobacco, but it may apply to other products, to varying degrees.

The Social Evolution of Tobacco Use

Up until the 1920s, tobacco was smoked primarily in pipes and in hand-rolled cigars, or it was chewed. Robert Proctor (2011, 31–35) reports that a revolution in tobacco preparation occurred in North Carolina in the mid-nineteenth century which led to the curing of tobacco leaves with charcoal-heated air through steel pipes or "flues." Leaves cured in this fashion had significantly lower alkalinity which made tobacco smoke much easier to inhale deep into the lungs. The flue-curing revolution made American tobacco a more potent experience that proved a major financial success. In the twentieth century, the market flourished with the introduction of disposable "safety matches," flammable paper wrappers, and Bonsack rolling machines that could pump out astronomical numbers of cigarettes on a daily basis. However, according to Proctor, these developments ultimately resulted in a medical catastrophe. "Flue curing may well be the deadliest invention in the history of modern manufacturing. Gunpowder and nuclear weapons have killed far fewer people" (2011, 34). In the twentieth century, worldwide consumption of tobacco led to the premature death of an estimated 100 million people. In the current century, "we . . . can expect a billion tobacco deaths if we continue on the present course" (p. 549).

Cancer by the Carton

In the nineteenth century, lung cancer was extremely rare. The US started tracking lung cancer deaths in 1914 when 400 cases were identified. However, with the huge popularity of cigarettes, it became increasingly prevalent, and reached epidemic proportions wherever cigarettes were widely used. In the US, the number of recorded deaths attributed to lung cancer peaked in 2005 at 163,500 (Proctor, 2011). Inferences about the link between smoking and health risks began to converge across different kinds of evidence. There had been clinical reports of the links between tobacco use and various lip and lung tumors in the late nineteenth and early twentieth centuries.

In the 1930s, an Argentinian oncologist, Angel Honorio Roffo, conducted experiments on animals to explore the link between carcinomas and the contents of tobacco smoke. He found that tar from tobacco smoke painted on the ears of rabbits produced tumors. This work was replicated on mice, and established that the lethal ingredient was the tar, as opposed to the nicotine. Following other approaches, researchers employed retrospective studies of hospital patients to link an elevated risk of current cancers to prior habits of cigarette use. In 1939, Franz H. Mueller (University of Cologne) linked cancers of the lung to previous cigarette use. In 1943, Shairer and Shöniger (University of Jena) drew the same conclusions from a better-designed study (Proctor, 2011, 226). Ironically, Nazi Germany was the first country in twentieth century Europe to undertake a sustained campaign against cigarette use, as outlined in Proctor's *Nazi War on Cancer* (1999). To preserve the vitality of the "master race," the German medical establishment undertook a cancer prevention campaign that included the promotion of healthy diets, natural foods, whole grain breads, and the banning of contaminants in food, such as pesticides, food dyes, and saccharin. The campaign extended to restricting worker exposure to such occupational carcinogens as asbestos, radon, and x-rays, and included a prolonged advertising campaign designed to suppress cigarette use.

In 1939, Fritz Lickint, published his 1100 page *Tabak und Organisus* (Tobacco and the Organism). Proctor describes it as "arguably the most comprehensive scholarly indictment of tobacco ever published" (1999, 184). It surveyed 8000 studies from the international literature linking cancers all along the "smoke alley" (lips, tongue, mouth, throat, esophagus, and lungs) to tobacco use. Lickint further tied tobacco use to arteriosclerosis, infant mortality, ulcers, and dozens of other maladies (p. 184). Finally, he claimed that nicotine made tobacco use addictive (comparing it to morphine addiction), and that non-smokers were at health risks from "passive smoking," that is, "second-hand smoke." Lickint believed that the curtailment of smoking would dramatically reduce cancer in Germany. The progressive aspects of Nazi public health policies were purged from memory by the hideous flip side of the preservation of the "master race"– the racial extermination of Jews and gypsies, and the euthanasia of persons judged unfit to live.

In postwar Britain and the US, a flood of new studies were was published, five alone in1950. The new studies were cohort or prospective studies that tracked tobacco use overtime before cancers appeared. In 1954, Doll and Hill published a preliminary report of the smoking habits of 40,000 British physicians initially contacted in 1951. They subsequently assessed the prevalence of death in this sample 29 months later, comparing the causes of death among smokers and nonsmokers. The Registrars General of the United Kingdom yielded 789 death reports, including 36 cases attributed to lung cancer. None of the nonsmokers succumbed to lung cancer, and the risk of cancer relative to the individuals' age group increased in proportion to the amount of their smoking. In a subsequent study published in 1956 after 53 months, there were 1714 deaths, including 84 attributed to lung cancer. All but one of the lung cancer deaths were in the smoking group. In 1954, Hammond and Horn published a study of over 187,766 men in the US. These were aged 50–69, and were followed up for a period of 3–5 years. Hammond and Horn discovered a similar association between a prior history of smoking and cancer (both lung and other forms) as well as other diseases (especially coronary heart disease). These health risks occurred in proportion to the level of smoking (Proctor, 2011, 225–30; US, 1964, 83–85).

A number of news reports brought these concerns to the public. In retrospect, one of the most effective was a short report by Roy Norr in *Reader's Digest* (1952), one of the most widely read publications in America: "Cancer by the Carton." Norr summarized the enormous increase in the incidence of cancer in American society, the opinions of leading medical experts linking this to tobacco use, and the need for action to educate the public about the risks of tobacco use.

In 1953, in response to public health concerns about the hazards of smoking, the industry engaged the services of the largest public relations firm in the world, Hill & Knowlton, to manage the clouds of suspicion over the industry. This resulted in collusion between all the major US tobacco companies in the development of an aggressive policy to contest the alleged linkage between tobacco and disease through a number of ingenious strategies.

- In January 1954, the industries' leading tobacco producers released the famous "Frank Statement" published in 448 newspapers nationwide. This announced the creation of the Tobacco Industry Research Committee which would be funded to investigate "all phases of tobacco use and health." The industry attracted highly respected scientists to lead the institute. The TIRC was renamed the Council for Tobacco Research in 1964 to create the illusion of distance from the industry (Glantz et al., 1996, 32–39).

- The industry fronted academic journals to publish research that was designed to air every potential cause of cancer except for tobacco (e.g., *Reports on Tobacco and Health Research*): asbestos, genetics, month of birth, reporting bias, measles virus, family factors, etc. (Michaels, 2008a, 7–8).
- The industry funded research in tobacco-friendly universities such as the Medical College of Virginia, in the heart of tobacco country, and cultivated the careers of senior scientists who were skeptical of the harm of tobacco (Proctor, 2011, 177–181).
- In the course of this funding bonanza, the industry recruited scores of scientists who would be employed as expert witnesses in torts for disease inflicted by tobacco use. The industry never lost a tort for damages from any of the hundreds of plaintiffs heard after the mid-fifties presenting with lung cancer, emphysema, or coronary heart disease (Player, 1998).
- Industry scientists also began to investigate the chemistry of tobacco in their own labs, and discovered its addictive qualities, as well as the carcinogenic effects of second-hand smoke. And while this private information accumulated in the labs of the producers, the companies continued to promote the healthy benefits of smoking, and to deny any links between tobacco use and disease (Glantz et al., 1996, 37ff; Proctor, 2011, 215–22).
- The industry marketed products that were said to be "milder," and promoted filtered products as a token of commitment to consumer health, although they never disclosed what risks the filters afforded protection from (TCLC, 2006, Part 3).
- Friends of the industry were able to attract money to front organizations such as the George C. Marshall Institute to provide industry a way to attack the work of its critics behind a façade (Oreskes & Conway, 2008, 60ff).
- The industry paid famous Hollywood performers to "place" cigarettes in their movies. For example, in 1983, Sylvester Stallone signed a contract to smoke Brown and Williamson brands (i.e., Kool & Belair) in five movies, for which he was to be paid $500,000. When the "product placement" in the movies appeared inconspicuous, the contract was cancelled and Stallone was paid $110,000 (Glantz et al., 1996, 366–67).
- Tobacco publicists acknowledged the allegations of harm, but insisted the question be posed in terms of the "controversy" over tobacco and harm, and aggressively lobbied news media to exercise impartiality by always insisting that both "sides" of the controversy be given equal attention (Michaels, 2008a, 11).
- The industry recruited scientists to reanalyze the original data of government and academic health researchers whose work supported the link between tobacco and health deficits, and to find ways to discredit their conclusions, a model followed for other studies of harmful products (Michaels, 2008a, 50, 52, 74–76, 103, 148, etc.)
- The industry financed the development of the "product defense industry" which specialized in taking doubt before juries in legal cases, and in lobbying elected officials, as well as government scientists on the industry perspective (Michaels, 2008a, 46ff.).

- Firms which flourished in the defense of tobacco reappeared to contest the scientific evidence for the causes and consequences of acid rain, ozone depletion, and toxic chemicals employed in various manufacturing processes (Oreskes & Conway, 2010).

The US Surgeon General Reports

It is just over 50 years since the publication of the First US Surgeon General's Report on *Smoking and Health* (US, 1964). Since that time, governments have undertaken public health policies to reduce the devastating effects of tobacco. The most recent report appeared in 2014, *The Health Consequences of Smoking—50 Years of Progress* (US, 2014). It estimated that in the US, from 1965 to 2014, there were over 20,000,000 preventable, premature deaths caused by tobacco use. A series of targeted public service programs were undertaken to reduce tobacco consumption. These included aggressive taxation, limitations of advertising, grotesque pictures of tobacco-induced illness on the covers of tobacco cartons, control of sales by age, smoking prevention in work places and public conveyances, etc. These have resulted in a reduction of smoking in the US from about 43% of adults in 1965 to 18% in 2012 (US, 2014, 17) (Table 13.1).

A Game-Changing Case: The Racketeering Case Against Tobacco

When the health risks of tobacco first came to light in the 1950s, hundreds of victims sued the companies for damages. Several legal theories emerged in these cases: the products were unfit to use, they were inherently dangerous and the advertising failed to alert users to the risks. Tobacco never settled a single case out of court,

Table 13.1 Premature deaths caused by smoking and exposure to second-hand smoke, 1965–2014 (US, 1964: 1): Cause of death totals

Smoking-related cancers: 6,587,000
Cardiovascular and metabolic diseases: 7,787,000
Pulmonary diseases: 3,804,000
Conditions related to pregnancy and birth: 108,000
Residential fires: 86,000
Lung cancers caused by exposure to second-hand smoke: 263,000
Coronary heart disease caused by exposure to second-hand smoke: 2,194,000
Total: 20,830,000

Source: Centers for Disease Control and Prevention, National Center for Chronic Disease Prevention and Health Promotion, Office on Smoking and Health, unpublished data

invested extensively in expert witnesses who denied that the products were dangerous, that the plaintiffs' illnesses were caused by something other than tobacco, and that, even if the products were dangerous, smokers already knew the risks. They appealed every adverse decision relentlessly and successfully (Rabin, 1992).

They were also committed to strangling the plaintiffs financially to prevent cases from ever going to trial through endless pre-trial motions and depositions. They never paid a penny in damages. The fees of the plaintiff lawyers were typically only paid contingent on a successful settlement. The only notable decision in this period was in the case of *Lartigue (1963)* where the court found that the defendant was responsible for causing the plaintiff's illness, but because at the time they did not know the harm of the products, they could not foresee the outcome, and as a result could not be held liable (Player, 1998, 312–13). In the second wave of cases in the 1980s, the plaintiffs raised the issue that the companies knew that the products caused cancer and that they were addictive. The plaintiffs argued that the industry might not be totally responsible for an individual's habit, but bore some portion of the damages. In *Cipollone v. Liggett (1983*), these arguments met with more success and the plaintiff's surviving husband was awarded $400,000 in damages. The defendant was assessed 20% of the responsibility, but in New Jersey tort law, no damages were payable when the plaintiff was over 50% responsible (Player, 1998, 318). However, thousands of documents were released through pretrial discovery that began to uncover what the companies knew and when they knew it.

The third wave of cases was brought by states seeking some relief from the inflated healthcare costs arising from tobacco diseases. This built on the expanding mountain of culpable industry documents obtained in pretrial depositions. A case against Liggett & Myers resulted in the first successful court action against a cigarette manufacturer. The company, on the edge of bankruptcy, acknowledged the harmfulness of the product, agreed to pay damages and further agreed to turn over its own internal documents which implicated the entire industry.

In 1998, the Attorneys General from 46 US states negotiated a Master Settlement Agreement that collected $368.5 billion dollars to be paid over the following 25 years to the states as compensation for their inflated public healthcare costs (Player, 1998, 329–31). The agreement also prohibited advertising to children. And the industry disbanded their public "research" programs which were designed solely from the beginning to sow doubt about the links between tobacco use and illness. At the same time, a disgruntled employee, Merrell Williams, started circulating tens of thousands of pages of internal company documents that reflected the internal research that the companies had been conducting for 40 years (Glantz et al., 1996, 7–8). These were sent to news organizations, politicians, and health scientists, principally Stanton Glantz, and formed the basis of *The Cigarette Papers* (1996). This dramatically altered the legal response to tobacco control.

The most important case to examine issues in light of these files was a civil case called *United States v. Philip Morris* brought by the US Department of Justice in 1999 against the major tobacco companies. In 2000, the DOJ won a ruling that permitted the government to seek damages under the Racketeer Influence and Corrupt Organizations Act (RICO). RICO was created to combat organized crime by permitting the government to seize the assets of criminal organizations. The DOJ filed 1400 pages of evidence of misconduct on the part of the tobacco manufacturers who had engaged in a decades-long conspiracy to:

1. Mislead the public about the risks of smoking
2. Mislead the public about the danger of second-hand smoke
3. Misrepresent the addictiveness of nicotine
4. Manipulate the nicotine delivery of cigarettes to stimulate addiction
5. Market cigarettes misleadingly characterized as "light" or "low tar," while knowing that those cigarettes were at least as hazardous as full-flavored cigarettes
6. Target young smokers to ensure lifelong dependency
7. Reject the production of safer cigarettes, i.e., products with lower levels of nicotine (PHLC, 2010; TCLC, 2006)

In 2006, Judge Kessler issued a 1683-page opinion that found on the evidence that the tobacco companies had violated civil racketeering laws by lying for decades about the health risks of smoking and marketing to children. The DOJ sought to punish the companies by seizing assets obtained by this misconduct. However, the appeal court denied the government's remedy of a disgorgement of profits of $280 Billion (California HDE, 2005).The evidence suggested that the tobacco industry funded extensive pseudoscientific research in an attempt to discredit the efforts of various regulatory agencies to document the effects of environmental tobacco smoke, including second-hand smoke (Muggli et al., 2001).

In the 2006 decision Judge Kessler found that *"each and every one of these defendants repeatedly, consistently, vigorously - and falsely - denied the existence of any adverse health effects from smoking, despite the massive documentation in their internal corporate files from their own scientists, executives, and public relations people that confirmed that there was little evidence supporting their claims. Specifically, Defendants knew there was a consensus in the scientific community that smoking caused lung cancer and other diseases by at least January 1964. Despite this internal knowledge, the Defendants embarked on a campaign of proactive and reactive responses to scientific evidence that was designed to mislead the public about the health consequences of smoking"* (*US v. Philip Morris*, 2012). The court went on to say that the defendants publicly denied and distorted the truth about the addictive nature of nicotine, and designed their cigarettes to deliver the nicotine "sufficient to create and sustain addiction." The remedies consisted of an order issued in 2006 to publish "corrective statements" in advertisements on television, in newspapers, on the companies' websites and on cigarette packages to describe how the companies had misled the public. A preliminary agreement on how this was to be done was reached in October 2017, eleven years after the initial order was issued (Campaign TFK, 2017). The industry continues to face individual lawsuits from persons who have been affected by lung cancer and/or other tobacco-related diseases. In Canada, the provinces are negotiating with tobacco manufacturers to seek relief from costs inflicted on provincial health schemes from illnesses related to tobacco use. But tobacco remains legal and none of the tobacco executives who had the *mens rea* for decades have faced any criminal liabilities. Even after being directed by the court during the *Philip Morris* trial to preserve all business records, 11 tobacco executives were found to have erased incriminating emails covering a two-and-a-half -year period prior to the initial verdict. The companies were fined $2.75 Million (Levin, 2004). Not the individuals.

Beyond Tobacco: Exxon, Global Warming, and "Agnotology"

In 2015, a report appeared in *Scientific American* that expressly drew a parallel between Exxon and its knowledge of climate change, and the earlier history of tobacco. "Exxon was aware of climate change, as early as 1977, 11 years before it became a public issue . . . This knowledge did not prevent the company (now ExxonMobil and the world's largest oil and gas company) from spending decades refusing to publicly acknowledge climate change and even promoting climate disinformation—an approach many have likened to the lies spread by the tobacco industry regarding the health risks of smoking" (Hall, 2015). The journalists of the primary investigation of the Exxon case at *Inside Climate News* painted a more nuanced picture. In 1977, James F. Black gave a talk to senior executives suggesting that the expanding utilization of fossil fuels could lead to significant increases in greenhouse gases that would begin to warm the earth's atmosphere significantly (Banerjee, Song & Hasemyer, 2015). Within 2 years, the company's research division had commissioned a tanker, the Esso Atlantic, to measure the rate at which the oceans were absorbing CO^2, which it did from 1979 to 1982. Exxon also employed a team of mathematicians to prepare estimates of climate change based on complex atmospheric models. The work of Exxon scientists was published in various refereed journals between 1983 and 1984, and thereafter. Exxon was the sole leading oil and gas producer to take climate change seriously, and to develop an expertise in climate science.

Other scientists at Exxon warned of the development of an enormous natural gas find off Indonesia. It contained 70% CO^2 and would become the single largest source of CO^2 release on the globe if developed; it was not (Goldenberg, 2015). However, when the international community advocated the first steps to reduce carbon consumption by an international treaty at the Kyoto Summit, the chairman of Exxon, Lee Raymond, opposed it. For the next eleven years, Exxon funded climate change skeptics. In 2008, under mounting pressure from activist stakeholders, the company announced that it would end support for . . .[the] dozens of organizations who were actively distorting the science" (Banerjee et al., 2015). Currently, the Attorney General of New York has taken legal action to obtain corporate documents to determine if the company undertook a campaign to mislead shareholders and the public about global warming (Flitter, 2017). A 2017 study of company documents presented a rather ambiguous case against ExxonMobil based on a comparison of the publications of its scientists and the internal documents of executive versus what it suggested in its "advertorials" in the New York Times. "We conclude that ExxonMobil contributed to advancing climate science—by way of its scientists' publications—but promoted doubt about it in its advertorials . . . We stress that the question is not whether ExxonMobil 'suppressed climate change research.' But rather how they communicated about it" (Supran and Oreskes, 2017).

The analogy between the tobacco case and the CO^2 case is not altogether convincing. Oreskes and Conway (2008, 2010) argue as though the "facts" behind climate change are completely incontrovertible and that there was a scientific consensus about them from the late 1970s. However, in a symposium on *Merchants of Doubt* (*Metascience,* 2012), scholars highly supportive of the research pointed out that it depicted science, particularly climate science, in a fashion that was inconsistent with studies of the actual practices of scientists in Science and Technology Studies, which emphasize the contingency, the boot-strapping logic, and idiosyncrasies of the discovery process. As Steve Yearly observes, "Oreskes and Conway are keen to emphasize the similarities between the work on these environmental and health topics and regular academic science . . . one cannot be a skeptic about the heliocentric solar system because the science is settled" (Yearly, 2012, 535) – implying that climate science is certainly *not* as settled as Newtonian physics. Yearly also points out that there has been a move away from science considered as an autonomous institution devoted to basic discovery to its increasing assignment in the post-WW2 state to enlarging the productivity of the economy, the military and medicine. And in the area of public health science, there is an increasing emphasis on risk assessment which necessarily involves public and political involvement in the regulatory process.

Assessing an optimum level for pesticide exposure, disposal of hazardous materials, etc. requires an estimation of *probable* safety levels, *probable* consequences and an evaluation of alternative solutions. These solutions "have to be offered in public forums where various interest groups have a legitimate role and where (the threat of) legal review is likely to be invoked" (p. 534).

David Mercer (2012, 537) argues in a similar vein. There is a tendency for "Oreskes and Conway's analysis to treat the boundaries between science, policy and regulation as clear and distinct," but in a democracy, where science is only possible by massive public investment, this is not the case. Furthermore, health science inevitably comes to play a role in governance, even though the science is not always "settled." The recent US report of global warming (CSSR, 2017) emphasizes that it has to develop policies based on two separate parameters: the *confidence* in the likelihood of change and the *impact* of the change should it occur. This approach recognizes the uncertainty of the measures and predictions, but unlike the tobacco "sound science movement" (Ong and Glantz, 2001), it does not freeze the regulatory agenda. In the case of global warming, the consequences of getting the policy wrong may prove to be catastrophic.

To return to the comparison with the tobacco case, a final point should be raised. "Sound science" counseled against regulation before the science was settled, but the advocates in the tobacco industry played a key role in creating the doubt. That was the rationale for promoting the term. And in the course of doing so, they lied to the public while millions of people died from the normal use of their products. To what extent is the charge comparable in the case of Exxon? To what extent had Exxon undermined effective public policies to protect the environment through its secrecy and misrepresentations to the public? Or, on the contrary, to what extent have decisions about public policies been hobbled by technical incompleteness, debates about data manipulation, and the slow process of accumulating observations over the last few years as the current consensus has emerged, and as the international coalitions were proposed and adopted? At this point, no one can say with certainty. The exposé of tobacco is based on the disclosure of millions of pages of internal incriminating documents. No comparable record exists for Exxon.

There was another insidious aspect of the hold of tobacco on politicians and the media that differentiates it from the Exxon case: it stifled free speech. When *"60 Minutes"* produced a program on tobacco culpability and industry conspiracy, the program was spiked. When Stanton Glantz published the leaked tobacco papers on the website of USF, a congressional subcommittee took the unprecedented step of de-funding his studies of tobacco and health. And when Sharon Eubanks was successfully leading a RICO investigation against Philip Morris, persons associated with the Bush Presidency tried to undermine her prosecution. Tobacco lobbyists and lawyers were behind all of these cases. In a republic predicated on free speech, the power of corporate actors to suppress criticism is injurious to the free exchange of ideas and, in this case, the negotiation of effective policies to protect public health.

We do not have to draw any conclusions about Exxon at this point, but there is a more general lesson. It is raised through the term, "agnotology," coined by Robert Proctor (Proctor & Scheibinger, 2008). Recalling Nietzsche, it might be called *the genealogy of ignorance*. Often, the absence of knowledge is not a natural condition of society, but an outcome of concerted, institutional efforts to suppress knowledge, sow confusion, disappear the past, suppress unwanted voices, and occlude competing world views. In this essay, we have attempted to enlarge the study of groupthink – which emphasizes how people come to give erroneous accounts of the world – to conditions where knowledge of reality is actively and institutionally suppressed or distorted. Tobacco "science" represents a compelling case study in agnotology.

References

Banerjee, N., Song, L., & Hasemyer, D. (2015). The road not taken: Exxon's own research confirmed fossil fuels' role in global warming decades ago. *Inside Climate News* online, https://insideclimatenews.org/content/Exxon-The-Road-Not-Taken. Retrieved 26 July 2019.

California HDE. (2005). *California healthline daily edition "supreme court refuses to hear appeal on past profits in doj racketeering case against tobacco companies"*, Online https://california-healthline.org/morning-breakout/supreme-court-refusesto-hear-appeal-on-past-profits-in-doj-racketeering-case-against-tobaccocompanies/. Retrieved 10 Nov 2017.

Campaign TFK. (2017). Tobacco companies must finally tell public the truth about their lethal product – 11 years after a court ordered it. *Press Release* on October 4, https://www.tobacco-freekids.org/press-releases/2017_10_04_corrective. Retrieved 4 Nov 2017

CSSR. (2017). *Climate science special report: Fourth national climate assessment*. Washington, D.C.: US Global Change Research Program. https://doi.org/10.7930/J0J964J6

Flitter, E. (2017, June 2). New York prosecutor says Exxon misled investors on climate change. *Reuters Business News*. https://www.reuters.com/article/ususa-climatechange-exxon/new-york-prosecutor-says-exxon-misled-investors-onclimate-change-idUSKBN18T1XK Retrieved 4 Nov 2017.

Glantz, S., Slade, J., Bero, L. P., Hanauer, P., & Barnes, D. (1996). *The cigarette papers*. Berkeley, CA: University of California Press.

Goldenberg, S. (2015, July 9) Exxon knew of climate change in 1981, email says – But it funded deniers for 27 more years. *The Guardian* online, https://www.theguardian.com/environment/2015/jul/08/exxon-climate-change-1981-climate-denier-funding. Retrieved 26 July 2019.

Hall, S. (2015). Exxon knew about climate change almost 40 yeas ago. *Scientific American*, Online October 26, https://www.scientificamerican.com/article/exxon-knew-about-climate-change-almost-40-years-ago/. Retrieved 26 July 2019.

Levin, M (2004, July 22). Judge orders Philip Morris, Altria to pay $2.75 Million. *Los Angeles Times*. http://articles.latimes.com/2004/jul/22/business/fi-smoke22. Retrieved 4 Nov 2017.

Mercer, D. (2012). Symposium comments "perspectives on global warming". *Metascience, 21*, 235–240. https://doi.org/10.1007/s11016-011-9639-9

Metascience. (2012). Perspectives on global warming. *Australasian Association for the History, Philosophy and Social Studies of Science, 21*, 531–559. https://doi.org/10.1007/s11016-011-9639-9

Michaels, D. (2008a). *Doubt is their product*. New York, NY: Oxford University Press.

Michaels, D. (2008b). Manufactured uncertainty: Contested science and the protection of the public's health and environment. In R. N. Proctor & L. Schiebinger (Eds.), *Agnotology: The making and unmaking of ignorance* (pp. 90–107). Stanford, CA: Stanford University Press.

Muggli, M. E., Foster, J. L., Hurt, R. D., & Repace, J. L. (2001). The smoke you don't see: Uncovering tobacco industry scientific strategies aimed against environmental tobacco smoke policies. *American Journal of Public Health, 91*(9), 1419–1423.

Norr, R. (1952, December). Cancer by the carton. *Reader's Digest*, 7–8.

Ong, E. K., & Glantz, S. (2001). Constructing 'sound science' and 'good epidemiology': Tobacco, lawyers and public relations firms. *American Journal of Public Health, 91*(11), 1749–1757.

Oreskes, N., & Conway, E. M. (2008). Challenging science: how climate science became a victim of the cold war. In R. N. Proctor & L. Schiebinger (Eds.), *Agnotology* (pp. 55–89). Stanford, CA: Stanford University Press.

Oreskes, N., & Conway, E. M. (2010). *Merchants of doubt*. New York, NY: Bloomsbury Press.

PHLC. (2010). *United States v. Philip Morris (D.O.J. Lawsuit)*. St. Paul, MN: Public Health Law Center at William Mitchel College of Law. http://www.publichealthlawcenter.org/topics/tobacco-control/tobacco-controllitigation/united-states-v-philip-morris-doj-lawsuit/. Retrieved 3 Nov 2017.

Player, T. S. (1998). After the fall: The cigarette papers, the global settlement, and the future of tobacco litigation. *South Carolina Law Review, 49*, 311–342.

Proctor, R. N. (1999). *The nazi war on cancer*. Princeton, NJ: Princeton University Press.

Proctor, R. N. (2011). *Golden holocaust: origins of the cigarette catastrophe and the case for abolition*. Berkeley, CA: University of California Press.

Proctor, R. N., & Schiebinger, L. (Eds.). (2008). *Agnotology: the making and unmaking of ignorance*. Stanford, CA: Stanford University Press.

Rabin, R. L. (1992). A Sociolegal history of tobacco tort legislation. *Stanford Law Review, 44*(4), 853–878.

Supran, G., & Oreskes, N. (2017, August 23). Assessing ExxonMobil's climate change communications (1977–2014). *Environmental Research Letters, 12*(8). http://iopscience.iop.org/article/10.1088/17489326/aa815f?fromSearchPage=true. Retrieved 5 Nov 2017.

TCLC. (2006). *The Verdict is in: Findings from United States v. Philip Morris*. Saint Paul, MN: Tobacco Control Legal Consortium.

U.S. (1964). *Surgeon general's report, Smoking and health: report of the advisory committee to the surgeon general of the public health service*. Washington, D.C.: USGPO.

U.S. (2014). *Surgeon general's report, The health consequences of smoking: 50 years of progress*. Washington, D.C.: USGPO.

U.S. v. Philip Morris. (2012). Judgment of United States District Court for the District of Columbia, Civil Action No. 99-2496 (GK), November 27.

Yearly, S. (2012). Symposium comments, "Perspectives on global warming". *Metascience, 21*, 531–535. https://doi.org/10.1007/s11016-011-9639-9.

Chapter 14
A Plea for Global Consideration of Human Brain Sex Differences

James W. Howell

Introduction

A woman looking at medical science today can find herself in a perplexing situation. She may have heard the recent criticisms that medical and biological research is mostly done with men and not with women. She may have heard that the excuse for this was related to budget issues. There was a reluctance to spend the money and the time adjusting research to female cycles and differences in the anatomy and physiology of males and not females and of men and not women. Sexual dimorphism exists throughout the human body. Any individual patient wants to get a diagnosis and treatment that is proper for who they are and appropriate to their age and condition.

Confounding this issue is a movement within some groups in science questioning sexual dimorphism. Somehow the proponents of this movement have managed to particularly focus on the human brain, as if this body part in some way had no interaction with the other parts of the body and managed to evolve at its own separate pace and manner.

As you will see in this chapter, this way of thinking can put patients in dangerous situations. When you make a systematic study of the various organs of the body, as you will see in the brief descriptions of some parts of the human body in this chapter, it becomes readily apparent that there are vital differences between the anatomy and physiology of the woman's body and that of the man.

It is also very true that there have been many destructive and false ideas advanced over time about supposed biological differences between men and women that are not based on science at all but either on folklore or sexist ideas such as that women are "too emotional" to serve in an executive capacity. This does not mean, of course,

J. W. Howell (✉)
Department of Psychiatry, University of Tennessee Health Science Center,
Memphis, TN, USA
e-mail: atenra@comcast.net

D. M. Allen, J. W. Howell (eds.), *Groupthink in Science*,
https://doi.org/10.1007/978-3-030-36822-7_14

that there are no *real* differences. The proponents of the movement to deny sexual dimorphism make up a dangerous groupthink force that attempts to stifle those who disagree with their doctrines by calling their opponents misogynists enemies who want to discriminate against women.

Other scientists such as Debra Soh try to make it clear that denying science will not in fact do anything to fight misogyny (Lehman and Soh, 2017). The misogynists, bigots, and people who wish to discriminate against women will always find ways to spread their hatred and regressive ideas. The denial of science and sexual dimorphism will just spread ignorance and put women in danger.

In her paper on sex differences in the cardiovascular systems of men and women, Virginia Huxley (2007) emphasized the importance of understanding the dimorphism of the two systems. This improves diagnostic systems, the recognition of sex-specific pathophysiology, and the development and implementation of proper treatment for each of the sexes. She emphasized the fundamental importance of realizing the fact that each cell in the body is either XX or XY from the time the organism is in the uterus, through prepuberty, to adulthood.

Margaret McCarthy, Arnold, Ball, Blaustein, and DeVries (2012) went further in discussing sex differences by presenting a description of nonexclusive categories that would help in developing experimental designs:

1. The first type is absolute sexual dimorphism. This includes two-component sets of particular behavioral, physiological, or morphological forms, one found in the male and one in the female. Copulatory behavior would be an example.
2. The second type exists along a continuum or sliding scale in which any given male or female can be found at any point, but the *average* of individuals would differ between the sexes. Odor detection and learning are examples of this.
3. The third type, and most complicated to understand, involves characteristics which might converge at some endpoint or diverge after some challenge. The neurophysiology that regulates one of these behaviors might be completely different in the male and the female. Sex-specific parental behavior could be an example and might manifest itself completely differently from one species to another.

In considering the effect of accepting the idea that there are sex differences, one particular assumption has had a deleterious effect. Too many of the criticisms of sexual dimorphism in humans are rooted in what McCarthy (2016) calls the pervasive assumption that "sex difference in neuroanatomy and neurophysiology is synonymous with a sex difference in behavior." Such an assumption in a particular case would have to be tested.

There is a growing body of literature concerning sexual dimorphism. Margaret McCarthy's papers on the subject are a great place to start familiarizing yourself with this literature, but other references include Shansky (2016), Plaff and Christen (2013). In 2015, the (NIH 2015) made it mandatory, because there are physiological and anatomical differences between the sexes, that all research use sex balanced cohorts and treat sex as a biological variable. This was reaffirmed in later years.

Global Considerations

In Lise Eliot's review of Gina Rippon's book, The Gendered *Brain: The New Science That Shatters the Myth of the Female Brain*, she made a statement that seems to indicate a lack of understanding of anatomy, physiology, or evolution: "The brain is no more gendered than the liver, kidneys, or heart."

First, this ignores the fact that every cell of these organs has an XX or XY chromosome pair, marking the sex of the individual.

Second, according to an extensive literature, there are sex difference effects in most organs of the body. A few details about the liver, kidneys, and heart are considered below.

Sex Differences in Human Gut and the Brain

The human gut is a particularly striking example of sexual dimorphism. The gut and the human brain work closely together. The gut has been implicated in contributing to intuitive decision making, affect, components of language, higher cognitive functions, motivation, emotion regulation, and gastrointestinal homeostasis. In addition, the intestinal microbes and host microbes work with the nervous system's interaction with the brain to form what many call the *enteric nervous system* (the ENS, sometimes referred to as the "second brain") (Mayer, 2011). There are pronounced differences in the dynamics of microbial growth and effects both over time and between men and women. This is true even when comparing diverse ethnic and widely separated cultural groups (de la Cuesta-Zuluaga et al., 2019).

Gut microbiota seem to regulate the synthesis and release of oxytocin, which has an effect on parturition and lactation.

Human Olfaction Sex Differences

Sensitivity to smell varies according to sex among children (Schriever et al., 2018). Although most investigators have agreed since at least 1899 (Toulouse and Vaschide) that the abilities of women for olfaction are superior to men, some studies that involve large samples suggested the abilities between the sexes do not differ all that much. However, a meta-analysis of thousands of men and women in existing studies focused on sex differences in identification, discrimination, and threshold confirmed that women's olfactory abilities are greater than those of men (Sorokowski et al., 2019).

Doty and Cameron (2009) suggested that one possible explanation for this finding is interactions between early experiences of smell perception in certain brain regions with circulating endocrine substances. This, combined with later hormonal mechanisms in an adult woman's life, could result in the superior olfactory perception. Another possible explanation is that men have lesser verbal skills than women making it easier for women to answer questions in the experimental process (Larsson, Finkel, & Pedersen, 2000, Oberg, Larsson, & Backman, 2002).

Renal Function Sex Differences

In both mice and humans, persistent differential gene expression between the sexes in kidney function includes drug and steroid metabolism as well as osmotic regulation in a study by Rinn et al. (2004).

Sex Differences in the Cardiovascular System

Cardiovascular data reflected in textbooks, handbooks, and relevant Internet sites usually come from 18- to 22-year-old healthy males. As mentioned, the reason given is that authors were avoiding the "confusing" problem of cycling that would have to be considered when including data from women. Women are found to have lower norepinephrine levels than men and a host of other differences of which medical professionals should be aware when treating pathologies related to the heart. Even when considering the three typical hallmarks of men's heart attacks as described in the medical literature, the fact is that only one in three women will experience these symptoms when they have a myocardial infarction. According to Virginia Huxley (2007) those hallmarks are:

1. Chest discomfort or uncomfortable pressure, fullness, squeezing, or pain in the center of the chest that lasts longer than a few minutes or that comes and goes.
2. Spreading pain to one or both arms, back, jaw, or stomach.
3. Cold sweats and nausea.

In fact, a woman having a heart attack may well have other symptoms such as vomiting or back or jaw pain. It is important that sex differences be recognized, included in medical training, and used to diagnose and treat disease (Huxley, 2007).

In 2010, John Konhilas published an extensive review of the literature in which he further discussed the differences men and women experience with heart disease, especially congestive heart failure (CHF).

Sex Differences in the Liver

Krebs et al. (2003) describe how in the liver, as elsewhere, there is a complex interplay of hormonal, developmental, and tissue-specific control of gene expression. This leads to tissues which are found in two distinct forms in males versus females. For example, sex-specific patterns of liver gene expression occur in the production of several enzymes involved in the metabolism of steroids and as well as for the metabolism of synthetic chemicals. The extent and duration of the activation of certain hepatic genes are dependent on the nature of growth hormone signaling as well as interactions with numerous other proteins within the cells. Krebs adds that hepatic sex differences may prove relevant to medical issues that vary with gender, such as differences in drug metabolism and the incidence of certain diseases, as well as to problems related to pregnancy.

Twin Studies

Although twin studies are not definitive because of the extreme difficulty of separating out purely genetic effects from gene-environment interactional factors, they clearly show that genetic differences (such as the presence or absence of a Y chromosome) can create differences in anatomy, physiology, the endocrine system, and behavioral tendencies (although not specific behaviors).

Conclusions

The primary message of this chapter is that future work in the study of sex differences should include a broad investigation of as many aspects of the animal body as possible. The limited number of global considerations outlined here underlines the importance of doing this. Of course, there are many other organs, systems, and body functions that could have been included. Additionally, the few that have been included here have not been discussed exhaustively.

The brain is not isolated. Parts of the body are acting on it and the brain, of course, serves to regulate and maintain the body. This should be an obvious conclusion even after this brief glance of the literature.

Debra Soh said on March 11, 2019, in *Quillette* that, "Denying science won't end sexism," and that the people rejecting sexual dimorphism actually are questioning the value of feminism. This reminds me of a quote by one of the earliest feminist writers, Mary Wollstonecraft, who, when writing about her experiences in her book, *The French Revolution*, said, "Every political good carried to the extreme must be productive of evil (1790)."

Bibliography

Arnold, A., & Breedlove, A. (1985). Organizational and activational effects of sex steroids on brain and behavior: A reanalysis. *Hormones and Behavior., 19*(4), 469–498. https://doi.org/10.1016/0018-506x(85)90043-X

Baron-Cohen, S., Knickmeyer, R., & Belmonte, M. (2005). Sex differences in the brain: Implications for explaining autism. *Science, 310*, 819–823.

Broere-Brown, Z., Baan, E., Schalekamp-Timmermans, S., Verburg, B., Jaddoe, V., & Steegers, E. (2016). Sex-specific differences in fetal and infant growth patterns: A prospective population-based cohort study. *Biol Sex Differ, 7*, 65.

de la Cuesta-Zuluaga, J., Kelley, S. T., Chen, Y., Escobar, J. S., Mueller, N. T., Ley, R. E., et al. (*2019*). Age- and sex dependent patterns of gut microbial diversity in human adults. *mSystems, 4*, e00261–e00219. https://doi.org/10.1128/mSystems.00261-19

Doty, R. L., & Cameron, E. L. (2009). Sex differences and reproductive hormone influences on human odor perception. *Physiology & Behavior, 97*, 213–228. https://doi.org/10.1016/j.physbeh

Greenberg, D., Warrier, V., Allison, C., & Baron-Cohen, S. (2018). Testing the empathizing-systemizing theory of sex differences and the extreme male brain theory of autism in half a million people. *PNAS, 115*(48), 12152–12157. https://doi.org/10.1073/pnas.1811032115

Huxley, V. H. (2007). Sex and the cardiovascular system: The intriguing tale of how women and men regulate cardiovascular function differently. *Advances in Physiology Education, 31*, 17–22. https://doi.org/10.1152/advan.00099.2006

Ingalhalikar, M., Smith, A., Parker, D., Satterthwaite, D., Elliott, M., Ruparel, K., et al. (2014). Sex differences in the structural connectome of the human brain. *Proceedings of the National Academy of Sciences, 111*(2), 823–828.

Jazin, E., & Cahill, L. (2010). Sex differences in molecular neuroscience: From fruit flies to humans. *Nature Reviews Neuroscience, 11*, 9–17.

Knickmeyer, R. C., Wang, J., Zhu, H., Geng, X., Woolson, S., Hamer, R. M., et al. (2014). Impact of sex and gonadal steroids on neonatal brain structure. *Cerebral Cortex, 24*(10), 2721–2731.

Konhilas, J. P. (2010). What we know and do not know about sex and cardiac disease. *Journal of Biomedicine and Biotechnology*, 562051. https://doi.org/10.1155/2010/562051

Kopsida, E., Stergiakouli, E., Lynn, P. M., Wilkinson, L. S., & Davies, W. The role of the Y chromosome in brain function. *The Open Neuroendocrinology Journal, 2*, 20–30. https://doi.org/10.2174/1876528900902010020

Krebs, C. J., Larkins, L. K., Price, R., Tullis, K. M., Miller, R. D., & Robins, D. M. (2003). Regulator of sex-limitation (Rsl) encodes a pair of KRAB zinc-finger genes that control sexually dimorphic liver gene expression. *Genes & Development, 17*(21), 2664–2674. https://doi.org/10.1101/gad.1135703

Lenroot, R. K., Gogtay, N., Greenstein, D. K., Wells, E. M., Wallace, G. L., Clasen, L. S., et al. (2007). Sexual dimorphism of brain developmental trajectories during childhood and adolescence. *NeuroImage, 36*(4), 1065–1073. https://doi.org/10.1016/j.neuroimage.2007.03.053

Leonard, C., Towler, S., Welcome, S., Halderman, L., Otto, R., Eckert, M., et al. (2008). Sex matters: Cerebral volume influences sex differences in neuroanatomy. *Cerebral Cortex, 18*(12), 2920–2931. https://doi.org/10.1093/cercor/bhn053

Luders, E., Gaser, C., Narr, K. L., & Toga, A. W. (2009, November 11). Why sex matters: Brain size independent differences in gray matter distributions between men and women. *The Journal of Neuroscience, 29*(45), 14265–14270.

Mayer, E. A. (2011, July 13). Gut feelings: The emerging biology of gut-brain communication. *Nature Reviews. Neuroscience, 12*, 453–466. https://doi.org/10.1038/nrn3071

McCarthy, M. M. (2016). Multifaceted origins of sex differences in the brain. *Philosophical Transactions of the Royal Society B: Biological Sciences, 371*, 20150106. https://doi.org/10.1098/rstb.2015.0106

McCarthy, M. M., Arnold, A. A., Ball, G. F., Blaustein, J. D., & DeVries, G. J. (2012, February 15). Sex differences in the brain: The not so inconvenient truth. *The Journal of Neuroscience, 32*(7), 2241–2247.

NIH (2015). Consideration of sex as a biological variable in NIH-funded Research. Notice Number: NOT-OD-15-102.

O'Conner, C., & Joffe, H. (2014). Gender on the brain: A case study of science communication in the new media environment. *PLoS One, 9*(10), e110830. https://doi.org/10.1371/journal.pone.0110830

Plaff, D. W., & Christen, Y. (Eds.). (2013). *Multiple origins of sex differences in brain: Neuroendocrine functions and their pathologies*. New York, NY: Springer.

Polderman, T. J., Benyamin, B., de Leeuw, C. A., Sullivan, P. F., van Bochoven, A., Visscher, P. M., et al. (2015). Meta-analysis of the heritability of human traits based on fifty years of twin studies. *Nature Genetics, 47*, 702. https://doi.org/10.1038/ng.3285

Rinn, J. L., Rozowsky, J. S., Laurenzi, I. J., Petersen, P. H., Zou, K., Zhong, W., et al. (June 2004). Major molecular differences between mammalian sexes are involved in drug metabolism and renal function. *Developmental Cell, 6*, 791–800.

Rippon, G. (2019). The Gendered Brain: The new neuroscience that shatters the myth of the female brain. New York, NY: Vintage Publishing.

Ruigrok, A., Salimi-Khorshidi, C., Lai, M., Baron-Cohen, S., Lombardo, M., Tait, R., et al. (2013). A meta-analysis of sex differences in human brain structure. *Neuroscience and Biobehavioral Reviews*. https://doi.org/10.1016/j.neubiorev.2013.12.004lumenthal

Savic, I. (Ed.). (2010). *Sex differences in the human brain, their underpinnings and implications*. Philadelphia, PA: Elsevier.

Schriever, V. A., Agosin, E., Altundag, A., Avni, H., Van, H. C., Cornejo, C., et al. (2018). Development of an international odor identification test for children: The Universal Sniff Test. *The Journal of Pediatrics, 198*, 265–272.e3. https://doi.org/10.1016/j.pes.2018.03.011

Shansky, R. M. (Ed.). (2016). *Sex differences in the central nervous system*. Philadelphia, PA: Elsevier.

Snell, D. M., & Turner, M. A. (2018). Sex chromosome effects on male-female differences in mammals. *Curr Biol, 28*(22), R1313–R1324. https://doi.org/10.1016/j.cub.2018.09.018

Soh, D. (2019). Science denial won't end sexism. Quillette

Sorokowski, P., Karwowski, M., Misiak, M., Marzak, M. K., Dziekan, M., Hummel, T., et al. (2019). Sex differences in human olfaction: A meta-analysis. *Frontiers in Psychology, 10*, 242. https://doi.org/10.3389/fpsyg.2019.0024

Toulouse, E., & Vaschide, N. (1899). Mesure de l'ordorat chez l'homme et chez la femme. *CompteRendus Social Biology*, 381–383.

Tyan, Y., Liao, J., Lin, Y., & Weng, J. (2017). Gender differences in the structural connectome of the teenaged brain revealed by generalized q-sampling MRI. *Science Digest*. https://doi.org/10.1016/j.ncil.2017.05.014

Wang, C. (2018). Decoding sex differences in the brain, one worm at a time. *Gender and the Genome, 2*(3), 76–80. https://doi.org/10.1177/2470289718789306

Wheelock, M. D., Hect, J. L., Hernandez-Andrade, E., Hassan, S. S., Eggebrect, A. T., & Thomason, M. E. (2019). Sex differences in functional connectivity during fetal brain development. *Developmental Cognitive Neuroscience, 36*, 100632.

Chapter 15
Ideological Blinders in the Study of Sex Differences in Participation in Science, Technology, Engineering, and Mathematics Fields

David C. Geary and Gijsbert Stoet

There is little question that there are sex differences in engagement in certain science, technology, mathematics, and engineering (STEM) fields. The U.S. National Science Foundation (NSF), for instance, reports that women are awarded 57% of all undergraduate STEM degrees (compared to 61% of non-STEM degrees) but with substantial differences across fields. Women earn the majority of degrees in the life and social sciences, but less than 20% of the degrees in computer science and engineering (http://www.nsf.gov/statistics/2015/nsf15311/tables.cfm). In other words, the sex differences in STEM degrees and in later occupational choices are largely in inorganic fields, those focused on understanding non-living things as contrasted with living things. These differences are practically important because they and more general differences in the type of occupations men and women enter contribute, in part, to the sex difference in earnings (Del Río & Alonso-Villar, 2015).

These sex differences and the social prestige of many STEM occupations have generated a cottage industry within academia, the popular media, and beyond. The movement is fueled by the zeitgeist among some feminist activists that there should be gender equality – equal *outcomes* regardless of any underlying sex differences in academic or occupational interests or in the patterns of cognitive strengths – for anything of monetary or social value. In this case, the focus is on identifying and eliminating the causes of the STEM discrepancies (e.g., Hill, Corbett, & St Rose, 2010). As an example of the resources devoted to achieving equality, since 2001 the NSF has invested more than $130 million into the ADVANCE program (Advancement

D. C. Geary (✉)
Department of Psychological Sciences, Interdisciplinary Neuroscience Program,
University of Missouri, Columbia, MO, USA
e-mail: GearyD@missouri.edu

G. Stoet
Department of Psychology, University of Essex, Colchester, Essex, UK
e-mail: g.stoet@essex.ac.uk

D. M. Allen, J. W. Howell (eds.), *Groupthink in Science*,
https://doi.org/10.1007/978-3-030-36822-7_15

of Women in Academic Science and Engineering Careers: http://www.nsf.gov/funding/pgm_summ.jsp?pims_id=5383) in an attempt to close the gap in STEM disciplines with similar efforts instituted in other Western countries (e.g., http://www.ecu.ac.uk/equality-charters/athena-swan/). Many of the activities funded by these initiatives make sense and are likely to be helpful in some ways, such as developing mentoring programs for women who are junior faculty in science and engineering in university settings although it raises ethical questions when the same mentoring programs are not provided for male junior faculty, as is case in the UK's Athena SWAN Swan's programs. There are, in addition, other themes regarding the sources of these differences that are based on weak evidence and a large dose of wishful thinking. The most questionable and perhaps the most favored of these are stereotype threat, implicit bias, and microaggression.

Stereotype threat allegedly occurs when one is confronted with tasks or situations that trigger negative stereotypes (e.g., that 'women are not as proficient at math as men') that in turn results in a preoccupation about performing in a way that confirms the stereotype (Spencer, Steele, & Quinn, 1999). Critically, the preoccupation is said to undermine actual performance even when there is no factual basis to the stereotype. Implicit bias is a related concept and involves an unconscious association between group membership (e.g., sex or race) and stereotypical positive or negative attributes that in turn can result, in theory, in prejudicial behavior toward individuals within that group (Greenwald, McGhee, & Schwartz, 1998; Greenwald, Poehlman, Uhlmann, & Banaji, 2009). Microaggressions are subtle behaviors (e.g., facial expressions) or statements that are not explicitly hostile but are nevertheless interpreted by the receiver as conveying contempt, stereotypical attitudes, or other negative beliefs. Examples of verbal microaggressions are provided by the University of California, Santa Cruz (e.g., 'You're a girl, you don't have to be good at math', https://academicaffairs.ucsc.edu/events/documents/Microaggressions_Examples_Arial_2014_11_12.pdf).

The basic argument is that some significant proportion of the sex differences in STEM fields – but only those in which men outnumber women – is thought to be caused by pervasive negative stereotypes about women's abilities in these fields that in turn undermine their performance. And, by poor treatment by STEM teachers and colleagues – microaggressions – that seeps from their unconscious belief in these same stereotypes to create unsupportive and even subtly hostile classrooms and work environments. These types of explanations fit well with the narrative of some gender activists: that the sex difference is largely due to social and cultural factors that undermine women's pursuit of degrees and occupations in STEM fields (Hill et al., 2010).

In any case, these concepts have been embraced by the mass media and beyond. Examples of this embrace include accusations in the *New York Times* that the wording of several SAT items will trigger stereotype threat and undermine girls' performance on the mathematics section of the test (Hartocollis, 2016) and self-help books to cope with one's own unconscious biases (Thiederman, 2015). On the face of it, there is nothing wrong with academic and mass media focus on these topics, as related to sex differences in STEM participation. The real issues concern the magnitudes of these effects on women's STEM participation and the foregone opportunities of not focusing on other factors that might have an even stronger impact on their participation.

Let us consider first the magnitude of stereotype threat on girls' and women's mathematics achievement. As noted, the concept is now widely known in popular culture and the first scientific publication on the topic has been cited more than 3000 times in Google scholar (Spencer et al., 1999), a seminal contribution by this measure. Accordingly, it is not surprising that there are now interventions to counter the hypothesized negative effects of stereotype threat on women's performance in STEM fields (e.g., Walton, Logel, Peach, Spencer, & Zanna, 2015). Given the prominence of the topic and the resources devoted to it, we carried out the first meta-analysis (i.e., statistical aggregation of experimental results across many studies) of the effect of stereotype threat on sex differences in mathematics performance (Stoet & Geary, 2012). We reasoned that if stereotype threat had a substantive effect on girls' and women's mathematics performance then the most basic experimental manipulation of the effect should replicate across studies.

The design is simple and includes four groups: one group of women and one group of men who take a mathematics test under typical testing conditions (control group), and groups that take the test under threat conditions (experimental group). The latter might involve telling participants that men typically do better on the mathematics test. In theory, men in the experimental and control conditions should perform about the same on the test, but women in the threat condition should perform worse than women in the control condition. One would think that there would be hundreds of studies that have used this basic design, but most of the replications in this field (social psychology) are 'conceptual' and not exact; conceptual is based on creating conditions that should replicate the basic idea (that threat will compromise women's performance) rather than replicate the exact experimental procedures. We found 20 studies that were very similar to the basic experimental design followed by Spencer et al. (1999), and only 11 of them replicated their effect. Of the 11 that found an effect, only 3 did not rely on a controversial statistical control that might exaggerate any such effect.

We could not definitively conclude from our analyses that stereotype threat does not exist, but we did question whether the magnitude of any such effect merited the scientific and popular press attention it was receiving. This of course is not likely to be a popular conclusion, based on the above-described interest in the phenomenon, and indeed it was not. We sent the manuscript to three or four journals before an editor would even send it for peer review, a pattern that we have found for nearly all of our subsequent sex differences studies that reached unpopular conclusions; one of us (Geary) has the same experiences in his work on biological sex differences and the other of us (Stoet) has the same experience in his other work on educational sex differences. In this case, one of these is a very prominent journal in the field of psychology and the editors took three months – and this was only after several inquiries regarding the status of the submission – before they informed us that it would not be sent for peer review, indicating that failures to replicate (follow-up experiments that cannot confirm an original finding) were not of interest to them; this was before the emergence of the replication crisis in social psychology and the attendant focus on replications. Editors rejecting manuscripts without peer review are common but this is typically done within one or at most two weeks, not three months. After the article was published, we were greeted by an angry response by several proponents of stereotype threat, not the dispassionate curiosity as to why the effect is sometimes found and sometimes not.

In a related analysis, Flore and Wicherts (2015) found a similar overall (small) effect, but when they corrected for publication bias – the tendency for positive but not negative results to be published – the effect essentially disappeared. This means that there is evidence for a small stereotype threat effect in the scientific literature, but because studies that do not find an effect tend not to get published in this literature, the real-world impact of stereotype threat is probably close to zero (see also Ganley et al., 2013; Picho, Rodriguez, & Finnie, 2013). Picho et al. (2013) also found evidence for publication bias but discounted its importance. At the time of the writing of this chapter, a large replication effort is being carried out, and we are optimistic that this and other similar research focusing on replicability can give a definite answer on the question of whether stereotype threat can undermine girl's and women's performance in mathematics and if so, determine the magnitude of this effect. It should be noted, though, that the largest study carried out thus far with nearly 1000 students found no effects (Ganley et al., 2013). This latter study is of particular relevance, because it was carried out with adolescents and school children. If stereotype threat discourages girls from pursuing math-intensive STEM coursework and careers, its effect should be evident in adolescence. The fact that a large and well-designed study could not find any effect, in our opinion, suggests either the effect does not exist or it is unmeasurably small.

Either way, the existing evidence indicates that stereotype threat has received outsized attention from educational policy makers and opinion makers. The bottom line is that there is at best a small and probably no effect at all of stereotype threat on women's mathematical performance. Thus, the considerable efforts at addressing this 'problem' will almost certainly have little if any effect on girl's and women's participation in inorganic STEM fields.

We suspect the same is true for implicit bias. For a variety of cultural and legal reasons, the level of explicit sexism has dropped considerably over the years in most school and work environments. But, girls' interest and women's participation in inorganic STEM fields has remained stubbornly low over the past 20 years (Hill et al., 2010). So, there are two options. One might conclude that explicit sexism is no longer keeping girls and women away from these fields and so something else must be contributing to these sex differences. Or, one can maintain the conceptual grasp on sexism as a causal factor and switch focus to an 'unconscious' subtle form of sexism that results from implicit bias (see Greenwald et al., 1998; Greenwald et al., 2009) and its behavioral companion, microaggression (Basford, Offermann, & Behrend, 2014).

Indeed, implicit bias has achieved a cult-like status in some academic circles and in the wider culture. There are now on-line tests to assess one's implicit bias in a number of areas, including sex differences in work and family. We are not doubting that people do have all sorts of implicit beliefs that may or may not be accurate. The issues here are whether we can rigorously and accurately assess these biases, and whether the strength of any such biases is sufficient to explain the sex differences in STEM fields. The assessment of implicit bias is often done using the implicit associations test (e.g., https://implicit.harvard.edu/implicit/user/agg/blindspot/indexgc.htm) whereby the strength of people's associations between sex (or race) and certain attributes, such as work or science, is assessed by a series of categorization tasks. The difference between the speed of categorizing certain attributes (e.g., scientist, engineer) to one sex or the other is taken as an index of implicit bias. Nosek, Banaji, and Greenwald (2002) found that people are generally quicker to associate men with science and women with literature, which is taken as an implicit bias against women in science, although they do note that their results may reflect, in part, the actual occupational sex differences in these areas. Even so, proponents argue that there could be a reciprocal relationship, whereby actual differences influence implicit biases that in turn dissuade girls and women from pursuing STEM fields (see Miller, Eagly, & Linn, 2015).

There is, however, vigorous debate regarding what exactly is being measured by these types of implicit tests (e.g., Greenwald, Nosek, Banaji, & Klauer, 2005; Greenwald, Banaji, & Nosek, 2015; Oswald, Mitchell, Blanton, Jaccard, & Tetlock, 2013; Rothermund & Wentura, 2004) and whether they actually influence behavior (Blanton et al., 2009). Assuming the tests are actually measuring bias (e.g., sexism, racism), the relation between these implicit attitudes and actual behavior is small at best (e.g., Oswald et al., 2013), although proponents argue that these small effects add up over time (Greenwald et al., 2015). The ways in which implicit attitudes are thought to influence real-world outcomes include promoting stereotype threat (Miller et al., 2015) and microaggressions (Sue, 2010). As we noted above for stereotype threat, there are serious concerns about the ability to accurately measure microaggressions, whether they are related to implicit bias at all, if it is a valid concept, and whether 'victims' of microaggression suffer long-term consequences, among other concerns about the concept itself (see Lilienfeld, 2017). These issues have not stopped the development of yet another cottage industry for programs designed to make people aware of and to stop this 'aggression' on college campuses, in the workplace, and in daily life; an internet search for 'microaggression intervention' will provide many examples.

As with stereotype threat, the concepts of implicit bias and microaggression have gained such traction because they fit the narrative that inequalities of any kind are the result of some form of oppression; the entire narrative itself is a derivative of the postmodern spin on Marxism (Hicks, 2004). In many cases, explicit oppression is hard to find and thus the retort to unconscious bias and fleeting behaviors (microaggression) that continually 'assault' and undermine the 'victims'. In this case, the victims are girls' and women's aspirations toward and performance in STEM fields, especially engineering, computer science, and the physical sciences. The logical response to this narrative is the development of interventions to reduce stereotype threat, implicit bias, and microaggressions. But, what if these factors have much smaller effects on girls and women than proponents argue? The associated time and resources devoted to addressing these problems will have little or no long-term effect on girls' interest in or women's participation in inorganic STEM fields.

So, what is really going on? As with any life outcome that is complicated and unfolds over many years or decades, multiple factors likely contribute to the sex differences in interest and participation in STEM fields. Whatever the mix, proponents of stereotype threat, implicit bias, microaggression and related concepts expect that as societies become more equal, these forms of 'oppression' will diminish and boys and girls and men and women will become equal for most if not all non-physical traits, including participation in STEM (Hyde, 2005). Contrary to this hypothesis, we have recently found that countries renowned for gender equality show some of the largest sex differences in interest in and pursuit of STEM degrees (Stoet & Geary, 2018). For instance, Finland excels in gender equality (World Economic Forum, 2015), its adolescent girls outperform boys in science literacy, and it ranks near the top in European educational performance (Programme for International Student Assessment, 2016; https://nces.ed.gov/surveys/pisa/). With these high levels of educational performance and overall gender equality, Finland is poised to close the sex differences gap in STEM. Yet, Finland has one of the world's largest sex differences in college degrees in STEM fields, and Norway and Sweden, also leading in gender equality rankings, are not far behind. This is only the tip of the iceberg, as this general pattern of increasing sex differences with national increases in gender equality is found throughout the world, and not just for participation in STEM fields (e.g., Lippa, Collaer, & Peters, 2010).

The recent uptick in interest in concepts such as stereotype threat, implicit bias, and microaggression may be a reaction to this general phenomenon. If sex differences are the result of structural barriers (e.g., lack of employment opportunities), explicit sexism, and restricted educational opportunities, as they once were in many developed nations, then as these impediments fade into history, the sex differences attributed to them should fade as well. And, in fact some of them have faded and even reversed, such that more women than men attend and graduate from college and women now have structural advantages (e.g., hiring practices) in STEM fields (Ceci & Williams, 2015; Williams & Ceci, 2015). Despite these changes, many sex differences remain or have become larger over time. The latter are serious problems for anyone with strong beliefs about purely or largely social influences on sex differences and if the obvious social causes have been addressed, then there must be other, subtle oppressive factors that are causing these differences; enter stereotype threat, implicit bias, microaggression, and related concepts.

In any event, we propose that what is actually happening is that with economic development and advances in human rights, including gender equality, people are better able to pursue their individual interests and in doing so more basic sex differences are more fully expressed (Geary, 2010). With respect to STEM, these differences are related in part to student's interests and relative academic strengths. Sex differences in occupational interests, for instance, are large and well-documented, and reflect a more basic sex difference in interest in things versus people (Su, Rounds, & Armstrong, 2009). Men prefer occupations that involve working with things (e.g., engineering, mechanics) and abstract ideas (e.g., scientific theory) and women prefer working with and directly contributing to the wellbeing of others (e.g., physician, teacher). The sex difference in interest in people actually reflects a more general interest in living things, which would explain why women who are interested in science are much more likely to pursue a career in biology or veterinary medicine than computer science (Lofstedt, 2003).

Although women and men are similar in intelligence, there are more specific cognitive and academic sex differences that influence educational and occupational choices (e.g., Geary, 1996). One of these differences is relative strengths in reading, mathematics, and science (Stoet & Geary, 2015). Students who are relatively better in reading-related areas (e.g., literature) than they are in science or mathematics (or visuospatial abilities), *independent* of their absolute level of performance relative to other students, are more likely to pursue college degrees in the humanities and enter non-science occupations, with the reverse for students who are relatively better in science and mathematics than literature (Humphreys, Lubinski, & Yao, 1993). This is where the results from Finland and elsewhere make sense. Although adolescent girls in Finland perform as well or better than their male peers in science, the gap is even larger in reading such that more Finnish girls have larger relative advantages in reading than science. Most adolescent boys in contrast are relatively better at science or mathematics than reading, independent of their absolute level of performance. Individuals with this pattern are likely to enter STEM areas, whether as research scientists or technicians, and there are more boys than girls with this pattern, worldwide (Stoet & Geary, 2015).

At the same time, there are substantive numbers of girls with relatively higher science or mathematics than reading achievement – 24% of Finnish girls – but proportionately fewer of these girls pursue STEM degrees than their male peers (Stoet & Geary, 2018). The gap between the number of adolescent girls with a STEM-biased academic pattern and the number of women who obtain a STEM degree in college is not likely due to stereotype threat, implicit bias, or related factors, because this gap increases with increases in national levels of gender equality. Early studies have shown that mathematically gifted women enter STEM fields less often than mathematically gifted men, not because of bias or microaggression, but because they have broader educational interests and thus consider a wider range of occupations than these men (Lubinski & Benbow, 1992). It seems to us that interventions focused on this group of girls (e.g., individual mentoring) holds much more promise for increasing the number of women in inorganic STEM professions than do currently vogue interventions that focus on rending the wider society of stereotypes, implicit bias, and microaggressions.

References

Basford, T. E., Offermann, L. R., & Behrend, T. S. (2014). Do you see what I see? Perceptions of gender microaggressions in the workplace. *Psychology of Women Quarterly, 38*, 340–349.

Blanton, H., Jaccard, J., Klick, J., Mellers, B., Mitchell, G., & Tetlock, P. E. (2009). Strong claims and weak evidence: Reassessing the predictive validity of the IAT. *Journal of Applied Psychology, 94*, 567.

Ceci, S. J., & Williams, W. M. (2015). Women have substantial advantage in STEM faculty hiring, except when competing against more-accomplished men. *Frontiers in Psychology, 6*, e1532.

Del Río, C., & Alonso-Villar, O. (2015). The evolution of occupational segregation in the United States, 1940–2010: Gains and losses of gender–race/ethnicity groups. *Demography, 52*(3), 967–988.

Flore, P. C., & Wicherts, J. M. (2015). Does stereotype threat influence performance of girls in stereotyped domains? A meta-analysis. *Journal of School Psychology, 53*, 25–44.

Ganley, C. M., Mingle, L. A., Ryan, A. M., Ryan, K., Vasilyeva, M., & Perry, M. (2013). An examination of stereotype threat effects on girls' mathematics performance. *Developmental Psychology, 49*, 1886–1897.

Geary, D. C. (1996). Sexual selection and sex differences in mathematical abilities. *Behavioral and Brain Sciences, 19*, 229–284.

Geary, D. C. (2010). *Male, female: The evolution of human sex differences* (2nd ed.). Washington, D.C.: American Psychological Association.

Greenwald, A. G., Banaji, M. R., & Nosek, B. A. (2015). Statistically small effects of the implicit association test can have societally large effects. *Journal of Personality and Social Psychology, 108*, 553–561.

Greenwald, A. G., McGhee, D. E., & Schwartz, J. L. (1998). Measuring individual differences in implicit cognition: The implicit association test. *Journal of Personality and Social Psychology, 74*, 1464.

Greenwald, A. G., Nosek, B. A., Banaji, M. R., & Klauer, K. C. (2005). Validity of the salience asymmetry interpretation of the implicit association test: Comment on Rothermund and Wentura (2004). *Journal of Experimental Psychology: General, 134*, 420–425.

Greenwald, A. G., Poehlman, T. A., Uhlmann, E. L., & Banaji, M. R. (2009). Understanding and using the implicit association test: III. Meta-analysis of predictive validity. *Journal of Personality and Social Psychology, 97*, 17–41.

Hartocollis, A. (2016, June 26). Tutors see stereotypes and gender Bias in SAT. *Testers See None of the Above.* http://www.nytimes.com/2016/06/27/us/tutors-see-stereotypes-and-gender-bias-in-sat-testers-see-none-of-the-above.html?_r=1

Hicks, S. R. (2004). *Explaining postmodernism: Skepticism and socialism from Rousseau to Foucault.* Scholary Publishing, Inc. Tempe, AZ.

Hill, C., Corbett, C., & St Rose, A. (2010). *Why so few? Women in science, technology, engineering, and mathematics.* Washington, D.C.: American Association of University Women.

Humphreys, L. G., Lubinski, D., & Yao, G. (1993). Utility of predicting group membership and the role of spatial visualization in becoming an engineer, physical scientist, or artist. *Journal of Applied Psychology, 78*, 250–261.

Hyde, J. S. (2005). The gender similarities hypothesis. *American Psychologist, 60*, 581–592.

Lilienfeld, S. O. (2017). Microaggressions: Strong claims, inadequate evidence. *Perspectives on Psychological Science, 12*, 138–169.

Lippa, R. A., Collaer, M. L., & Peters, M. (2010). Sex differences in mental rotation and line angle judgments are positively associated with gender equality and economic development across 53 nations. *Archives of Sexual Behavior, 39*, 990–997.

Lofstedt, J. (2003). Gender and veterinary medicine. *The Canadian Veterinary Journal, 44*, 533–535.

Lubinski, D., & Benbow, C. P. (1992). Gender differences in abilities and preferences among the gifted: Implications for the math/science pipeline. *Current Directions in Psychological Science, 1*, 61–66.

Miller, D. I., Eagly, A. H., & Linn, M. C. (2015). Women's representation in science predicts national gender-science stereotypes: Evidence from 66 nations. *Journal of Educational Psychology, 107*, 631–644.

Nosek, B. A., Banaji, M. R., & Greenwald, A. G. (2002). Harvesting implicit group attitudes and beliefs from a demonstration web site. *Group Dynamics: Theory, Research, and Practice, 6*, 101–115.

Oswald, F. L., Mitchell, G., Blanton, H., Jaccard, J., & Tetlock, P. E. (2013). Predicting ethnic and racial discrimination: A meta-analysis of IAT criterion studies. *Journal of Personality and Social Psychology, 105*, 171–192.

Picho, K., Rodriguez, A., & Finnie, L. (2013). Exploring the moderating role of context on the mathematics performance of females under stereotype threat: A meta-analysis. *The Journal of Social Psychology, 153*, 299–333.

Rothermund, K., & Wentura, D. (2004). Underlying processes in the implicit association test: Dissociating salience from associations. *Journal of Experimental Psychology: General, 133*, 139–165.

Spencer, S. J., Steele, C. M., & Quinn, D. M. (1999). Stereotype threat and women's math performance. *Journal of Experimental Social Psychology, 35*, 4–28.

Stoet, G., & Geary, D. C. (2012). Can stereotype threat explain the sex gap in mathematics performance and achievement? *Review of General Psychology, 16*, 93–102.

Stoet, G., & Geary, D. C. (2015). Sex differences in academic achievement are not related to political, economic, or social equality. *Intelligence, 48*, 137–151.

Stoet, G., & Geary, D. C. (2018). The gender equality paradox in STEM education. *Psychological Science, 29*, 581–593.

Su, R., Rounds, J., & Armstrong, P. I. (2009). Men and things, women and people. *Psychological Bulletin, 135*, 859–884.

Sue, D. W. (2010). *Microaggressions in everyday life: Race, gender, and sexual orientation.* Hoboken, NJ: Wiley.

Thiederman, S. (2015). *3 keys to defeating unconscious bias.* San Diego, CA: Cross-Cultural Communications.

Walton, G. M., Logel, C., Peach, J. M., Spencer, S. J., & Zanna, M. P. (2015). Two brief interventions to mitigate a "chilly climate" transform women's experience, relationships, and achievement in engineering. *Journal of Educational Psychology, 107*, 468–485.

Williams, W. M., & Ceci, S. J. (2015). National hiring experiments reveal 2: 1 faculty preference for women on STEM tenure track. *Proceedings of the National Academy of Sciences USA, 112*, 5360–5365.

World Economic Forum. (2015). *The global gender gap report 2015.* Geneva, Switzerland: World Economic Forum.

Chapter 16
Groupthink in Sex and Pornography "Addiction": Sex-Negativity, Theoretical Impotence, and Political Manipulation

Nicole Prause and D J Williams

Concepts of excessive sexuality have existed for hundreds of years, but have recently turned profitable. The concept of profiting from treating sex as addictive was invented in the early 1980s with the publication of Carnes' (1983) clinical observations titled, *Out of the Shadows: Understanding Sexual Addiction.* Despite the fact that no science existed to support the model at the time, "addiction" was the first chosen framework. Speculatively, this model of sexual behavior would be most profitable: "addiction" treatments can command inpatient resources in contrast to typical time-limited, outpatient approaches for problems of compulsivity or relationship discord. Gradually, a diverse variety of academics, professionals, policy-makers, and lay people have become increasingly concerned about sexual behavior that is commonly interpreted to be "out of control." While sexual "addiction" emerged largely due to cultural anxieties following the sexual revolution (Irvine, 1995), it gained momentum in large part due to its medicalization. Media accounts of celebrities who claimed to succumb to this supposed disorder fanned fashionable flames (Reay, Attwood, & Gooder, 2013). As the sex addiction industry became more firmly established, the target then widened to include viewing pornography, or more precisely, visual sexual stimuli (VSS). Currently, sex (and pornography)"addiction" are commonly discussed as separate, yet somewhat overlapping, clinical and political issues. However, the argument for the application of an addiction model to both sexual frequency and VSS rests on the same basic assumptions, shares the same logic, and is often promoted by the same believers.

The scientific method is designed to produce knowledge that is objective and valid. Science requires falsifiable hypotheses generated by the proposed model,

N. Prause
Liberos LLC, Los Angeles, CA, USA

D J Williams (✉)
Social Work, & Criminology, Idaho State University, Pocatello, ID, USA

Center for Positive Sexuality (Los Angeles), Los Angeles, CA, USA
e-mail: willdj@isu.edu

D. M. Allen, J. W. Howell (eds.), *Groupthink in Science*,
https://doi.org/10.1007/978-3-030-36822-7_16

then conducting carefully controlled studies with the ability to disprove (falsify) each hypothesis. This is a very high standard because every model prediction must hold true for the model to retain support. In the social and behavioral sciences, in particular, researchers must carefully consider broader social and cultural contexts that may influence the research process and interpretation of findings. Considering sociocultural influence on research questions requires careful exploration of potential extraneous variables, and alternative theories that could help explain patterns of behaviors. After such thorough examination, when data consistently fail to disprove the hypothesis, then support for the model is warranted. A model is never considered entirely "proven" because it is always subject to future falsification. In short, rigorous science, along with high quality scholarship more generally, demands considerable skepticism and critical analysis. Thus, the role of the scientist is primarily as a debunker, attempting to identify empirical fail points of proposed models. When one model fails, another, better-fitting model must be considered.

Consistent with other reviews (i.e., Ley, 2012, 2018; Ley, Prause, & Finn, 2014; Prause & Fong, 2015; Williams et al., 2017; Voros, 2009), we find that the addiction model as applied to sex and VSS viewing fails to meet scientific criteria for model support. Although only one hypothesis generated by the addiction model would need to be falsified to reject the model, many hypotheses generated by the addiction model have been falsified. These falsifications have been replicated by independent laboratories. Thus, "sex addiction" should not be considered a valid model, much less a diagnosis of pathology. A frequent objection by therapists is that debating the "addiction" model is merely becoming distracted by labels (see below). This reflects a basic misunderstanding of science. What you "call it" actually refers to the model being tested and defines how best to help.

Sexual scientists recognize the high complexity of frequent sexual behaviors and have parsed many models that could describe these behaviors, including non-pathology models (Walton, Cantor, Bhullar, & Lykins, 2017). In this chapter we focus on the scientific rejection of the "addiction" model of frequent sex and VSS viewing as contrasted by its perseverance in popular parlance. We hope to contribute to the current discussion concerning fundamental philosophical and methodological problems associated with the application of an addiction model, particularly as promoted by groupthink that runs afoul of basic principles of science. We draw attention to the impact of widespread sociohistorical sex-negativity, the need to consider broader theoretical explanations, and the political strategy for somewhat disparate institutions to adopt the veneer of science to promote their respective self-interests.

Sex Negativity and Sociohistorical Considerations

Despite the fact that sexual norms, and thus also laws and moral judgments concerning sexuality, vary tremendously across cultures and historical time periods (Bullough, 1976; Hayes & Carpenter, 2012; Popovic, 2006), there has been a lack of recognition of sociosexual diversity within sexology (Bhugra, Popelyuk, & McMullen, 2010). Bullough (1976) classified various cultures as more or less sex negative or sex positive. Sex-negativity is characterized by sexual asceticism, a narrow range of socially accepted sexual behaviors, lack of openness to sexuality, and sociosexual scripts preoccupied with risk and danger. Sex-positivity, or positive sexuality, acknowledges risk and danger, yet also recognizes the importance of sexual pleasure and wellbeing, embraces sexual diversity, and encourages open communication. Positive sexuality acknowledges personal and cultural diversity regarding sexuality and focuses less on sexual "deviance," and more on the ethics of various sexual practices (Williams, Christensen, & Capous-Desyllas, 2016).

There is little doubt that much of Western society, historically, has been thoroughly sex-negative (for an example, see Le Bodic, 2009 and Malan & Bullough, 2005 for a history of masturbation). American culture, in particular, continues to struggle with all types of sociosexual matters. The United States has been painfully slow to acknowledge and support the rights of lesbian, gay, bisexual, and transgender (LGBT) persons (i.e., Adam, 2003; Huebner, Rebchook, & Kegeles, 2004; Scott, 1998); support women's reproductive choices and provide access to contraception (i.e., Deckman & McTague, 2014; Harrison, 2005); and fully accept a range of consensual erotic and sexual practices (i.e., Ortmann & Sprott, 2012; Rubin, 1984). Furthermore, a review of contemporary U.S. sexual offending policy found that policy is terribly costly, sometimes increases injustice, and is largely fueled by myths rooted in widespread sex-negativity, rather than the large body of existing research (Williams, Thomas, & Prior, 2015).

It is not surprising that sexual literacy is a widespread problem. Sex education is mandated in schools in fewer than half of the U.S. states, and only 13 states require information to be medically accurate (Guttmacher Institute, 2012). At the same time, the federal government in recent decades has largely funded abstinence-only programs, particularly during the Bush administration, despite meta-analytic research showing that such programs are ineffective (Kirby, 2007). Sex education scholars have also pointed out that current sex education programs may unknowingly perpetuate a hegemonic sexuality with racial, class, and gender inequalities built into them (Connell & Elliott, 2009; Hobaica & Kwon, 2018; Hoefer & Hoefer, 2017). In focus groups concerning the effects of VSS viewing, a primary concern is that groupthink drives discussants to attempt to prove their righteousness by being critical of VSS (Iantaffi, Wilkerson, Grey, & Rosser, 2015).

Scientists and clinicians, of course, function within, and are influenced by, the broader sociohistorical context. In a climate of widespread sex-negativity, federal funding for scientific research on sexuality has generally been quite scarce, with virtually no funding for projects that consider positive possibilities of sexuality. Projects concerning sexuality at all that receive federal funding from the National Institutes of health have been uniquely attacked politically merely for possessing content on sexuality (Epstein, 2006). Curiously, it has only been recently that public health scholars have begun to consider seriously the potential psychosocial health benefits of sexuality and the importance of sexual pleasure (Anderson, 2013; Diamond & Huebner, 2012; Satcher, Hook III, & Coleman, 2015). When considering health generally, scientists and clinicians have, for quite some time, followed the World Health Organization (WHO) recommendation that good health is more than simply the absence of disease, but includes positive dimensions, such as quality of life, life satisfaction, and overall wellbeing. However, the acceptance of similar positive constructs into definitions of sexual health has been slow. Moreover, while defining sexual health is shaped by sociohistorical events (Edwards & Coleman, 2004), there is often a lag time between accepted operational definitions of constructs and the widespread application of constructs within clinical practice.

Here We Go Again! Changing Discourse from "Badness" to "Sickness"

Two decades ago, Irvine (1995) traced how the social process of medicalization led to the invention of sex addiction. This same social process has occurred previously with other notable sexual "disorders," such as masturbation and homosexuality. At the heart of medicalization is the use of language. While therapists argue that diagnostic labels assist validating patients' experiences, data show this is far from a universal experience, with as many diagnosed feeling devalued as helped by their label (Perkins et al., 2018). In their classic work on the medicalization of deviance, generally, Conrad and Schneider (1992) documented how discourses on deviant behavior have shifted from interpretations of "badness" to reinterpretation as "sickness." In considering a range of scholarship on sexuality, Hammack, Mayers, and Windell (2013) reported that sickness script changed in the 1970s to a "species" script following the removal of homosexuality in the DSM in 1973, and then to a "subject" script in the 1990s when scholarship diversified (including the emergence of queer theory). In their review on the interpretation of sexual deviance, De Block and Adriaens (2013) discuss the historical difficulties that the field of psychiatry has had, and continues to have, in classifying and understanding sexual behaviors. In considering sociohistorical issues and the diversification of scholarship, this has become more challenging. Indeed, specific terms do make a difference because of the scripts in which they are embedded. In addressing sexual variation, is there a different connotation between "deviance" and "diversity"?

Helping Professions and Culturally Biased "Evidence"

The public may assume that contemporary helping professions, including psychology, counseling, social work, and marriage and family therapy, use interventions that are informed by a sound body of research and evidence. The American Counseling Association (ACA) *Code of Ethics* (2014, p. 10) states: "When providing services, counselors use techniques/procedures/modalities that are grounded in theory and/or have an empirical or scientific foundation." Note, having a "scientific foundation" is an option, not a requirement, for counselor practice. Related fields try to avoid regulation with even weaker requirements. The American Psychological Association (APA) remains neutral, offering empirically supported treatment as one option, rather than a requirement (Elmore, 2016). A push by some psychologists to science-based interventions caused so much tension within APA that a schism formed and clinical science emerged (McFall, 1991). While valid debates exist concerning how to best implement ESTs, such as avoiding trademarked therapies (Rosen & Davison, 2003) and treatments less effective for minority clients (Bernal & Scharro-del-Rio, 2001), the case for distrusting clinical judgment over data remains extensive (Meehl, 1957; Miller, Spengler, & Spengler, 2015). Therapists' confidence in their own outcomes with patients typically far exceed their actual positive impact (Waller & Turner, 2016) and often do no better, or have outcomes even worse, than untrained paraprofessionals (Berman & Norton, 1985). Therapists raise many objections to following science-based treatments, including beliefs that feelings cannot be measured, beliefs that they are more important than the therapy used, and preferring to use their "gut" instead of evidence (Gyani, Shafran, Rose, & Lee, 2015).

Marriage and family therapy (MFT) practitioners especially rejected empirically supported interventions, with many refusing to leave their "clinical intuition" for science-backed treatments. A review of their flagship *Journal of Marital and Family Therapy* showed quantitative content, especially clinical trials, actually decreased from 2005 to 2014 (Parker, Chang, & Thomas, 2016). Specifically, MFT authors instructed researchers "should avoid attitudes that can reflect the belief that they know better than clinical practitioners who have been working in the field for decades" (Dattilio, Piercy, & Davis, 2013, p. 10). Unfortunately, longitudinal data show that years of experience as a therapist actually are associated with decreased efficacy with patients (Dunkle & Friedlander, 1996; Erekson, Janis, Bailey, Cattani, & Pedersen, 2017; Goldberg et al., 2016). MFTs continue to be disconnected from, and resistant to, implementing science-based treatments (Withers, Reynolds, Reed, & Holtrop, 2017). Indeed, science is not mentioned in any part of the MFT Commission on Accreditation (Crane, Wampler, Sprenkle, Sandberg, & Hovestadt, 2002). This is partially a self-selection problem, where MFT students select their program in large part due to a perceived fit with their personal religious beliefs (Hertlein & Lambert-Shute, 2007). However, the lack of training in human sexuality at such programs also appears to increase the problem.

The helping professions, as a whole, require very little, if any, training on human sexuality. For example, while the Council on Social Work Education (CSWE, 2008, 2015) includes sexual orientation (along with age, class, color, culture, gender, gender identity and expression, immigration status, political ideology, race, religion, and sex) in its statement on human diversity, there is no requirement for training on sexuality at any level (bachelor, master, doctoral) of education. A content analysis of popular social work textbooks found a glaring absence of discussion about sexual diversity (Prior, Williams, Zavala, & Milford, 2016). Further, most MFT faculty do not have any focused training in human sexuality (Zamboni & Zaid, 2017). As a result, MFT comfort with sexual topics has not improved over decades (Dermer & Bachenberg, 2015). Specifically, a majority of MFT practitioners surveyed reported discomfort counseling homosexual clients. Perhaps not surprising, then, it is easy to see why many well-intentioned professionals, functioning in a longstanding socio-historical climate of sex-negativity, uncritically accept and promote an addiction framework of sexual behavior and VSS viewing, despite sociocultural biases, which helping professions supposedly oppose, inherent in sex/VSS addiction concepts and screening instruments (see Joannides, 2012; Williams, 2017). Of course, helping professionals are authority figures and are viewed as being experts on the issues for which they provide services. Unfortunately, this is not always true when it comes to matters pertaining to sexuality. When there are new opportunities to provide services (and profit), it can be easy for groupthink to occur and medicalization promoted by helping professionals to expand.

Religion Masquerading as Public Health and Neuroscience

Religion is a significant force in the sex and VSS viewing addiction movement. Dominant Western religious organizations have a long history of opposition to various sexual practices (i.e., those that are not monogamous, married, vanilla; Rubin, 1984) and VSS viewing (Thomas, 2013). Recent research has found that there is a strong positive relationship between religiosity and perceived VSS addiction even when the actual amount of VSS viewing is controlled (Grubbs, Exline, Paragament, Hook, & Carlisle, 2015). In their review of the literature, Grubbs and Perry (2018) found that moral incongruence about VSS viewing is common and is associated with greater distress about VSS viewing, more frequently reported problems with VSS viewing, and an increased likelihood of perceived addiction to VSS viewing. Sociological studies by Thomas (2013, 2016) documented religious institutions' shifting narratives regarding the effects of VSS viewing from being a problem of social deviance (1950s and 1960s) to a problem of temptation and sin (1970s), and finally, now almost exclusively (beginning in the 1980s), to a problem of addiction that can have negative public health effects on society. Subsequently, using data from popular religious magazines combined with national survey data, Thomas, Alper, and Gleason (2017) have traced how religious anti-VSS viewing narratives apparently become internalized among those within such religious traditions to function as a form of self-fulfilling prophecy with respect to marital satisfaction. Some have noted that this has made some strange coalitions, such as anti-pornography feminists lecturing in religious spaces and filing anti-pornography legislation together (Whittier, 2014). Limited coalitions between traditionally oppositional groups serve to decrease issue-specific opposition (Pullum, 2017). In this case, therapists want to make money, religious groups want to regulate sexual expression, and feminists want to limit (perceived) harm to women. The movement regularly claims secular roots to the public, but these religious alliances have been revealed repeatedly in both personal (e.g., Allen, 2015) and political (e.g., Campbell, 2018) biases.

The recent shifting of discourse from religious to public health (scientific) discourse is purposeful to persuade both public and professional opinion to accept the sex/VSS viewing model. The strategy is to make the addiction model appear to be constructed based on objective, scientific evidence. This, of course, reflects the same classic pattern of medicalization (Conrad & Schneider, 1992) and lends an "objective" measure of social control to unsanctioned sexual behavior (Voros, 2009).

Sexy Neuroscience

Attempts to appeal to authority when health is the topic make scientists the authority of claimed knowledge. Being told that scientists completely understand a phenomenon has been shown to increase the layperson's confidence in their own (inaccurate) knowledge (Sloman & Rabb, 2016). The field of neuroscience is especially widely touted for its documented ability to deceive consumers of health information. Viewing brain images in the context of health statements increases untrained individuals' beliefs in the information presented (McCabe & Castel, 2008), and this occurs without increasing their actual knowledge of neuroscience (Ikeda, Kitagami, Takahashi, Hattori, & Ito, 2013). Others have suggested that it is not the brain images per se that increase false confidence, but rather the presence of any neuroscience-sounding information, whether or not it was relevant to the research described (Hook & Farah, 2013). Thus, confidence may be most likely bolstered by the mention of neuroscience concepts when the actual science is most weak. This is a lucrative strategy. Using brain information to push addiction models has been shown to increase acceptance of treatment (see Figure 1 in Racine, Sattler, & Escande, 2017). Sex addiction clinicians appear anxious to appeal to neuroscience authority. The International Institute for the Treatment of Trauma and Addictions, an organization that licenses sex addiction therapists, advertised a talk on the "neuroscience" of sex by a speaker who actually was not a neuroscientist (IITAPllc, 2014). Rather, the speaker had self-published his only text on the topic for the Latter Day Saints' concerning how to use religion to overcome the evils of pornography. He later published a letter to the editor claiming to critique our study, which was so bizarre, rambling, and obviously uninformed about basic principles of neuroscience that we declined the journal's offer to respond to it. Climate scientists have faced similar challenges from the presentation of fake experts (Hansson, 2018).

There are conditions under which this bias may be reduced. Studies in which the participant was encouraged to question the presented neuroscience, such as using descriptions like "Can Brain Scans Detect Criminals?" reduced the bias to accept information presented with brain images (Schweitzer, Baker, & Risko, 2013). However, participants were less likely to believe direct critiques of neuroscience data rather than glowing, positive reviews of neuroscience data (Popescu, Thompson, Gayton, & Markowski, 2016). Where scientists accurately characterize data as having falsified the addiction model of sex, activists confidently claim that the addiction model is "proven," despite that science can only support a model. Combine poor public discrimination of neuroscience evidence with confirmation bias of a sex-negative society, and it is not difficult to understand the political traction of various groups that are promoting such a false narrative.

The primacy of brain data is a problem that extends into the field of neuroscience. Descriptions of neuroscience data as "underlying" or "explaining" sexual behaviors represents a classic error of biological reductionism. In reality, science is integrative, with biology, behavior, social, and other levels of analysis often equally important in model testing (Cacioppo, 2002). The best model holds up across these levels of analysis. This is partly why psychology has been anxious to grab the designation of the "hub science" that can best integrate these sources of information (Cacioppo, 2007). The ability to document differences in proposed groups by brain activations provides no evidence that a particular group necessarily has a disease.

Addiction Is the Wrong Model

While some people clearly are distressed by their sexual behaviors, it is important to identify the best model. The best model is one that best characterizes and predicts future behaviors. Thus, there are many models of high-frequency sexual behaviors. These include a number of non-pathological models (Walton et al., 2017), including the high sex drive and/or social shame model. These are empirically separable (Prause, 2017). While falsification of behavior models is a core tenet of science, it bears explanation. The therapists claiming to treat "sex addicts" describe differentiating models as irrelevant for treatment and reflecting merely different "names" for the same behaviors (Carnes & Love, 2017). Such fundamental misunderstandings of science are of concern for the type of care patients are likely to receive. Indeed, there is currently no random-assignment, controlled trial for sex or porn addiction as of this writing. Websites concerning "porn addiction" are especially likely, relative to other behavioral issue websites, to recommend religious absolution and complete abstinence as a goal (Rodda, Booth, Vacaru, Knaebe, & Hodgins, 2018). The most popular conceptualization by clinicians has been the "sex addiction" model, which is curious given that it has the weakest empirical support.

The specifics of an addiction model can, of course, vary a bit between scientists. However, most scientists agree that key features of any addiction include compulsions to seek the drug/behavior, a loss of control of the behavior or consumption, a withdrawal state (Koob & Le Moal, 2008), involvement of neural reward systems, and neuroadaptations over time that promote craving over liking (Robinson & Berridge, 2000). While an addiction model includes components of compulsivity and impulsivity, those ("compulsion" and "impulsivity") also are recognized as separable, distinct models from addiction (Prause, 2017).

By applying the falsification criterion to models of frequent sexual behaviors, the "addiction" model has been falsified (Prause, Steele, Staley, Sabatinelli, & Hajcak,

2016; Prause, Janssen, Georgiadis, Finn, & Pfaus, 2017). That is, several of the predictions made by an addiction model have failed in experiments. These experiments have been replicated and extended by independent laboratories, which is the gold standard for falsification.

Both the American Psychiatric Association (2013) and the World Health Organization International (WHO) specifically excluded "sex addiction" from their nomenclature (within *Diagnostic and Statistical Manual of Mental Disorders*, or DSM, and the *International Classification of Diseases*, or ICD). "Porn addiction" also was excluded from the ICD-11 (Grant et al., 2014). Notably, the ICD-11 is considering whether or not to add "compulsive sexual behavior" at this time. ICD currently requires ruling out "Distress that is entirely related to moral judgments and disapproval about sexual impulses." As no study to date has ever tested any patient sample that meets these requirements, it is unclear to whom the diagnosis would refer. From the first nationally representative study, 2.3% of men and 0.2% of women in the Netherlands reported feeling that they might be sexually compulsive (National Institute for Public Health, 2017). Given that this assessment did not rule out individuals with concerns due to moral judgments, it appears likely that such problems may not be experienced by any portion of the population. More succinctly, such tiny numbers appear within the error variance of self-description. Notably, the oft-repeated prevalence guess of one sex and pornography addiction therapist for these difficulties (Carnes, 2013) turned out to be 2.6 (men) to 30 (women) times higher than suggested by actual data from nationally representative samples.

Perhaps the most common scientific misperception pushed by anti-pornography organizations is that dopamine involvement is the same as addiction (Ley, 2018). For example, alarming titles such as "Technology gives us dopamine...highly addictive!" (Sprout, 2017) and "Sex releases the highest levels of dopamine naturally available, equal to morphine & nicotine" (Wilson, 2018) are touted to gain political support for an addiction model. Both statements are false. Dopamine is involved in many functions, including learning, salience, and movement (Schultz, Stauffer, & Lak, 2017). Dopamine is not specific to addiction. Further, dopamine has never been compared by titers with substances; in fact, null-hypothesis statistics could never support the conclusion that conditions are "equal." Certainly, there is strong evidence that increases in dopamine availability increase sexual behaviors just as sexual behaviors themselves increase the activity of dopamine. These are necessary, but not sufficient, conditions for addiction (see above). Dopamine activity would need to be involved to support an addiction model, but dopamine is altered in many behaviors with no relationship to any proposed addiction.

Withdrawal hypotheses appear to lack empirical support. Even with substances, withdrawal is not consistently a required feature, such as for inhalants (Hasin et al., 2013). Similarly, behavioral addiction clinicians sometimes advocate removing the requirement of withdrawal for behaviors (Van Rooij & Prause, 2014). However, clinicians have argued that "sex addiction" patients exhibit withdrawal. For example, Goodman (2001) argued that withdrawal is a component of "sex addiction" but that withdrawal need not be evidenced physiologically. In direct contradiction, the withdrawal symptoms reported by other clinicians (Karila et al., 2014) include only and explicitly physiological symptoms, with 70% of patients claiming experiences of "nervousness, insomnia, sweating, nausea, increased heart rate, shortness of breath, and fatigue." The field of psychophysiology is well-equipped to document all of these claimed symptoms; yet none have been documented to date. Given that there also are currently no data on human sexual deprivation states in non-pathology, this hypothesis from the addiction model can reasonably be described as having no supportive data.

Conclusion

Concerns around sexual behavior, including sex film viewing, appear largely driven by social forces. These forces include monetary gain (i.e., therapists and politicians), religious (i.e., Latter Day Saints and evangelicals), and ideological (i.e., feminists). To reach the goal of pathologizing these sexual behaviors, such groups have conspired to appropriate a false framework of "health" behaviors, which requires promoting an appearance of science. We have demonstrated that such collaborative adversarial movements (Whittier, 2014) led to gross overestimates of prevalence, basic misunderstanding of scientific model testing, mischaracterizations of neuroscience, appeals to fake authorities, and intentional disregard of disconfirming data. In fact, data suggest the best thing for individuals who report distress about their sexual behaviors is likely to do nothing. Curiously, a study of individuals who believed that they were "sex addicts" found that 100% of women (*N* = 68) and 95% of men (*N* = 167) spontaneously resolved their concerns without treatment over a 5-year period, and most were resolved within the first year of expressing the concern (Konkolÿ, Thege, Woodin, Hodgins, & Williams, 2015).

So how do we respect some individuals' distress about their own particular sexual behaviors given the current socio-cultural situation? First, we use standardized, validated assessments of accepted diagnoses. For example, depression is mistakenly described as "comorbid" with "porn addiction" where a primary diagnosis of depression is likely more appropriate and parsimonious. Many empirically supported depression treatments exist that accommodate sexual features, but no sex addiction ESTs exist. Second, psychoeducation is essential. Education is an important component of most sexual interventions. However, due to widespread sex negativity and poor sex education in the United States, there is extensive misinformation on the Internet, especially regarding what is "normal." Third, advocate for patients who are being misled, such as by calling attention to clinicians who refuse to base treatments on rigorous science (McFall, 1991). Patients may struggle to distinguish between qualified clinicians and those who are simply reproducing sex-negative discourses of pathology via neuroscience jargon. Also, many patients appear unaware that clinicians are not required to provide treatments with any scientific support. Scientists engaging in social media can provide information more directly to people with concerns (Bik & Goldstein, 2013). For those rightfully concerned about organized social attacks to providing this information online, it is useful to consult guides that excuse scientists from corresponding with activists online (Lewandowsky & Bishop, 2016).

Unfortunately, groupthink on the topic of sex and pornography "addiction" is surprisingly common. There remains a glaring need for scientists and practitioners to remember that Western society remains saturated in a socio-cultural climate of sex-negativity. Proponents of the sex/pornography addiction movement are (often intentionally) influenced by their own broader interests (i.e., monetary, religious, ideological). Current social scripts concerning commonly disapproved sexual behaviors and identities reflect a long history of following a "badness" (religious) to "sickness" (public health) central theme. Finally, as we have documented herein, actual controlled, peer-reviewed neuroscientific investigations fail to support an addiction model.

References

Adam, B. D. (2003). The defense of marriage act and American exceptionalism: The "gay marriage" panic in the United States. *Journal of the History of Sexuality, 12*, 259–276.

Allen, S. (2015, October 20). *"Porn kills love": Mormons' anti-smut crusade*. Retrieved April 19, 2018, from https://www.thedailybeast.com/articles/2015/10/20/porn-kills-love-mormons-anti-smut-crusade

American Counseling Association. (2014). *Code of ethics*. Alexandria, VA: Author.

American Psychiatric Association. (2013). *Diagnostic and statistical manual of mental disorders (DSM-5®)*. Washington, D.C.: American Psychiatric Pub.

Anderson, R. M. (2013). Positive sexuality and its impact on overall well-being. *Bundesgesundheitsblatt, 56*, 208–214. https://doi.org/10.1007/s00103-012-1607-z

Berman, J. S., & Norton, N. C. (1985). Does professional training make a therapist more effective? *Psychological Bulletin, 98*, 401–407. https://doi.org/10.1037/0033-2909.98.2.401

Bernal, G., & Scharro-del-Rio, M. R. (2001). Are empirically supported treatments valid for ethnic minorities? Toward an alternative approach for treatment research. *Cultural Diversity & Ethnic Minority Psychology, 7*(4), 328–342.

Bhugra, D., Popelyuk, D., & McMullen, I. (2010). Paraphilias across cultures: Contexts and controversies. *Journal of Sex Research, 47*, 242–256. https://doi.org/10.1080/00224491003699833

Bik, H. M., & Goldstein, M. C. (2013). An introduction to social media for scientists. *PLoS Biology, 11*(4), e1001535.

Bullough, V. L. (1976). *Sexual variance in society and history*. Chicago, IL: University of Chicago Press.

Cacioppo, J. (2007). Psychology is a hub science. *APS Observer, 20*(8).

Cacioppo, J. T. (2002). Social neuroscience: Understanding the pieces fosters understanding the whole and vice versa. *The American Psychologist, 57*(11), 819–831.

Campbell, A. (2018, February 8). *Kansas senate uses fake science to declare porn a public health crisis*. Retrieved April 19, 2018, from https://www.huffingtonpost.com/entry/kansas-senate-porn-resolution_us_5a7c5bc9e4b0c6726e101d66

Carnes, P. (1983). *Out of the shadows: Understanding sexual addiction*. Minneapolis, MN: CompCare.

Carnes, P. (2013). *Don't call it love: Recovery from sexual addiction*. New York, NY: Bantam.

Carnes, S., & Love, T. (2017). Separating models obscures the scientific underpinnings of sex addiction as a disorder. *Archives of Sexual Behavior, 46*(8), 2253–2256.

Connell, C., & Elliott, S. (2009). Beyond the birds and the bees: Learning inequality through sexuality education. *American Journal of Sexuality Education, 4*, 83–102. https://doi.org/10.1080/15546120903001332

Conrad, P., & Schneider, J. W. (1992). *Deviance and medicalization: From badness to sickness*. Philadelphia, PA: Temple University Press.

Council on Social Work Education (CSWE). (2008). *Educational policy and educational standards*. Alexandria, VA: Author.

Council on Social Work Education (CSWE). (2015). *Final 2015 educational policy (EP)*. Alexandria, VA: Author.

Crane, D. R., Wampler, K. S., Sprenkle, D. H., Sandberg, J. G., & Hovestadt, A. J. (2002). The scientist-practitioner model in marriage and family therapy doctoral programs: Current status. *Journal of Marital and Family Therapy, 28*(1), 75–83.

Dattilio, F. M., Piercy, F. P., & Davis, S. D. (2013). The divide between "evidenced-based" approaches and practitioners of traditional theories of family therapy. *Journal of Marital and Family Therapy, 40*(1), 5–16.

De Block, A., & Adriaens, P. R. (2013). Pathologizing sexual deviance: A history. *Journal of Sex Research, 50*, 276–298. https://doi.org/10.1080/00224499.2012.738259

Deckman, M., & McTague, J. (2014). Did the "war on women" work? Women, men, and the birth control mandate in the 2012 presidential election. *American Politics Research, 43*, 3–26. https://doi.org/10.1177/1532673X14535240

Dermer, S., & Bachenberg, M. (2015). The importance of training marital, couple, and family therapists in sexual health. *Australian and New Zealand Journal of Family Therapy, 36*(4), 492–503.

Diamond, L. M., & Huebner, D. M. (2012). Is sex good for you? Rethinking sexuality and health. *Social and Personality Psychology Compass, 6*, 54–69. https://doi.org/10.1111/j.1751-9004.2011.00408.x

Dunkle, J. H., & Friedlander, M. L. (1996). Contribution of therapist experience and personal characteristics to the working alliance. *Journal of Counseling Psychology, 43*, 456.

Edwards, W. M., & Coleman, E. (2004). Defining sexual health: A descriptive overview. *Archives of Sexual Behavior, 33*, 189–195.

Elmore, A. (2016). Empirically supported treatments: Precept or percept? *Professional Psychology, Research and Practice, 47*(3), 198–205.

Epstein, S. (2006). The new attack on sexuality research: Morality and the politics of knowledge production. *Sexuality Research and Social Policy Journal of NSRC, 3*, 1–12. https://doi.org/10.1525/srsp.2006.3.1.01

Erekson, D. M., Janis, R., Bailey, R. J., Cattani, K., & Pedersen, T. R. (2017). A longitudinal investigation of the impact of psychotherapist training: Does training improve client outcomes? *Journal of Counseling Psychology, 64*(5), 514–524.

Goldberg, S. B., Rousmaniere, T., Miller, S. D., Whipple, J., Nielsen, S. L., Hoyt, W. T., et al. (2016). Do psychotherapists improve with time and experience? A longitudinal analysis of outcomes in a clinical setting. *Journal of Counseling Psychology, 63*(1), 1–11.

Goodman, A. (2001). What's in a name? Terminology for designating a syndrome of driven sexual behavior. *Sexual Addiction and Compulsivity, 8*(3–4), 191–213.

Grant, J. E., Atmaca, M., Fineberg, N. A., Fontenelle, L. F., Matsunaga, H., Reddy, Y. C. J., et al. (2014). Impulse control disorders and "behavioural addictions" in the ICD-11. *World Psychiatry: Official Journal of the World Psychiatric Association, 13*(2), 125–127.

Grubbs, J. B., Exline, J. J., Paragament, K. I., Hook, J. N., & Carlisle, R. D. (2015). Transgression as addiction: Religiosity and moral disapproval as predictors of perceived addiction to pornography. *Archives of Sexual Behavior, 44*, 125–136. https://doi.org/10.1007/s10508-013-0257-z

Grubbs, J. B., & Perry, S. L. (2018). Moral incongruence and pornography use: A critical review and integration. *Journal of Sex Research* (online first). https://doi.org/10.1080/00224499.2018.1427204

Guttmacher Institute. (2012). *State policies in brief: Sex and HIV education*. New York, NY: Author.

Gyani, A., Shafran, R., Rose, S., & Lee, M. J. (2015). A qualitative investigation of therapists' attitudes towards research: Horses for courses? *Behavioural and Cognitive Psychotherapy, 43*, 436–448.

Hammack, P. L., Mayers, L., & Windell, E. P. (2013). Narrative, psychology and the politics of sexual identity in the United States: From "sickness" to "species" to "subject". *Psychology and Sexuality, 4*, 219–243. https://doi.org/10.1080/19419899.2011.621131

Hansson, S. O. (2018). Dealing with climate science denialism: Experiences from confrontations with other forms of pseudoscience. *Climate Policy, 1*, 1–9.

Harrison, T. (2005). Availability of emergency contraception: A survey of hospital emergency department staff. *Annals of Emergency Medicine, 46*(2), 105–110. https://doi.org/10.1016/j.annemergmed.2005.01.017

Hasin, D. S., O'Brien, C. P., Auriacombe, M., Borges, G., Bucholz, K., Budney, A., et al. (2013). DSM-5 criteria for substance use disorders: Recommendations and rationale. *The American Journal of Psychiatry, 170*(8), 834–851.

Hayes, S., & Carpenter, B. (2012). Out of time: The moral temporality of sex, crime, and taboo. *Critical Criminology, 20*, 141–152. https://doi.org/10.1007/s10612-011-9130-3

Hertlein, K. M., & Lambert-Shute, J. (2007). Factors influencing student selection of marriage and family therapy graduate programs. *Journal of Marital and Family Therapy, 33*(1), 18–34.

Hobaica, S., & Kwon, P. (2018). "This is how you hetero:" sexual minorities in heteronormative sex education. *American Journal of Sexuality Education, 12*, 423–450. https://doi.org/10.1080/15546128.2017.1399491

Hoefer, S. E., & Hoefer, R. (2017). Worth the wait? The consequences of abstinence-only sex education for marginalized students. *American Journal of Sexuality Education, 12*, 257–276. https://doi.org/10.1080/15546128.2017.1359802

Hook, C. J., & Farah, M. J. (2013). Look again: Effects of brain images and mind-brain dualism on lay evaluations of research. *Journal of Cognitive Neuroscience, 25*(9), 1397–1405.

Huebner, D. M., Rebchook, G. M., & Kegeles, S. M. (2004). Experiences of harassment, discrimination, and physical violence among young gay and bisexual men. *American Journal of Public Health, 94*, 1200–1203. https://doi.org/10.2105/AJPH.94.7.1200

Iantaffi, A., Wilkerson, J. M., Grey, J. A., & Rosser, B. R. (2015). Acceptability of sexually explicit images in HIV prevention messages targeting men who have sex with men. *Journal of Homosexuality, 62*, 1345–1358. https://doi.org/10.1080/00918369.2015.1060066

IITAPllc. (2014, February 21). *Dr. Don Hilton speaking about the neuroscience of pornography #addiction. #IITAPSymposium*. Retrieved from https://twitter.com/iitapllc/status/436897536075239424

Ikeda, K., Kitagami, S., Takahashi, T., Hattori, Y., & Ito, Y. (2013). Neuroscientific information bias in metacomprehension: The effect of brain images on metacomprehension judgment of neuroscience research. *Psychonomic Bulletin & Review, 20*(6), 1357–1363.

Irvine, J. M. (1995). Reinventing perversion: Sex addiction and cultural anxieties. *Journal of the History of Sexuality, 5*, 429–450.

Joannides, P. (2012). The challenging landscape of problematic sexual behaviors, including "sexual addiction" and "hypersexuality". In P. Kleinplatz (Ed.), *New directions in sex therapy: Innovations and alternatives* (pp. 69–84). New York, NY: Routledge.

Karila, L., Wéry, A., Weinstein, A., Cottencin, O., Petit, A., Reynaud, M., & Billieux, J. (2014). Sexual addiction or hypersexual disorder: different terms for the same problem? A review of the literature. *Current pharmaceutical design, 20*(25), 4012–4020.

Kirby, D. (2007). Abstinence, sex, and STD/HIV education programs for teens: Their impact on sexual behavior, pregnancy, and sexually transmitted disease. *Annual Review of Sex Research, XVIII*, 143–177.

KonkolÿThege, B., Woodin, E. M., Hodgins, D. C., & Williams, R. J. (2015). Natural course of behavioral addictions: A 5-year longitudinal study. *BMC Psychiatry, 15*, 4.

Koob, G. F., & Le Moal, M. (2008). Review. Neurobiological mechanisms for opponent motivational processes in addiction. *Philosophical Transactions of the Royal Society of London. Series B, Biological Sciences, 363*(1507), 3113–3123.

Le Bodic, C. (2009). Masturbation and therapy: The example of treatment for perpetrators of sexual abuse. *Sexologies, 18*, 255–258. https://doi.org/10.1016/j.sexol.2009.09.003

Lewandowsky, S., & Bishop, D. (2016). Research integrity: Don't let transparency damage science. *Nature, 529*(7587), 459–461.

Ley, D. (2012). *The myth of sex addiction*. Lanham, MD: Rowman & Littlefield.

Ley, D. (2018). The pseudoscience behind public health crisis legislation. *Porn Studies* (online first). https://doi.org/10.1080/23268743.2018.1435400

Ley, D., Prause, N., & Finn, P. (2014). The emperor has no clothes: A review of the "pornography addiction" model. *Current Sexual Health Reports, 6*, 94–105. https://doi.org/10.1007/s11930-014-0016-8

Malan, M. K., & Bullough, V. (2005). Historical development of new masturbation attitudes in Mormon culture: Silence, secular conformity, counterrevolution, and emerging reform. *Sexuality and Culture, 9*(4), 80–127.

McCabe, D. P., & Castel, A. D. (2008). Seeing is believing: The effect of brain images on judgments of scientific reasoning. *Cognition, 107*(1), 343–352.

McFall, R. M. (1991). Manifesto for a science of clinical psychology. *The Clinical Psychologist, 44*(6), 75–88.

Meehl, P. E. (1957). When shall we use our heads instead of the formula? *Journal of Counseling Psychology, 4*(4), 268–273.

Miller, D. J., Spengler, E. S., & Spengler, P. M. (2015). A meta-analysis of confidence and judgment accuracy in clinical decision making. *Journal of Counseling Psychology, 62*(4), 553–567.

National Institute for Public Health and the Environment. (2017). Groupthink in Sex and Pornography "Addiction": Sex-Negativity, Theoretical Impotence, and Political Manipulation. In H. de Graaf Ciel Wijsen, (Ed.), *Sexual health in the Netherlands*. New York: Springer.

Ortmann, D. M., & Sprott, R. (2012). *Sexual outsiders: Understanding BDSM sexualities and communities*. Lanham, MD: Rowman & Littlefield.

Parker, E. O., Chang, J., & Thomas, V. (2016). A content analysis of quantitative research in journal of marital and family therapy: A 10-year review. *Journal of Marital and Family Therapy, 42*(1), 3–18.

Perkins, A., Ridler, J., Browes, D., Peryer, G., Notley, C., & Hackmann, C. (2018). Experiencing mental health diagnosis: A systematic review of service user, clinician, and carer perspectives across clinical settings. *The Lancet Psychiatry*. https://doi.org/10.1016/s2215-0366(18)30095-6

Popescu, M., Thompson, R. B., Gayton, W., & Markowski, V. (2016). A reexamination of the neurorealism effect: The role of context. *Journal of Science Communication, 15*(6), A01.

Popovic, M. (2006). Psychosexual diversity as the best representation of human normality across cultures. *Sexual and Relationship Therapy, 21*, 171–186. https://doi.org/10.1080/14681990500358469

Prause, N. (2017). Evaluate models of high-frequency sexual behaviors already. *Archives of Sexual Behavior, 46*(8), 2269–2274.

Prause, N., & Fong, T. (2015). The science and politics of sex addiction research. In L. Comella & S. Tarrant (Eds.), *New views on pornography: Sexuality, politics, and the law*. Santa Barbara, CA: Praeger.

Prause, N., Janssen, E., Georgiadis, J., Finn, P., & Pfaus, J. (2017). Data do not support sex as addictive. *The Lancet Psychiatry, 4*(12), 899.

Prause, N., Steele, V. R., Staley, C., Sabatinelli, D., & Hajcak, G. (2016). Prause et al. (2015) the latest falsification of addiction predictions. *Biological Psychology, 120*, 159–161.

Prior, E. E., Williams, D. J., Zavala, T., & Milford, J. (2016). *What do(n't) American undergraduate social work students learn about sex? A content analysis of sex positivity*. University of Windsor, http://www1.uwindsor.ca/criticalsocialwork/HBSEtextbooks

Pullum, A. (2017). Foul Weather Friends: Enabling Movement Alliance through an Intentionally Limited Coalition. *Social Currents, 5*(3), 228–243. https://doi.org/10.1177/2329496517725329
Racine, E., Sattler, S., & Escande, A. (2017). Free will and the brain disease model of addiction: The not so seductive allure of neuroscience and its modest impact on the attribution of free will to people with an addiction. *Frontiers in Psychology, 8*, 1850.
Reay, B., Attwood, N., & Gooder, C. (2013). Inventing sex: The short history of sex addiction. *Sexuality and Culture, 17*, 1–19. https://doi.org/10.1007/s12119-012-9136-3
Robinson, T. E., & Berridge, K. C. (2000). The psychology and neurobiology of addiction: An incentive–sensitization view. *Addiction, 95*(8), 91–117.
Rodda, S. N., Booth, N., Vacaru, M., Knaebe, B., & Hodgins, D. C. (2018). Behaviour change strategies for internet, pornography and gaming addiction: A taxonomy and content analysis of professional and consumer websites. *Computers in Human Behavior, 84*, 467–476.
Rosen, G. M., & Davison, G. C. (2003). Psychology should list empirically supported principles of change (ESPs) and not credential trademarked therapies or other treatment packages. *Behavior Modification, 27*(3), 300–312.
Rubin, G. (1984). Thinking sex: Notes for a radical theory of the politics of sexuality. In C. Vance (Ed.), *Exploring female sexuality* (pp. 267–319). Boston, MA: Routledge.
Satcher, D., Hook III, E. W., & Coleman, E. (2015). Sexual health in America: Improving patient care and public health. *JAMA, 314*, 765–766.
Schultz, W., Stauffer, W. R., & Lak, A. (2017). The phasic dopamine signal maturing: From reward via behavioural activation to formal economic utility. *Current Opinion in Neurobiology, 43*, 139–148.
Schweitzer, N. J., Baker, D. A., & Risko, E. F. (2013). Fooled by the brain: Re-examining the influence of neuroimages. *Cognition, 129*(3), 501–511.
Scott, J. (1998). Changing attitudes toward sexual morality: A cross-national comparison. *Sociology, 32*, 815–845.
Sloman, S. A., & Rabb, N. (2016). Your understanding is my understanding: Evidence for a community of knowledge. *Psychological Science, 27*(11), 1451–1460.
StaciSprout. (2017, September 24). *Technology gives us dopamine...highly addictive*! Retrieved from https://twitter.com/Stacisprout/status/912173274599014400
Thomas, J. N. (2013). Outsourcing moral authority: The internal secularization of evangelicals' anti-pornography narratives. *Journal for the Scientific Study of Religion, 52*, 182–206. https://doi.org/10.1111/jssr.12052
Thomas, J. N. (2016). The development and deployment of the idea of pornography addiction within American evangelicalism. *Sexual Addiction and Compulsivity, 23*, 182–195. https://doi.org/10.1080/10720162.2016.1140603
Thomas, J. N., Alper, B. A., & Gleason, S. A. (2017). Anti-pornography narratives as self-fulfilling prophecies: Religious variation in the effect that pornography viewing has on the marital happiness of husbands. *Review of Religious Research, 59*, 471–497. https://doi.org/10.1007/s13644-107-0301-x
Van Rooij, A., & Prause, N. (2014). A critical review of "internet addiction" criteria with suggestions for the future. *Journal of Behavioral Addictions, 3*(4), 203–213.
Voros, F. (2009). The invention of addiction to pornography. *Sexologies, 18*, 243–246. https://doi.org/10.1016/j.sexol.2009.09.007
Waller, G., & Turner, H. (2016). Therapist drift redux: Why well-meaning clinicians fail to deliver evidence-based therapy, and how to get back on track. *Behaviour Research and Therapy, 77*, 129–137.
Walton, M. T., Cantor, J. M., Bhullar, N., & Lykins, A. D. (2017). Hypersexuality: A critical review and introduction for the "sexhavior cycle". *Archives of Sexual Behavior, 46*, 2231–2251. https://doi.org/10.1007/s10508-017-0091-8
Whittier, N. (2014). Rethinking coalitions: Anti-pornography feminists, conservatives, and relationships between collaborative adversarial movements. *Social Problems, 61*(2), 175–193.

Williams, D. J. (2017). The framing of frequent sexual behavior and/or pornography viewing as addiction: Some concerns for social work. *Journal of Social Work, 17*, 616–623. https://doi.org/10.1177/1468017316644701

Williams, D. J., Christensen, M. C., & Capous-Desyllas, M. (2016). Social work practice and sexuality: Applying a positive sexuality model to enhance diversity and resolve problems. *Families in Society, 97*, 287–294. https://doi.org/10.1606/1044-3894.2016.97.35

Williams, D. J., Thomas, J. N., & Prior, E. E. (2015). Moving full-speed ahead in the wrong direction? A critical examination of US sex offender policy from a positive sexuality model. *Critical Criminology, 23*, 277–294. https://doi.org/10.1007/s10612-015-9270-y

Williams, D. J., Thomas, J. N., Prior, E. E., Wright, S., Sprott, R., et al. (2017). Sex and pornography "addiction": An official position statement of the Center for Positive Sexuality (CPS), National Coalition for sexual freedom (NCSF), and the alternative sexualities Health Research Alliance (TASHRA). *Journal of Positive Sexuality, 3*, 40–43.

Wilson, G. (2018, March 9). *Sex releases the highest levels of dopamine naturally available, equal to morphine & nicotine. Sex & addictive drugs (meth, cocaine) activate the same reward center neurons, which differ from other natural rewards. He should read Hilton's article.* Retrieved from https://twitter.com/YourBrainOnPorn/status/972119573502701568

Withers, M. C., Reynolds, J. E., Reed, K., & Holtrop, K. (2017). Dissemination and implementation research in marriage and family therapy: An introduction and call to the field. *Journal of Marital and Family Therapy, 43*(2), 183–197.

Zamboni, B. D., & Zaid, S. J. (2017). Human sexuality education in marriage and family therapy graduate programs. *Journal of Marital and Family Therapy, 43*(4), 605–616.

Chapter 17
The Tyranny of the Normal Curve: How the "Bell Curve" Corrupts Educational Research and Practice

Curt Dudley-Marling

Does the good of the many outweigh the good of the one? –
(Spock's mother, Star Trek IV [Nimoy, n.d.])

The idea that human behavior distributes more or less "normally" along the lines of a bell-shaped curve (the *normal curve*) has achieved the level of common sense in American popular culture as well as educational and social science research. It is generally assumed that various human traits cluster around the mean of a more or less *normal* distribution and, for many traits and abilities, people may be defined in terms of their relationship to the mean (or average). For traits like body size and temperament and mental health, for instance, average is typically presented as the ideal (i.e., normal) and people who fall outside the boundaries of normal for these traits are at risk for being stigmatized as *abnormal*. For traits like intelligence, appearance and athleticism, on the other hand, above average is most desirable while below average for these traits may lead to lower social status. Overall, the lens of normality affects how we see ourselves and others and how we organize our institutions including the institution of schooling.

The ideology of the normal curve is a foundational principle of modern schooling. The assumption that human behavior tends to fall along the boundaries of a bell curve, with most people clustering around the mean, affects how schools are organized, how students are taught and evaluated, who is included (and excluded) from the "normal" classroom curriculum, and how educational research is conducted and interpreted—particularly how educational research is used to inform classroom practice. There are, however, fundamental problems relying on norm-based research as a basis for educational decision-making. For starters, only truly random events distribute *normally*, and the behavior of human beings, unlike the roll of the dice or the flip of a coin, is never truly random. Moreover, making claims about individuals

C. Dudley-Marling (✉)
Lynch School of Education, Boston College, Chestnut Hill, MA, USA
e-mail: curt.dudley-marling@bc.edu

D. M. Allen, J. W. Howell (eds.), *Groupthink in Science*,
https://doi.org/10.1007/978-3-030-36822-7_17

based on group membership ignores the reality that the profiles of individuals frequently do not conform to group norms as I show below. The common practice of using data derived from norm-based research to make claims about individual students is an instance of the ecological fallacy that "admonishes us against making inferences about specific individuals based on aggregate data collected from the group to which those individuals belong" (Hlebowitsh, 2012, p. 2).

The normal curve—as applied to the behavior, traits, and abilities of humans—is a myth (Dudley-Marling & Gurn, 2010), an example of scientific groupthink that distorts the meaning of educational research, leading to practices that fail to meet the needs of individuals or subgroups of students whose profiles depart from group norms (e.g., kindergarteners, three-year olds, etc.). In this chapter, I critique the use of the normal curve as a foundation for educational research. I begin by briefly reviewing the research evidence showing that human behavior does not, in fact, distribute normally. This is followed by a discussion of how the ideology of the normal curve distorts educational research and practice. For instance, the use of "the norm" as a reference point for the behavior of individuals creates a vehicle of exclusion for students situated outside the boundaries of "normal" by conflating human differences with deviance. Moreover, the use of the norm as a proxy for group behavior effaces individual differences, obscuring a fundamental insight of the disability studies movement: it is normal to be different. Overall, modern schooling is saturated with the ideology of the normal curve which, by serving the mythical *normal* or *average* child, often meets the needs of no one in particular. Finally, this chapter considers the possibilities of an alternate lens for viewing human behavior that acknowledges the natural variability within groups of people (i.e., "it's normal to be different") as a foundation for organizing schools and conducting educational research.

Humans Are Not *Normal*

Herrnstein and Murray (1994), in their controversial text, *The Bell Curve*, described the normal curve as "one of nature's more remarkable uniformities" (p. 557). This perspective is widely shared by social scientists, educators, and the general public. As it turns out, however, a substantial body of evidence indicates that the normal curve is a poor representation of social reality that has led to "misguided educational theories, inferences, policies, and practices" (Walberg, Strykowski, Rovai, & Hung, 1984, p. 88).

Sir Francis Galton, one of the first people to advocate the use of the normal curve as a model of human diversity, also provided one of the earliest challenges to the universality of the normal curve. When Galton set out to gather a variety of empirical data to demonstrate the utility of the normal curve he found that, contrary to his expectations, the data for human traits like height, weight, strength, and eyesight failed to produce perfect normal distributions (Micceri, 1989). Similarly, Karl Pearson, a pioneer of modern statistical methods, concluded that, based on his own observations, a wide-range of phenomena—many cited as textbook examples of normality—did not produce normal distributions (Micceri, 1989). David Wechsler (1935) and Lee Cronbach (1970), major figures in the history of psychological assessment, also cautioned that psychological phenomena do not inherently distribute normally (Fashing & Goertzel, 1981). Geary (1947) went even further, recommending that all statistics textbooks begin with the statement, "Normality is a myth; there never was, and never will be, a normal distribution" (p.241). Although Geary (1947) conceded this statement was a bit of hyperbole, he argued that researchers should never take normality for granted. Indeed, over time, researchers have identified numerous examples of what Bradley (1968) called "bizarre distributions" of human behavior that depart substantially from a normal, bell-shaped distribution.

Despite these challenges to the normal curve as a representation of human behavior, the normal curve continues to exert a powerful influence on educational researchers and practitioners and social scientists more generally (Micceri, 1989). It may be that these individuals have been unduly influenced by the assumption that objective, well-designed achievement and ability tests *necessarily* produce normal distributions that are presumed to be representative of human behavior. Educators may assume, for example, that learning outcomes are normally distributed because achievement scores are presumed to distribute normally. However, achievement tests are "by tradition, custom, or conscious purpose . . . designed to produce such manifest distributions and are not necessarily indicative of the underlying latent [normal] distributions" (Walberg et al., 1984. p. 88). Moreover, the tendency of achievement and ability test data to distribute normally is, to some degree, "simply a mathematical and statistical effect" (Sartori, 2006, p. 415). Standardized educational tests, for example, rely on summated scaling techniques by which persons taking tests attempt to answer a large number of items and receive total scores corresponding to the number of items they answer correctly. This type of measurement has an inherent bias towards a normal distribution in that it is essentially an averaging process, and the central limit theorem indicates that distributions of means tend to be normally distributed (Fashing & Goertzel, 1981; Sartori, 2006). In other words, the average of averages tends to produce normal distributions even if the variables being measured do not distribute normally.

Even given the theoretical bias of objective tests toward normal distributions there is empirical evidence indicating that actual test scores "are seldom normally distributed" (Nunnally, 1978, p. 160). Micceri (1989), for example, examined the distributional characteristics of 440 large-sample achievement and psychometric measures obtained from journal articles, research studies, and national, state, and district tests. Major sources of test data included the California Achievement Test, the Comprehensive Test of Basic Skills, Stanford Reading Tests, Scholastic Aptitude Test (SAT), and the Graduate Record Exam (GRE). In all, Micceri's sample included 46 different test sources and 89 different populations. His analysis indicated that all 440 distributions he examined were "significantly non-normal" (p. 156). It seems that even educational tests designed to produce normal distributions do not necessarily produce such distributions in practice.

The evidence strongly indicates that only truly random events, like the throw of the dice or the flip of a coin, produce normal distributions. Human behaviors are always socially and culturally mediated and, therefore, never occur randomly, a conclusion supported by an overwhelming body of theory and research. Yet the myth of the normal curve as a model of human behavior continues to exert a powerful influence on theory and practice in education and the social sciences, an instance of scientific groupthink that misrepresents the human experience.

In the following sections I consider how the expectation that human behaviors distribute along the lines of a normal curve misleads educational researchers and practitioners.

How the Ideology of the Normal Curve Distorts Educational Research, Theory, and Practice

The expectation that human behaviors tend to distribute along the lines of bell-shaped, normal curve corrupts how educational researchers interpret their data and how policy makers and practitioners make use of these data. In the sections below, I consider how the myth of the normal curve subverts educators' understanding and use of data from research based on both descriptive and inferential statistics.

The Meaning of "Average"

Educational researchers and policy makers—and even the general public—find means (or averages) useful for describing student characteristics, including the academic performance of various groups and subgroups as well as trends in student achievement over time. For example, student achievement test data by school, school district—or even state or country—are routinely offered up as rough estimates of how well students are achieving in various jurisdictions. Further, disaggregating achievement test data by race or SES over a span of years is often used as a measure of how well schools are addressing historic inequities that have plagued American education and society more generally.

The utility of statistical averages as general indicators of student performance within and across various jurisdictions or within particular groups and subgroups is, however, dependent on the degree to which the mean is a reasonable proxy for the performance of particular groups, that is, a significant proportion of the given population clusters about the mean (the distribution is *normal*). However, the actual distribution of target populations is rarely known by practitioners or policy makers who use these data and, in any case, as the discussion above indicates, human behaviors cannot reasonably be expected to distribute along the lines of a normal curve. Student achievement, for example, is mediated by a host of factors including the curriculum, class size, teacher experience and expectations, and socioeconomic conditions, none of which is random, a prerequisite for producing a normal, bell-shaped distribution.

Even if achievement test data for groups or jurisdictions did, in fact, distribute along the lines of a bell curve—and, again, this is highly unlikely given the non-randomness of human behavior—the use of the statistical mean to describe the performance of groups of students would still obscure the variation that is always present within any human population. Critics of American education, for example, frequently cite international comparisons to support their claim that U.S. schools are failing to meet the nation's needs. *The Global Report Card*, a website created by the George W. Bush Institute, for instance, states that "the majority of American students are falling behind their international counterparts" and "the consequences to our country could be dramatic" ("The Global Report Card," 2014).The widely cited *Programme for International Student Assessment* (PISA) seems to support this claim. The latest PISA report indicates that U.S. schools rank 25th among OECD countries on various measures of academic achievement (PISA, 2015). While the PISA data certainly invite further scrutiny by policy makers, the relatively poor ranking of U.S. schools, based on statistical averages, masks the considerable variation within and across U.S. schools. For instance, data from the National Assessment of Educational Progress (NAEP), often referred to as the "nation's report card" on the health of American schools, show considerable variability within and across states. For instance, NAEP data indicate that, on average, Massachusetts schools significantly outperform schools in Louisiana in both reading and mathematics achievement (NAEP, 2013). Yet, there are many low-performing schools in Massachusetts and high-performing schools in Louisiana, facts obscured by state averages. Moreover, it is certain that the highest achieving schools in Louisiana outperform the lowest achieving schools in Massachusetts. It may even be the most successful schools in Lousiana outperform the most successful schools in Massachusetts. And, of course, the average performance of particular schools reveals little about the achievement of individual students.

The focus on the average performance of students across nations, states, school districts, and individual schools also masks how factors like poverty affect student achievement. Berliner's (2013) analysis of data from international comparisons, for instance, shows that U.S. students attending schools with relatively low poverty rates do very well compared to their counterparts in other countries. He concludes that, "it is quite clear that America's public school students achieve at high levels when they attend schools that are middle- or upper-middle-class in composition" (p. 7). On the other hand, children and youth attending schools where more than 50% of the children live in poverty do not do nearly as well and students attending schools where at least 75% of the student body is eligible for free and reduced price lunch do even worse. In these schools "academic performance is not merely low: it is embarrassing" (Berliner, 2013, p. 7). Nearly 20% of American children attend these high-poverty schools. But even Berliner's analyses of PISA data can be misleading since high achievers will likely be found in the lowest functioning schools—

and not all children are well served in even the most affluent, highest performing schools.

Some of these problems can be avoided by disaggregating data by groups (SES, for example) or using descriptive statistics that are more sensitive to the variability in any data set (e.g., quartile ranges). But, in the end, the fidelity of descriptive statistics is a function of the underlying distribution and, even then, group averages offer little insight into the behavior, characteristics or abilities of individual students. Writing over 80 years ago in the *Journal of Comparative Psychology*, Knight Dunlap (1935) warned of reporting data on the basis of what he referred to as the "average animal . . . an animal which is entirely mythical" (p. 1). Dunlap observed that in his "list of Great Experiments in Bad Psychology there is one research study in which the average value presented as significant is a value which every person in the experiment conspicuously avoided" (p. 2). Put differently, the statistical average for any particular group of people may apply to no one person in the group. In the context of educational research, the reliance on means to represent groups always risks mischaracterizing individual students, confounding curricular and policy decisions made on the basis of these data.

The Meaning of Mean Differences

Descriptive statistics like averages can be useful for highlighting trends in education or drawing attention to particular issues even if such measures tend to efface individual differences. However, absolute differences between and within groups and subgroups do not necessarily signify meaningful (i.e., non-random) differences. On the NAEP fourth-grade reading rankings for states, for instance, Massachusetts ranks first, Connecticut fourth, and the state of Washington ranks tenth, but it is quite possible that these differences are due to random factors and are, therefore, not meaningful (that is, not *statistically significant*). Nor do absolute differences in mean performance over time permit educational researchers to make strong claims about the efficacy of particular curricular innovations. In order to determine whether mean differences in academic performance between states are "significant" or if targeted instructional interventions are efficacious, educational researchers typically make use inferential statistics.

Consider the example of "best practices," a primary focus of much educational research aimed at identifying effective, evidence-based instructional practices for use in the classroom. The U.S. Department of Education's What Works Clearinghouse, for example, "reviews the existing research on different *programs*, *products*, *practices*, and *policies* in education . . . to provide educators with the information they need to make evidence-based decisions" (i.e., what *works*) (What Works Clearinghouse, 2017). Specifically, the What Works Clearinghouse focuses on "high-quality research," including the use of appropriate statistical analyses that, presumably, permits strong causal claims about the efficacy of particular instructional methods. Typically, this involves some sort of statistical test of mean differences such as analysis of variance, t-tests, and so on that enable researchers to make assertions about the relative effectiveness of specific interventions assuming researchers have designed studies that eliminate alternative explanations (rival hypotheses) for their results through the use of control groups, group matching, random assignment to groups, and so on.

However, the strongest claim that can be made for even the most carefully designed intervention studies is that particular interventions worked *on average*. In the typical case where specific educational programs or strategies have been found to be effective compared to one or more alternative interventions there is always variability in the data; specifically, no educational intervention has been found to be effective for all students and, indeed, there are always students in comparison groups whose achievement exceeds the mean performance of the experimental groups.

Effect size, a measure educational and other social science researchers routinely compute to determine the meaningfulness of statistically significant differences, is illustrative. Effect size is a useful metric since trivial differences between and within groups can sometimes achieve statistical significance especially with large sample sizes. For instance, an intervention that produced a trivial *improvement* in IQ of just one point could prove to be statistically significant given a sufficiently large sample size. Effect sizes provide a way to gauge the meaningfulness of statistically significant differences and, in the case of an IQ difference of a single point, the effect size would be quite small and, therefore, not meaningful.

Ultimately, effect size, given in standard deviation units, is a measure of variability although it is rarely interpreted that way. An effect size of 0.8, for example, which is considered "large" in social science research (Cohen, 1969), means that, in the theoretical case of a normal distribution, scores for 79% of the control group fall below the mean for the experimental or treatment group. A "large" effect size of 0.8 also means, however, that, again theoretically, 21% of the control group scored higher than the mean for the treatment group. A well-designed study of a reading intervention with a sufficiently large sample size that produced an effect size as large as 0.8 (standard deviation units) would almost certainly qualify as a *best practice*, for example, even though, in this hypothetical case, over 20% of the students in the control condition outperformed the average for the experimental group. Again, this is in the theoretical case where experimental and comparison groups produce normal distributions. In reality, where we can expect non-normal distributions for almost any group of students, the proportion of students for whom the intervention "worked" is, at best, uncertain. What is certain, however, is that even the strongest claims that can be made in support of the most effective educational practices must be qualified with reference to the variability that is always present in any student population, that is, no intervention will work for all of the children all of the time and even the most effective practice may not *work* for a significant proportion of students.

Making assumptions about the potential effectiveness of any practice for individual students based on group means is an instance of an ecological fallacy, an error in reasoning common in how researchers, practitioners, and policy makers interpret data from educational research (Hlebowitsh, 2012). For example, based on the assumption that best practices work for all or most students, teachers are being directed to teach curricula based on evidence-based practices (Every Student Succeeds Act [ESSA], 2015) with little consideration of students for whom *best practices* are not effective. If students fail to achieve in the presence of best practices the common assumption is that the problem lies in the student who lacks the ability or effort to succeed *normally* (see Dudley-Marling, 2004 for discussion of the social construction of learning failure). Additionally, in the all-too-frequent case where best, evidence-based practices are implemented prescriptively (e.g., Finn, 2009) teachers' professional discretion is circumscribed, making them less effective with students who do not conform to the norm (see Allington, Johnston, & Day, 2002).

Like the descriptive measure of average, tests of mean differences are based on the faulty assumption that human traits and behaviors distribute along the lines of a normal, bell-shaped distribution with most people clustering about the mean. The fetishization of the mean has the effect of masking the range of human differences that are always present in any population of students, perverting educational decision-making in the process.

Conclusion: It Is Normal to be Different

Recalling the quote at the beginning of this chapter, the idealization of the mean (or average), by obscuring the variability that is always present in any population of students, privileges the "good of the many," students presumed to be more or less average, over "the good of the one," students for whom the mean is a poor representation of their ability or performance. Normative data from even the most comprehensive and well-designed studies routinely mislead educators regarding the needs of individual students who tend not to conform to normative descriptions. This is a case of not being able to see the individual trees for the forest.

The antidote to the "tyranny of the normal curve" is for educators to shift their gaze from measures of normative tendencies to measures of variance. Difference is the norm when it comes to human affairs and this insight ought to change how we conduct and interpret educational research and how we assess and teach students. What about the students for whom "best practices" are not effective, for example? And, more to the point, what about the individual students sitting at desks and tables in elementary and high school classrooms across the country? What do they look like and what sort of instruction do they respond to? Toward this end schools need to create affordances for teachers to provide individual support and direction for students including the assessment of individual student needs and progress monitoring. Recognizing the variability that exists in any group of students also highlights the importance of encouraging teachers to draw on their professional knowledge and experience in support of student learning. It is worth noting that the conceit that there are *best*, research-based practices that should dictate praxis is not limited to education. The implementation of the best practice service model in medicine and counseling, for example, is widespread with the effect that the professional judgment of physicians and counselors is increasingly devalued.

"Best practices" and other data derived from norm-based research (and assessment) should, at best, be suggestive. Mandating "best practices" because they are research based ignores both the reality of individual needs and the critical importance of teachers' professional judgment. It also effaces the serious limitations of norm-based research practices. In reality the *best* practice is to reject the normal curve as a representation of human behavior. When it comes to the human experience, there is no such thing as a normal curve. It is difference that is the norm.

References

Allington, R. L., Johnston, P. H., & Day, J. P. (2002). Exemplary fourth-grade teachers. *Language Arts, 79*, 462–466.

Berliner, D. C. (2013). Effects of inequality and poverty vs. teachers and schooling on America's youth. *Teachers College Record, 115*(12). Date accessed: 2/17/2015 http://www.tcrecord.org/library/abstract.asp?contentid=16889

Bradley, J. V. (1968). *Distribution-free statistical tests*. Englewood Cliffs, NJ: Prentice Hall.

Cohen, J. (1969). *Statistical power analysis for the behavioral sciences*. New York, NY: Academic Press.

Cronbach, J. L. (1970). *The essentials of psychological testing*. New York, NY: Harper & Row.

Dudley-Marling, C. (2004). The social construction of learning disabilities. *Journal of Learning Disabilities, 37*(6), 482–489.

Dudley-Marling, C., & Gurn, A. (2010). Troubling the foundations of special education: Examining the myth of the normal curve. In C. Dudley-Marling & A. Gurn (Eds.), *The myth of the normal curve* (pp. 9–23). New York, NY: Peter Lang.

Dunlap, K. (1935). The average animal. *Journal of Comparative Psychology, 19*, 1–3.

Every Student Succeeds Act (ESSA) of 2015, Pub.L. No. 114-95. (2015). Retrieved from: https://www.gpo.gov/fdsys/pkg/BILLS-114s1177enr/pdf/BILLS-114s1177enr.pdf on January 13, 2016.

Fashing, J., & Goertzel, T. (1981). The myth of the normal curve: A theoretical critique and examination of its role in teaching and research. *Humanity and Society, 5*(1), 14–31.

Finn, P. J. (2009). *Literacy with an attitude: Educating working-class children in their own self-interest*. Albany, NY: SUNY.

Geary, R. C. (1947). Testing for normality. *Biometrika, 34*, 209–242.

George W. Bush Institute. (2014). *The global report card*. Available at globalreportcard.org

Herrnstein, R. J., & Murray, C. (1994). *The bell curve: Intelligence and class structure in American life*. New York, NY: Free Press.

Hlebowitsh, P. (2012). When best practices aren't: A Schwabian perspective on teaching. *Journal of Curriculum Studies, 44*(1), 1–12.

Micceri, T. (1989). The unicorn, the normal curve, and other improbable creatures. *Psychological Bulletin, 105*(1), 156–166.

National Assessment of Educational Progress (NAEP). (2013). *The nation's report card*. Washington, D.C.: National Center for Educational Statistics.

Nimoy, L. (Director), & Nimoy, L. (Writer). (n.d.). *Star trek IV – The voyage home* [Video file].

Nunnally, J. C. (1978). *Psychometric theory*. New York, NY: McGraw-Hill.

OECD. (2015). *PISA: Results in focus*. Available at https://www.oecd.org/pisa/pisa-2015-results-in-focus.pdf

Sartori, R. (2006). The bell curve in psychological research and practice: Myth or reality? *Quality and Quantity, 40*(3), 407–418.

Walberg, H. J., Strykowski, B. F., Rovai, E., & Hung, S. S. (1984). Exceptional performance. *Review of Educational Research, 54*(1), 87–112.

Wechsler, D. (1935). *The range of human abilities*. Baltimore, MD: William & Wilkins.

What Works Clearinghouse. (2017). *Find what works based on the evidence*. https://ies.ed.gov/ncee/wwc/. Accessed 15 Aug 2017.

Chapter 18
KETEK

John M. Norwood, Elizabeth Schriner, and Ah Young Wah

Background

The following interaction was not atypical in the 1990s and 2000s during the heyday of the pharmaceutical industry: "Hello, Doctor, I am your pharmaceutical representative for an exciting new drug. It has many, many positive aspects and has minimal to no side effects or drug interactions. May I have your commitment that you will prescribe this product?" That interaction could have, in fact, occurred several times daily in any physician's office. Into that milieu appeared Ketek (generic: telithromycin). The first in a new class of antibiotics, it was expected to be a blockbuster drug and a source of significant profit for its manufacturer. In one of the greatest scandals in the history of the U.S. Food and Drug Administration, enthusiastic approval of the medication led shortly to horror and deceit. Ketek no longer remains on the market today, but reverberations from its stormy background continue.

J. M. Norwood (✉)
Medicine-Infectious Disease, University of Tennessee College of Medicine, Memphis, TN, USA
e-mail: jnorwoo2@uthsc.edu

E. Schriner
Division of Quality of Life (QoLA), St. Jude Children's Research Hospital, Memphis, TN, USA

A. Y. Wah
Regional One Health – East Campus, Memphis, TN, USA

D. M. Allen, J. W. Howell (eds.), *Groupthink in Science*,
https://doi.org/10.1007/978-3-030-36822-7_18

FDA's Accelerated Approval Process

Historically, the FDA has been extraordinarily conservative after a pregnant Australian woman was given thalidomide in the 1950s and the fetus developed severe birth defects (Hamburg, 2012). For a drug to be approved, it must demonstrate that it is safe and effective in laboratory studies, animal models, and three phases of clinical trials in humans. From this data, detailed and complex statistical analyses can predict outcomes of release into general medical practice. These studies are done by pharmaceutical companies under the oversight of the United States FDA. If a product is successful in these trials, the sponsor may submit a new drug application (NDA). Once approved, the drug enters Phase IV clinical trials and is available for the general medical community; ongoing monitoring is required for years. This protracted review process is designed to allow ample time for investigation of the new agent. During the 1980s and 1990s, however, the human immunodeficiency virus (HIV) epidemic in the United States forced the FDA to speed up the process of drug approval given the urgent need to provide treatment for people with acquired immunodeficiency syndrome (AIDS) (Center for Disease Control, 2011). Given the success of HIV treatment regimens, the FDA accelerated approval of other drugs, which led to the removal of multiple medications from the market after significant problems were discovered post-release. For example, Vioxx, a well-known anti-inflammatory medication, was discontinued for public use after allegations of drug-related heart attacks and strokes surfaced. By the time of its removal, Merck had already sold billions of dollars of the medication worldwide (McIntyre & Evans, 2014).

Ketek (Generic: Telithromycin) Development

Unfortunately, the worsening resistance of bacterial infections in the late twentieth century has created an ongoing crisis in the availability of safe and effective antibiotic therapy. Erythromycin, a standard treatment for community-acquired pneumonia, a common bacterial infection, was introduced in 1957. It was mostly used for cases of pneumonia if the patient was allergic to penicillin or for cases involving organisms that would not be treatable with penicillin. Second generation macrolides, such as azithromycin and clarithromycin, were developed later by Pfizer and Abbott as similar but better tolerated antibiotics—with fewer drug interactions and a slightly broader spectrum of activity. These antibiotics prevent the development of certain key bacterial proteins by binding to bacterial structures called ribosomes (Fernandes, 2016). Telithromycin, brand name "Ketek," was manufactured by Hoechst Marion Roussel pharmaceuticals (later Sanofi-Aventis) as the first agent in a class of macrolide-like medications, which symbolized an exciting advancement in the war on antibiotic resistance. Ketek was made semi-synthetically by chemically adjusting the structure of erythromycin. Its structure allowed for binding at two points on the bacterial ribosome instead of one, which helped to prevent the development of bacterial resistance and benefited the effectiveness of the medication (Sanofi-Aventis, 2015).

Ketek Approval Delays in the United States Sanofi-Aventis submitted its Ketek new drug application (NDA) to the FDA on February 28, 2000, seeking consent for four indications (community-acquired pneumonia, acute bacterial sinusitis, acute bacterial exacerbation of chronic bronchitis, and pharyngitis), including a claim of effectiveness for drug-resistant Streptococcus pneumoniae. Shortly afterwards, Ketek was approved by the European Medicines Evaluation Agency. In April 2001, the FDA conducted its initial review of Ketek and its Anti-Infective Drugs Advisory Committee voted to deny approval for three of the four indications. The committee requested more safety and efficacy data for these claims, as early evidence in animal models revealed possible liver, heart, and visual side effects. Sanofi-Aventis responded in July 2002 with multiple Phase I studies and three Phase III studies, including the "Randomized, Open-Label, Multicenter Trial of the Safety and Effectiveness of Oral Telithromycin (Ketek) and Amoxicillin/Clavulanic Acid (Augmentin) in Outpatients with Respiratory Tract Infections in Usual Care Settings," also known as Study 3014 (Von Eschenbach, 2007). More than 1800 physicians enlisted in Study 3014, many of them new to clinical investigation. For each patient the provider enrolled, he or she earned up to $400. By the end of the recruitment period, more than 24,000 patients had enrolled (McGoey, 2012).

Here the details of Ketek's background grow murky, and many of the resulting lawsuits and congressional hearings focused their investigations on the events surrounding Study 3014. During these investigations, several healthcare providers and clinic personnel received punishments ranging from lost licenses and fines to prison time. There are still concerns about the level of involvement of the "big fish"—Sanofi-Aventis and the FDA. Did the pharmaceutical company submit fraudulent data knowingly? What prevented the FDA from effectively functioning during this process? Many lives were destroyed by Ketek, and so much of what happened next may have been preventable.

Ketek Enters the Market David Ross was one of the FDA physicians who reviewed Ketek's NDA in 2000 and denied approval pending further data. He reported receiving Study 3014, amongst other materials, in July 2002, and then attended a second federal advisory committee in January 2003 to discuss its findings. Around this time, a handful of FDA employees became aware of issues regarding Study 3014's data integrity. However, according to the testimony of FDA Commissioner Dr. Andrew von Eschenbach, inspections had only occurred at three of Study 3014's 1800 sites at the time of the second advisory committee's review. Small pockets of poorly-run clinical sites are not unusual. Therefore, Dr. Ross and the other members of the second advisory committee were not notified of Study 3014's integrity issues. In his later statement to the House Committee on Energy and Commerce, Dr. von Eschenbach (2007) defended this action:

> To avoid compromising any ongoing investigation, it is Agency policy not to publicly disclose even the existence of a pending investigation. Therefore, we could not discuss the data integrity issues of Study 3014 at the public Advisory Committee meeting. However, we also believed, based on the best information available to us, that the concerns applied to only one site out of more than 1800. It is not unusual for data from some sites to be eliminated from a study but to accept data from the other sites. At the time, there was less information about the other sites under investigation.

Unaware of Study 3014's faults, the committee voted 11-1 in favor of Ketek approval. Two weeks later, upon conclusion of its audits involving the first three clinical sites it investigated, the FDA issued an "approvable letter" to the drug manufacturer, which noted unresolved data integrity issues associated with Study 3014 and concerns about incomplete foreign safety data (von Eschenbach, 2007). When the advisory committee convened in March 2003 to discuss other matters, the FDA administrators briefly mentioned that an approvable letter had been issued to Sanofi-Aventis requesting "more information about data from Europe and Latin America" and that final approval also depended on open "inspectional issues" from Study 3014 (von Eschenbach, 2007). The manufacturer responded to the approvable letter in October 2003. As Dr. von Eschenbach (2007) described:

> The October 2003 submission addressed issues of Study 3014 and included post-marketing reports for spontaneous adverse events for approximately four million prescriptions for patients in other countries where Ketek had already been approved. Upon completing the review of the sponsor's October submission, including the findings from the additional audits of clinical trial sites summarized in a March 2004 memorandum from the Division of Scientific Investigations, *the Agency decided that it could not rely on Study 3014* to support approval of Ketek because of the systemic failure of the sponsor's monitoring of the clinical trial to detect clearly existing data integrity problems. Accordingly, Study 3014 was dropped for consideration in making the decision whether to approve Ketek. The Agency considered data from other clinical trials and the international post-marketing experience to conclude there was adequate evidence of safety.

Thus, on April 1, 2004, Ketek graduated to Phase IV trials and was released for public use. The drug was given three indications: acute bacterial sinusitis, acute exacerbation of chronic bronchitis, and mild to moderate community acquired pneumonia in adults. Ketek's official launch by Sanofi-Aventis advertised it as one of the most important innovations in antibiotic therapy. By 2005, its sales reached $193 million (Mathews, 2006).

Concerns Emerge Regarding Ketek-Associated Liver Damage

Seven months after its approval (February 2005), Ketek's success received its first blow when 26-year-old construction worker Ramiro Obrajero Pulquero walked into a North Carolina emergency room vomiting blood. Doctors diagnosed him with acute liver failure, but could not explain from where the young man had contracted it. He died three days later. His wife was shocked by the sudden nature of his death: "He was a healthy man, strong, and then suddenly we were watching him slip away"

(Mathews, 2006). The only abnormal event at the time of his admission appeared to be a recent nasal infection, treated with a cutting-edge antibiotic. Purported as an outlier by the FDA and Sanofi-Aventis, Mr. Obrajero's story did not reach the headlines. However, by January 2006, Dr. Kimberly Clay and colleagues from the same North Carolina hospital identified two other cases like Mr. Obrajero's. They submitted their findings for the March 2006 issue of the *Annals of Internal Medicine* (Clay et al., 2006). In an unheard-of move, Dr. Harold Sox, editor of the *Annals*, released the report online two months early. "I can't think of a specific instance where we have published a case report like this early," Dr. Sox said. Dr. John Hanson, one of the study's co-authors, added in an interview (Smith, 2006):

> We were stunned by the fact that we saw three cases in one medical center in a very short period of time. It was startling.

Though both Dr. Sox and Dr. Hanson recognized the possibility of coincidence, they felt compelled to report this finding to the wider medical community. "The sooner doctors know about this, the sooner they can take it into account in deciding whether to use the drug," Dr. Sox argued (Smith, 2006).

Shortly before the article's release, higher-ups in the FDA learned of Dr. Clay's findings and conducted an emergency meeting regarding Ketek's safety. The agency issued a public announcement on January 20, 2006, the same day Dr. Clay's report was published online. Incredibly, the announcement cited safety statistics from Study 3014 (despite being officially considered "unreliable" per Dr. von Eschenbach's statement) and supported the drug's approval (Ross, 2007).

FDA Internal Debate over Ketek Safety Critics of the Ketek scandal highlighted the inconsistencies in the FDA's position, which appeared to be less in the public's best interest and more in the interest of procuring revenue for the pharmaceutical company. At least four FDA officials—Dr. David Graham (who issued the earliest warnings about Vioxx, too), Dr. Charles Cooper, Dr. David Ross, and Dr. Rosemary Johann-Liang—provided emails and other statements expressing concerns over Ketek's safety to the *New York Times* in June 2006. Referring to Ketek's approval, Dr. Graham wrote: "It's as if every principle governing the review and approval of new drugs was abandoned or suspended where [Ketek] is concerned" (Harris, 2006). He continued:

> The FDA views industry as its client, and that's the only explanation here. The agency saw that it needed to align its interests with the company's, and the company's interest was 'get this drug approved.'

Dr. Cooper added concerns over the FDA's gratuitously forgiving relationship with Sanofi-Aventis: "Given [the company's] track record in which they have proven themselves to be nontrustworthy, [...] we have to consider the possibility that [the staff at Sanofi-Aventis] are intentionally doing a poor job of collecting the postmarketing data to protect their drug sales" (Harris, 2006).

Appalled at the "very serious" problems revolving around Ketek, Sen. Charles Grassley (R-IA) (Harris, 2006) noted later:

> It's no surprise to learn that the F.D.A. didn't listen to Dr. Graham [and Dr. Cooper] on the dangers of Ketek. The F.D.A. has made it their business to discredit [those] who aren't willing to cater to the drug companies.

Grassley told NPR interviewers: "There's got to be respect for the scientific process; and dissident scientists, that have a point of view that might not be the party line, have to be respected" (Silberner, 2006).

In response to the furor from its internal debate and Dr. Clay's article, the FDA did send out a "Dear Doctor" letter about Ketek-associated liver toxicity in June 2006. Over the next year, Ketek prescriptions plummeted and the FDA issued increasingly stronger warnings (Edwards, 2011). Details surrounding the FDA's growing repudiation of Ketek differ radically depending on who tells the story. To some, not only are the discredited clinical sites responsible for Ketek's subsequent fatalities, but the FDA and Sanofi-Aventis should have been held accountable, too. In February 2007, congress decided it would help clear up the matter. As hearing after hearing concluded, the seriousness of the situation was obvious. People were dying, and something had to be done.

David Ross and NEJM April 2007 In the *New England Journal of Medicine*'s April 2007 issue, David Ross, a former medical officer at the FDA and now a director for the Department of Veterans Affairs, published his perspective on the events surrounding Ketek's fall from grace. In it, he not only claimed to have evidence of fraudulent and ineffective clinical trials, he also indicated that the FDA had been aware of it since before Ketek's approval (Ross, 2007). He reported that FDA managers, in cahoots with Sanofi-Aventis personnel, were negligent in presenting Study 3014 to the second federal advisory committee without mentioning that the study's integrity was under criminal investigation. Specifically, Ross provided a timeline of misconduct and evidence of seemingly purposeful obfuscation, including e-mails and other internal pressure tactics in both the FDA and Sanofi-Aventis. He recalled a meeting with Dr. von Eschenbach in which the commissioner compared the FDA to a football team and threatened to "trade" any players that discussed Ketek's issues outside of the agency (Harris, 2007).

FDA Response April 2007 In the same *New England Journal of Medicine* issue, several key FDA administrators published a response to Ross' accusations. "Although the FDA did not rely on Study 3014 to support approval, we reviewed the study for safety findings that would have counted 'against the drug,' as is consistent with good review practice," noted Dr. Janice Soreth (Soreth, Cox, Kweder, Jenkins, & Galson, 2007). These administrators, like von Eschenbach, defended the public announcement made in January 2006. Dr. John Jenkins, director of the FDA's office of new drugs, told interviewers that the rate of liver-related problems looked "not all that different than we would see for other antibiotics for similar infections" (Mathews, 2006).

The overwhelming public response to Ross' article, however, was one of concern and mistrust. It was eventually revealed that five of the six authors of the FDA rebuttal received consulting fees from Sanofi-Aventis, according to a Wall Street Journal exposé. The sixth was an Aventis employee at the time of Study 3014″ (Mathews, 2006). It is too easy to imagine that such connections could have created bias; yet, whatever their motives, key FDA personnel continued to support Ketek.

FDA Investigation With such disagreement between Dr. Ross and the 2007 FDA rebuttal letter, what is the real story? Investigations by the agency and Sanofi-Aventis uncovered obvious "bad guys"—i.e. clinical sites that fabricated patient data and forged paperwork—who were prosecuted and fined or imprisoned. Yet, how could Sanofi-Aventis be unaware of such incredible breaches of research protocol? How could FDA administrators not realize the magnitude of the brewing crisis? Are the FDA's critics correct and the agency is now more interested in promoting the interests of Big Pharma instead of public health?

To ensure compliance with the Code of Federal Regulations (CFR), FDA employees conduct intermittent inspections of clinical trial locations. At the conclusion of these inspections, the FDA issues Form 483, which itemizes observations or areas that need to be addressed. Once higher FDA officials receive Form 483, they may send the clinical site a Warning Letter if they deem the observations serious violations. If the site supervisor's response to this letter is inadequate, the FDA opens an official investigation and sends a Notice of Initiation of Disqualification Proceedings and Opportunity to Explain (NIDPOE). When discrepancies involving Study 3014 arose, the FDA sent out these letters to several individuals, including Dr. Keith Pierce and Dr. Maria Anne Kirkman-Campbell.

Dr. Pierce's NIDPOE is an excellent example of the violations involving Study 3014. In it, he is charged with "repeatedly and deliberately submitting false information to the sponsor in a required report" (NIDPOE issued to Pierce, 2010). Specifically, his FDA observer noted the following issues involving the radiologist who was supposed to determine patient eligibility for the study:

1. The signatures on the 'radiologist interpretation worksheet' were forged, unbeknownst to the radiologist.
2. Several patients enrolled in the study did not qualify according to a comparison of the radiologist's initial report (which often showed findings like normal sinuses) and the 'radiologist interpretation worksheet' (which, for the same patient, listed mucosal thickening and even 'total sinus opacity' instead).
3. The radiologist reported potential for bias—he was asked to 'reread' some of the x-rays with the clinical investigator standing over his shoulder.

In addition, a chart review for some of the enrolled subjects revealed that their cases deviated from the study protocol. For instance, two patients received Rocephin and ciprofloxacin (both antibiotics), which were specifically prohibited during the trial duration. Another violation included failure to maintain accurate patient histories and medications (NIDPOE issued to Pierce, 2010).

Cisneros and Kirkman-Campbell Dr. Kirkman-Campbell's NIDPOE revealed similar, if not more extensive, deceit. In many ways, she became the face of the

Ketek scandal. Ann Marie Cisneros, a compliance officer from the clinical trial company Pharmaceutical Products Development (PPD) who monitored clinical sites for Sanofi-Aventis, testified about Study 3014's flaws and her investigation of Dr. Kirkman-Campbell before a congressional subcommittee on February 13, 2007. There were warning signs of fraud even before Cisneros personally visited Kirkman-Campbell's office, Cisneros admitted. For instance, the practice had enrolled over 400 patients, an enormous number considering it was located in Gadsden, Alabama (with a population just north of 36,000). No participants withdrew from the trial. Kirkman-Campbell's entire staff and most of her family were part of these highly-dedicated participants. Cisneros also unearthed consent forms that appeared to be forgeries (patients were enrolled at times and on days the office was closed) and patients with no history of conditions relevant to the study would suddenly manifest qualifying symptoms. She e-mailed her findings to her superiors at PPD and Sanofi-Aventis in 2002 (McGoey, 2012). Less than two years later, *the same year Ketek was approved for public use*, Kirkman-Campbell was sentenced to 57 months in prison and ordered to pay $925,000 in restitution to Sanofi-Aventis NIDPOE issued to Kirkman-Campbell, 2006). Again, critics question how such a gigantic misstep was possible—how it was that the FDA actively participated in a criminal investigation involving Ketek's safety data and still permitted its release to the general public.

When she testified before congress, Cisneros was stalwart about the deliberate obfuscation of falsified findings: "Mr. Chairman, I knew it. PPD knew it. And Aventis knew it" (House of Representatives, 2008). Douglas Loveland, one of the FDA criminal investigators who was assigned to the Ketek trial, supported Cisneros' statement but explained why Sanofi-Aventis could never be legally responsible for what happened. At the time of Cisneros' investigation, Sanofi-Aventis did respond to Cisneros' concerns, albeit ineffectively. If they had not, the cover-up could have clearly been prosecuted. However, the pharmaceutical company had records of the actions it took after Cisneros' investigation. Incredibly, Loveland explained, math was to blame for the company's failure to identify imminent catastrophe (House of Representatives, 2008):

> When you get into a traffic accident, you call a traffic cop. [Aventis] came in and they said, 'we have indicators of fraud,' and they called a mathematician. A mathematician didn't know what fraud looked like, and he couldn't identify it. He looked at all the data, couldn't figure out a rule to apply to the data set, came back and said, 'I don't see fraud.' They took that to convince themselves that two of the most serious allegations raised by Ms. Cisneros and by other PPD folks weren't indicators of fraud.

The next mistake Sanofi-Aventis made, Loveland testified, was to issue a "blizzard" of memos to the clinical sites involved in fraud. These memos were meant to address the glaringly obvious patterns of falsified information—the convenient diagnoses, inadequate histories, crossed-out or white-out forms, etc. After signing these memos, the clinical sites were considered "rehabilitated" and their cooperation was forwarded to the relevant oversight agencies. When questioned about their fraud-detecting processes, Sanofi-Aventis agreed its mechanisms were imperfect

(House of Representatives, 2008). Sloppiness, Loveland contended, led to the same flawed decision-making process as intentional fraud: a pharmaceutical company rushed their data (and any investigations of the merits of this information) and patients died. Fortunately for Sanofi-Aventis (and unfortunately for Loveland and his colleagues), the legal system does not equate the two missteps. The pharmaceutical company was acquitted of wrongdoing.

FDA Involvement and Response In 2011, a judge upheld Sanofi-Aventis' legal immunity (Edwards, 2011). The FDA, on the other hand, descended into a bitter civil war. After Dr. von Eschenbach's "teamwork" analogy, Dr. Ross and several of his colleagues left the agency. "Without significant changes to our drug safety system and FDA, we are certain to see more Keteks," Ross argued at his congressional hearing (House of Representatives, 2007). David Graham made a similar statement when his testimony helped force Merck to withdraw Vioxx. Graham supported Ross' brutal evaluation of the FDA's problems, as did Rep. Bart Stupak (D-MI): "One must ask, if the FDA is not protecting its client, the American people, whose interest is being protected?" (Richwine, 2007).

In his testimony, Dr. Ross alleged that Dr. von Eschenbach made at least 11 false statements to the House Oversight and Investigation subcommittee (House of Representatives, 2007). Though the FDA refuted these allegations in a letter to congress, Dr. von Eschenbach resigned in 2009 (Mundy, 2008). Despite the motivation for improvement one assumes these events would inspire, an even larger scandal involving the FDA surfaced a year later. A former employee for Cetero Research, a firm that conducted pharmaceutical trials internationally, reported record tampering and falsification of test data. From April 2005 to August 2009, Cetero participated in 1400 drug trials, all of which were suspect. At least 100 drugs had been approved based on these studies. Even today, the FDA refuses to release the names of these medications and many of them are still consumed regularly by patients worldwide (ProPublica, 2013).

Conclusion

So there it is—a story of murder and deceit. From the time of its approval in 2004 and David Ross' article in 2007, Ketek was prescribed over five million times. Over the past decade, numerous lawsuits have arisen, alleging negligent misrepresentation, defectively designing a medication, failure to warn consumers, deceptive advertising, and more. Questions remain—why was Ketek allowed to remain on the market, what role did Sanofi-Aventis and the FDA play in obfuscating the study flaws and safety data, and will the improvements made after the scandal be effective in preventing similar catastrophes?

One thing is clear: bad science has far-reaching consequences for patients, physicians, pharmaceutical companies, and researchers. Physicians rely on the FDA and pharmaceutical companies to provide evidence of efficacy and safety. Prescribing habits depend heavily on this data. As mentioned earlier, the Ketek scandal destroyed many lives. Healthcare providers unwittingly gave patients medication that killed them. Consumers trusted the FDA to protect them from dangerous products, not just ineffective ones. Everyone involved in Ketek's development, from the FDA to Sanofi-Aventis, underwent intense scrutiny. Several lost jobs or confidence in their employers. Some were even imprisoned.

However, experts cannot agree whether more stringent review processes and clinical trial guidelines will help or hurt the situation. The Ketek case represents a constant source of tension in medical research between new therapies and safety issues. In his book, *Antibiotics: The Perfect Storm*, Dr. David Shlaes (2010) explains:

> The science of discovering new antibiotics is exceedingly challenging and the economics of antibiotics are becoming less and less favorable. The regulatory agencies like the FDA are contributing to the problem with a constant barrage of clinical trial requirements that make it harder, slower and more costly to develop antibiotics. The pharmaceutical industry, under extraordinary financial pressures, is consolidating at historic rates leaving fewer and fewer large companies standing. The antibiotic market is not as promising as markets for treatment of chronic diseases like high cholesterol or chronic depression or high blood pressure. For those diseases which we cannot cure, the drugs must be taken for long periods of time, frequently for a lifetime. Antibiotics, which actually cure disease, are only taken for days or weeks.

Pharmaceutical companies must recuperate their costs for developing their products, and the development process is extremely expensive. Dr. Shlaes argues (and many healthcare providers and researchers agree) that making the clinical trial process even more complex could dry up the pharmaceutical pipeline for antibiotics. Ultimately, patients and providers may have to decide whether the benefits of these medications outweigh the risks, including the sometimes fatal outcomes surrounding innovation. To Mrs. Obrajero, David Ross, Ann Marie Cisneros, and the numerous other individuals whose lives were forever altered by Ketek, this choice may not seem like much of a choice at all.

The timeline of the rise and fall of Ketek:

- *February 2000*: Aventis submits NDA for Ketek, the first ketolide antibiotic.
- *June 2001*: The FDA declines to approve Ketek for certain indications and requests more safety and efficacy data.
- *October 2001*: Sanofi-Aventis begins enrolling patients in Study 3014. By January 2002, Dr. Marie Anne Kirkman Campbell has already recruited 287 patients.
- *February 2002*: Sanofi-Aventis manager Nadine Grethe gets an email from Pharmaceutical Products Development, which coordinated the clinical trial. The e-mail warns of potential fraudulent activity at Dr. Campbell's location.
- *July 2002*: Sanofi-Aventis submits the completed results of Study 3014 to the FDA, including 407 patients from Dr. Campbell's location.
- *October 2002*: An FDA inspector visits Dr. Campbell's site and notes several protocol violations. Shortly afterwards, inspectors visit Dr. Carl Lange in Illinois and Dr. Egisto Salerno in San Diego. These three providers enrolled the greatest number of patients and all had major safety issues in their data.

- *January 2003*: Dr. David Ross and the second advisory committee meet to consider the Study 3014 data, unaware of the ongoing fraud investigation. The panel votes 11–1 to approve Ketek. The FDA issues an "approvable letter."
- *April 2003*: Dr. Campbell is indicted for fraud and sentenced to 57 months in prison.
- *April 2004*: The FDA approves Ketek, officially not relying on Study 3014 for safety data.
- *February 2005*: Ramiro Obrajero Pulquero dies from Ketek-associated liver failure.
- *January 2006*: Dr. Kimberly Clay of the Carolinas Medical Center publishes about Mr. Obrajero and other possible liver complications in the *Annals of Internal Medicine*. The same day, the FDA issues a public safety announcement citing safety data from Study 3014.
- *April 2006*: The FDA has received 110 reports of adverse events associated with Ketek, including 23 cases of acute liver injury, 12 cases of liver failure, and four deaths, as well as blurred vision and other problems.
- *June 2006*: Four FDA safety investigators express their concerns over Ketek in the *New York Times*. Eventually, the FDA agrees to send out a "Dear Doctor" letter to alert providers about possible liver injury in cases involving Ketek.
- *February 2007*: One day before a congressional hearing on its handling of Ketek, the FDA finally issues a black box warning, the strongest type of safety guidance, for the antibiotic.
- *April 2007*: David Ross publishes his perspective on the FDA's involvement in the Ketek scandal in the *New England Journal of Medicine.* The FDA publishes a response letter in the same issue (Fig. 18.1).

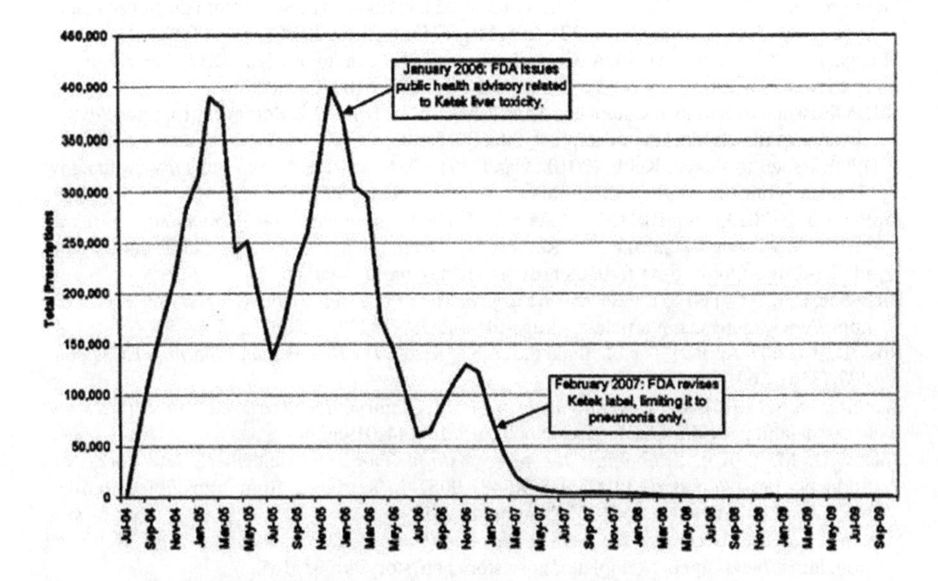

Fig. 18.1 Number of Ketek prescriptions over time. Edwards (2011)

References

Centers for Disease Control and Prevention. (2011, January 10). *HIV and AIDS timeline*. Retrieved from https://npin.cdc.gov/pages/hiv-and-aids-timeline

Clay, K. D., Hanson, J. S., Pope, S. D., Rissmiller, R. W., Purdum, P. P., & Banks, P. M. (2006, March 21). Brief communication: Severe hepatotoxicity of Telithromycin: Three case reports and literature review. *Annals of Internal Medicine, 144*(6), 415–420. https://doi.org/10.7326/0003-4819-144-6-200503210-00121

Edwards, J. (2011, February 18). FDA Approved an Antibiotic Based on Bogus Data – But the Courts Don't Care. *CBS News*. Retrieved from https://www.cbsnews.com/news/fda-approved-an-antibiotic-based-on-bogus-data-but-the-courts-dont-care/

Fernandes, P. (2016, August 22). The solithromycin journey – It is all in the chemistry. *Bioorganic & Medicinal Chemistry, 24*(24), 6420–6428. https://doi.org/10.1016/j.bmc.2016.08.035

Hamburg, M. (2012, February 7). *50 years after thalidomide – Why regulation matters*. FDA. Retrieved from https://blogs.fda.gov/fdavoice/index.php/2012/02/50-years-after-thalidomide-why-regulation-matters/

Harris, G. (2006, July 19). Approval of antibiotic worried safety officials. *New York Times*. Retrieved from https://www.nytimes.com/2006/07/19/health/19fda.html

Harris, G. (2007, June 11). Potentially incompatible goals at FDA. *New York Times*. Retrieved from https://www.nytimes.com/2007/06/11/washington/11fda.html

House of Representatives, 110th Cong. (2007). *The adequacy of FDA to assure the safety of the nation's drug supply. Hearings before the subcommittee on oversight and investigations of the committee on energy and commerce.*

House of Representatives, 110th Cong. (2008). *Ketek study fraud: What did Aventis know. Hearings before the subcommittee on oversight and investigations of the committee on energy and commerce.*

Mathews, A. W. (2006, May 1). Fraud, errors taint key study of widely used Sanofi drug. *Wall Street Journal*. Retrieved from https://www.wsj.com/articles/SB114644463095840108

McGoey, L. (2012). The logic of strategic ignorance. *The British Journal of Sociology, 63*(3), 553–576. https://doi.org/10.1111/j.1468-4446.2012.01424.x.

McIntyre, W. F., & Evans, G. (2014). The Vioxx® legacy: Enduring lessons from the not so distant past. *Cardiology Journal, 21*(2), 203–205. https://doi.org/10.5603/CJ.2014.0029

Mundy, A. (2008, Dec 15). FDA Commissioner Eschebach to Resign. *Wall Street Journal*. Retrieved from https://www.wsj.com/articles/SB122938610079708825

NIDPOE issued to Kirkman Campbell, Anne. (2006, May 18). FDA. Retrieved from http://www.circare.org/fdawls3/kirkman-campbell_20060518.pdf

NIDPOE issued to Pierce, Keith. (2010, March 17). FDA. Retrieved from https://www.fda.gov/RegulatoryInformation/FOI/ElectronicReadingRoom/ucm206820.htm

ProPublica. (2013, April 15). *FDA let drugs approved on fraudulent research stay on the market*. Retrieved from https://www.propublica.org/article/fda-let-drugs-approved-on-fraudulent-research-stay-on-the-market

Richwine, L. (2007, Feb 13). *FDA reviews urge action to fix drug safety*. Reuters. Retrieved from https://www.reuters.com/article/us-drugs-fda-s-idUSN1322731520070214

Ross, D. B. (2007, April 9). The FDA and the case of Ketek. *The New England Journal of Medicine, 2007*(356), 1601–1604.

Sanofi-Aventis. (2015). *Ketek: Highlights of prescribing information*. Retrieved from https://www.accessdata.fda.gov/drugsatfda_docs/label/2015/021144s019lbl.pdf

Shlaes, D. M. (2010). *Antibiotics: the perfect storm*. Dordrecht/Heidelberg/New York, NY: Springer. https://doi.org/10.1007/978-90-481-9057-7. Retrieved from https://bfosinfo.files.wordpress.com/2010/09/9048190568antibiotics.pdf

Silberner, J. (2006, December 16). *FDA to leave antibiotic Ketek on the market*. NPR. Retrieved from https://www.npr.org/templates/story/story.php?storyId=6635165

Smith, M. (2006, January 20). Three severe liver damage cases linked to ketolide antibiotic." *Medpage Today*. Retrieved from https://www.medpagetoday.com/gastroenterology/generalhepatology/2525

Soreth, J., Cox, E., Kweder, S., Jenkins, J., & Galson, S. (2007, April 19). Ketek – the FDA perspective. *The New England Journal of Medicine, 356*(16), 1675–1676.

Von Eschenbach, A.C. (2007, March 22). *The future of FDA's drug safety program*. FDA. Retrieved from https://wayback.archive-it.org/7993/20170723044140/https://www.fda.gov/NewsEvents/Testimony/ucm154072.htm

Chapter 19
Wildlife Contraception and Political Cuisinarts

Jay F. Kirkpatrick and John W. Turner Jr.

Introduction

New ideas, particularly in the sciences, often elicit strong responses. These run the gamut from rational to dogmatic. This is true even for ideas that have been proven and validated. A variety of organizations, all with sizable constituencies and bearing burdens founded in culture, politics, economics and bureaucracy often feel threatened by new advances because of possible impact on the agendas that serve their own memberships. While their concerns differ, the approach to discredit the new ideas is boringly similar: undermine the idea with purposeful distortions, out of context arguments, irrelevant comparisons and refusal to accept published science. But the results are always the same. At worst the public pushes back from the advances, and at best it becomes ambivalent.

Prior to human intervention, wildlife populations were controlled by the natural processes causing mortality. When animal populations exceeded the carrying capacity of their environment, the environment degraded and resident species died from starvation and disease. Coincidently, the high population density led to a decrease in reproductive success because in animals the age of first breeding was delayed, fewer offspring were produced and juvenile mortality increased.

Historically humans have imposed artificial mortality control upon wild populations through regulated hunting, trapping and poisoning. This was accepted as a normal and essential aspect of human survival. It remains a significant part of human culture and continues to be the primary management tool for some species. However, increasing urbanization, the withdrawal of private lands from the public hunting

---

J. F. Kirkpatrick (Deceased)
The Sience and Conservation Center, Billings, MT, USA

J. W. Turner Jr. (✉)
Department of Physiology & Pharmacology, University of Toledo College of Medicine, Toledo, OH, USA
e-mail: John.Turner@utoledo.edu

D. M. Allen, J. W. Howell (eds.), *Groupthink in Science*,
https://doi.org/10.1007/978-3-030-36822-7_19

domain, regulatory prohibitions on the use of poisons and trapping, low fur prices and changing public attitudes about lethal wildlife control have reduced the effectiveness of human-induced mortality control as a management tool. We presently face exploding populations of some highly adaptable or protected species but without acceptable management tools for protecting associated environment and animals alike. These events and factors are generally recognized as the impetus behind the emergence of the concept of wildlife fertility control (Asa & Porton, 2005; Rutberg, 2013). The question was how to make it a reality. It seemed that the simplest and least controversial approach to solving the new problems of wildlife management would be the application of existing human hormonal contraceptives to wildlife. Well, nothing is so simple, and the scientists who embarked on this journey to develop new technology and begin applying it might just as well have become involved in the global warming, gay marriage, gun control and universal healthcare issues.

An almost humorous dimension of this is that those same scientists had entered eagerly into this endeavor simply to solve a societal problem. They knew from the start that this endeavor, successful or not, was not a profit-making venture. It was an effort to face the fact that the ever-expanding human population was compressing wildlife space into limited islands of habitat. The options for quelling this rising tide were three: kill, remove (to where?) or slow down reproduction rates. The first was considered unacceptable, the second would run out of space and the third stood alone as logical (Kirkpatrick & Turner, 1985, 1991).

The pursuit of this arcane science, i.e. wildlife contraception, started with hormonal steroids such as used in human birth control, but the key technological breakthrough occurred about 1990 when vaccine-based contraception replaced traditional steroid-based approaches. Very quickly success with a porcine zona pellucida (PZP)–based vaccine was demonstrated in wild horses (Kirkpatrick, Liu, & Turner 1990), white-tailed deer (McShea et al., 1997; Turner, Liu, & Kirkpatrick, 1992), feral burros (Turner, Liu, & Kirkpatrick, 1996), captive exotic species in zoos (Kirkpatrick, Zimmermannn, Kolter, Liu, & Turner, 1995) and a bit later with African elephants (Fayrer-Hosken, Grobler, Van Altena, Kirkpatrick, & Bertschinger, 2000) and bison (Duncan, King, & Kirkpatrick, 2013). To the surprise and chagrin of the researchers, objections were raised. The two species that evoked the loudest cries were wild horses and urban deer.

Wild Horses

In the case of wild horses, opposition initially arose within wild horse advocacy groups, notably large and politically active organizations. These groups based their objections not on specific scientific arguments, but rather on the wishful thinking that a large, fecund adaptable wild species could be left unmanaged on public lands used for a wide spectrum of purposes, mostly driven by economic interests. A major complicating factor was the passage of the Free-Roaming Wild Horse and Burro Act of 1971, which imparted almost complete protection to these animals without a hint of effective management.

Predictably, these highly fecund wild horse populations grew from an estimated 17,000 in 1971 to somewhere between 60,000 and 80,000 by the early 1980s. With a myopic view of reality, the interest groups argued for no management under the delusion of self-regulation (which translates into range destruction and starvation), or by predation (despite the absence of effective predation on wild horses in most horse ranges). They also argued that if the economically valuable cattle and sheep were removed from public lands, there would be more habitat for wild horses. However, despite horses representing less than 10% of mouths grazing public land, their lack of economic value made them a ready target.

The opening barrage of opposition to horse population management was not very successful from a legislative standpoint, but litigation and a variety of legal actions became the norm and consequently stalled progress in contraceptive management. The federal government, largely represented by the Bureau of Land Management, installed in 1973 a management system known as Adopt-A-Horse, in which large numbers of horses were captured through helicopter round-up and then removed from the range for adoption of younger ones by the public. Horse injury and mortality were common, and tensions grew between the government and advocacy groups, fueling more litigation. Aside from the questionable humane aspects of this approach, it was neither logistically nor economically successful in keeping up with reproduction on the range (Bartholow, 2008). Lagging adoptions resulted in "surplus" horses that had to be quartered, fed and cared for, and currently there are more than 60,000 wild horses in long-term holding facilities. The annual cost to the taxpayer was more than $75 million in 2013 (De Seve & Boyles-Griffin, 2013) and has continued to rapidly rise to the present.

This management inadequacy combined with encouragement for population control by the National Academy of Sciences provoked some moderate interest by the BLM in fertility control. Between 1977 and the present, the agency has provided varying levels of financial support for the advancement and application of contraceptive technology. However, as time went by, outside demands to expand the application of fertility control became more strident. Intransigence and even opposition to fertility control grew within the agency (National Academy of Science Reports, 1980 and 2013). In fact, despite a clear statement in the 2013 NAS Report that the BLM needed to apply contraception intensively, little change in application rate has occurred to date.

In order to understand the lack of an organized front in moving to a new BLM management paradigm, one has to examine the administrative structure of BLM. Each of the ten western states with wild horses has a state office under the administration of a politically appointed state director. Quite often these directors are appointed for their ability to manage (facilitate) economic uses of public lands (e.g., livestock grazing, mining, energy development and a plethora of recreational uses). Also, each state director is more or less a free agent, and unless their policies are outright illegal, no one in Washington can challenge them. Some state directors were open-minded and sympathetic to the wild horse plight and some were not, thus there was no coordinated forward movement across the west.

Within each state there are numerous herd management areas (HMAs), each with its own personnel with the responsibility for managing the horses in their HMA. Often consensus on this subject did not exist across HMAs, even within a particular state. Some opposition came from the HMA field managers and was culturally based. A spoken theme delivered to the scientists on numerous occasions by these field managers and crew explained that "we don't do it that way out here; we do it with saddle-horses and ropes." They failed to mention the helicopters that were central to round ups, but their point was clear. This cultural perspective impeded progress.

The Washington and Reno offices of the BLM, which ostensibly oversee all dimensions of the wild horse program, were more or less detached from the realities of the field operations. They too had their conflicts with which to deal. For example, several ranching families throughout the west made millions of dollars annually rounding up wild horses under contract to the BLM. These contracted operations merely mocked the fertility control approach in the early years, but as its application spread, they became vocal opponents. Fertility control was an approach that might cut into the considerable public dollars flowing into their businesses. Some published newsletters complaining about fertility control, and in the Washington (DC) and Reno offices there were those who were sympathetic to keeping the contracted services happy.

As the horse number grew, few state BLM offices paid much attention to the DC/Reno oversight of the program. In 2009 the Washington office sent out a memo to all state offices and HMAs making it clear that when a round-up occurred, any horses to be returned to the range were to be treated with a contraceptive vaccine. A week after the memo went out, an HMA in one western state simply went on the electronic media to declare that this approach did not work, and they would not use it.

Additional cultural and political resistance developed in the central offices. By 2012 one very effective contraceptive vaccine (PZP) was federally approved by EPA and the registration was held by the world's largest animal welfare organization. This particular organization had a history of conflict with the BLM (including instances of litigation), and old wounds were opened. Thus, the DC/Reno offices began to reject fertility control or at least make it difficult to apply, largely because they were disaffected with the organization that held the vaccine registration. One excuse was that BLM did not have the money with which to train BLM personnel to use the vaccine, as required by EPA. Another was that they had problems storing and preparing the vaccine, despite the routine nature of that. A third argument was that too much federal paperwork was required for site-specific permission to use it.

A different version of discontent came from the ranching community. Once again there was little in the way of agreement in this realm. A large segment of the ranching industry, represented primarily by those who used the public lands for grazing, opposed fertility control because they wanted horse removal rather than stewardship. Some in the ranching community were more sympathetic and supported fertility control. A good example of the former was seen with litigation in

2015 by a group of Nevada ranchers who demanded that all horses rounded up be permanently removed, which would indirectly prevent contraceptive use. Various iterations of this approval have been applied on the basis that federal law provides an upper limit for horse numbers on each herd area.

The law requires that a given population exceeding its assigned appropriate management level (AML) be reduced to that level and maintained there or below it. BLM has attempted to do this almost exclusively by removal of horses and has failed overall. The program-wide horse numbers on the range in 2019 are rapidly approaching 90,000 in the face of an agency goal of 35,000. This situation exists despite BLM's own funding of research yielding significant PZP vaccine improvements (e.g., Turner et al., 2008; Turner, Liu, Flanagan, Bynum, & Rutberg, 2002) and the regular pleas of the science community for the past 25 years to incorporate aggressive program-wide vaccine contraception into wild horse management.

A good example of this was published in 2013 in the widely read journal *Science* (Garrott & Oli, 2013). Unfortunately, and despite such appeals, since 2017 the agency has taken a mantra-like stance of "remove to AML, before any contraception." This position creates a quandary, since AML has been unavailable for many HMA's despite the effort. The fact is that a coincident combination approach of some (e.g., 50%) "catch/removal" and some (e.g., 50%) "catch/contraception/release" is the solution supported by data-based modelling. This information in various forms has been provided to the agency since 2012. At this point the cost either way is monumental.

As a retrospective on how damaging culture and politics can be to scientific progress and outcome application, it is noteworthy that the National Park Service began using vaccine contraception as the lone management tool for the wild horse population on Assateague Island National Seashore in 1994 and has successfully continued this form of management to the present (Kirkpatrick & Turner, 2008). While identical vaccine application eventually occurred in select small wild horse populations in the western United States, it required 8 years of regular pestering. It has been highly successful but has required the concerted effort of a few committed BLM field managers and local citizens. In other words, the BLM is not embracing it.

In deference to the agency, many herd areas (HMAs) contain horse numbers in the many hundreds that are not readily accessible by darting. However, the BLM has known since 2004 (because BLM funded the research) that a one-injection vaccine with 1–2 years of effectiveness was available for treating the many gathered mares that were returned to the range, thus preventing thousands of foals. BLM instead treated only as a small percentage, expressing various "reasons" but again not embracing contraception. The long delay in BLM approval and the continued limited acceptance of contraception in DC and Reno again have reflected the power of misinformation and personal, cultural and political bias.

It is worth noting that the relative autonomy at the local and state level of the agency has more enabled status quo rather than progress in horse population management. On the other hand it is not fair to fault the many employees who are doing the best they can in the face of the local realities they deal with, i.e., ranchers, horse advocates, habitat advocates, recreationists, anti-government souls, loonies and the paperwork and logistics of multi-tasking land stewardship. As with any organization, some folks are dedicated and some are just seeing a job. However, the byzantine nature of the agency does not foster timely progress. As is the case with most giant organizations, bureaucracy is the gun with which the agency shoots itself in the foot.

Going back to the subject of logic regarding wild horse control, it is ironic that with only a few exceptions, the wild horse advocacy groups reversed track by 2010 and began to support fertility control. This reversal was based on their realizing that the only three choices were (1) range destruction/starvation, (2) round up and removal or (3) fertility control. Predation, self-regulation and disappearance of livestock were simply never going to happen. Thus, they embraced fertility control by default. That reversal, while friendly to the fertility control paradigm, only seemed to increase the polarization with the larger BLM (if the advocates like it, we do not!)

The optimistic beginning to a perceived solution for regulating wild horse populations by a small group of scientists trying to find a better and more humane future for innocent animals morphed into a cultural and political nightmare. No one was prepared for the firestorm that came from their efforts, and to date the solution remains within reach but unrealized. In April 2019 a document focused on "A Path Forward for Management of BLM's Wild Horses and Burros" was put forth by a coalition of 12 organizations of varying purpose to provide Congress and BLM with a clear picture of issues, approaches and a long-term view for addressing this crisis. Thus, the effort continues.

Urban Deer

The controversy surrounding urban deer fertility control is less convoluted than with horses but far more intense. Again, it caught the scientists by surprise. What could possibly be controversial about inhibiting reproduction in urban deer that are eating shrubbery, causing car accidents and damaging the remaining urban woodlands?

The possible application of fertility control for controlling urban deer populations via a contraceptive vaccine was first broached in 1988 at a Princeton conference, and reactions by managing agencies ranged from frowns to amusement. The managing entities consisted of state fish and game agencies, which by law are responsible for wildlife management in their respective states. Soon after the conference, several organizations (including a New Jersey arboretum, a public park in Philadelphia and a group of small communities on Long Island, NY) began lobbying for fertility control. The state agencies sobered a bit and began pushing back.

Initially their arguments against urban deer fertility control centered on a list of hypothetical biological consequences and to a lesser extent on the cultural philosophy that hunting was the only solution (Turner, 1997). Based on these objections, states in which projects were proposed (NJ, PA and NY) simply refused to issue permits to conduct any trials. Subsequently, Turner et al. (Turner et al., 1992) demonstrated that the PZP vaccine (same as used in horses) provided excellent contraceptive efficacy in captive white-tailed deer. Captive studies continued, and researchers requested permission to perform field trials in Metro parks where hunting is prohibited.

By this time, an unspoken undercurrent was developing in state wildlife agencies that contraceptive management of deer living in urban communities and city parks could somehow become a threat to recreational hunting. Driving that concern in part were declining hunting-license sales across the United States and the potential further loss of revenue if deer contraception expanded. While the agency revenue loss would be significant, the potential loss of ancillary revenue related to hunting would be enormous. Hunters buy weapons and gear, stay in motels, put gas into their vehicles, dine in restaurants, purchase ammunition, etc. This concern led the commercial facets of the hunting industry to take a stand against fertility control. The state agencies in turn blurred the lines between urban deer and truly wild deer in the forests. Opposition grew, and urban deer kept eating ornamental shrubbery.

However, states do not have jurisdiction over wildlife on federal lands, so the scientists found several federal field sites for testing the idea of managing urban deer without the need for state approval. The first was a trial at the Smithsonian Institute's Conservation and Research Center in Front Royal, VA. The trial was successful and generated useful data (McShea et al., 1997). The second test occurred in a group of small communities on Fire Island National Seashore (FIIS), in NY. This was a National Park Service (NPS) unit and beyond the legal jurisdiction of the state. As plans progressed, however, the state raised strident objections, all based on "biological" issues. By this time, counterparts in PA and NJ had also refused to allow fertility control to move forward and were beginning to coordinate their objections. It was clear that the issue was a powder keg and that other states were going to join in the effort to prevent urban deer fertility control.

Despite this, the project on FIIS went forward because of the federal classification. The New York Department of Environmental Conservation (DEC), realizing that the project seemed inevitable, threatened the NPS with a lawsuit to stop the project. The NPS, through its regional science office, responded with a terse message that challenged NY to see who really did have authority there. Cooler heads prevailed in Albany and the project went forward. To illustrate the degree of threat seen by state agencies, it is notable that the head of the New Jersey fish and game agency threatened to sue New York for allowing the project to get underway. No action was taken, but it indicated the seriousness with which states viewed fertility control as a threat.

The NPS and even the scientists were also soon informed of a possible lawsuit by a collection of hunting groups on Long Island. While nothing came of that, it signaled the entrance of the larger hunting community into the fray. In the end the project went forward and after 17 years of fertility control the deer population in these communities was reduced by 70% without the removal of a single deer (Naugle, Rutberg, Underwood, Turner, & Liu, 2002; Rutberg, Naugle, Turner, Fraker, & Flanagan, 2013, Rutberg, Naugle, & Verret, 2013; Rutberg & Naugle, 2008). The published data were to become a thorn in the side of all the concerned state agencies. By 1993 the state agencies publicly opposed deer contraception. At the Third International Conference on Fertility Control in Wildlife (Denver, CO), the agencies showed up in force. They were careful to not emphasize the subject of hunting in city parks, instead focusing on modeling (not data-based) with a bias against contraception.

Despite this opposition, a third major project was born at the National Institute of Standards and Technology (NIST) in Gaithersburg, MD. This one also had a rocky start. NIST is a facility of the U. S. Department of Commerce and once again outside the jurisdiction of the state of Maryland. Maryland Department of Natural Resources (DNC) strongly objected and when NIST refused to allow them to have a hunt on the one-square mile, heavily populated (6000 employees) research facility, the Maryland agency went to the Congressional Sportsman's Caucus. NIST officials and the U. S. Department of Commerce refused to give in and petitioned the U. S. Solicitor General's office for a clarification of the law. The results were predictable; Maryland had no wildlife management authority on the NIST campus. The project went forward and more data were forthcoming and published (Rutberg, Naugle, Thiele, & Liu, 2004).

However, Maryland DNR remained persistent. As the project started, they threatened to ring the facility with agency personnel and shoot any deer leaving the grounds, which are surrounded by heavily traveled highways and residential areas (a suburb of Washington, DC). At that point a local animal welfare organization pointed out that this would make a wonderful media opportunity for the evening news. Maryland backed off temporarily.

Approximately 2 years into the project, Maryland DNR asked for a meeting with the research team and NIST officials and asked if they could conduct a test on the health of the deer. It is worth mentioning that when the project went forward, DNR was invited to participate and take blood samples or make any measurements they deemed valuable. They declined. Many questioned why Maryland DNR waited 2 years to seek permission to kill 50 deer and "assess their health." At that point the research-team veterinarian asked the Director of the Maryland DNR if, when he took his dog to the veterinarian, the dog had to be killed to assess its health. Thereafter no further communications of note occurred between NIST and Maryland DNR.

As might be expected, the researchers developing and testing the PZP vaccine were having their own share of frustration in the face of what seemed illogical resistance to its use. Because of the public notoriety of the deer contraception subject, they experienced many interviews and spoke at numerous public community meetings, stressing their purpose that deer fertility control focus was for parks, preserves and communities where hunting was illegal. A reporter at one of these interviews said he was told state agencies were concerned that fertility control is a threat to hunting. Author Kirkpatrick smiled and after a brief pause said "If those folks think that some guys with dart guns can control state wild deer populations, they must be smoking something really good."

Through the 1990s, the attacks directed at urban deer fertility control by state fish and game agencies were largely based on scientific questions. Chief among these questions and almost identical to ones asked by opponents of PZP for horses were

(1) possible passage of the vaccine through the food chain, (2) possible extension of the breeding season with energetic consequences to the females, and (3) possible genetic effects. In no case were data or evidence of any kind offered to support the concerns. Coincidentally, through the three ongoing projects, an extensive database was generated that answered the questions for deer. The vaccine antigen could not survive the digestive tract. Extension of the breeding season was minimal and did not cause notable energetic loss. In fact, the weight of treated deer improved relative to deer that became pregnant and faced a summer of lactation.

Finally, when compared to the genetic effects of hunting, where the largest and most robust animals were selected against (for their antlers), contraception was a bargain. As numerous biological questions were gradually answered by the ongoing research (Kirkpatrick & Turner, 1995), the demand for the fertility control approach grew in the public sector and public meetings on the subject became more strident and were eventually tinged with hostility as people spoke their views. Unfortunately for all involved, the entrance of animal welfare/protection groups on the side of fertility control led to a deep polarization with the state agencies, which continued to selectively quote and ignore science as it suited their goals (Kirkpatrick & Turner, 1997; Rutberg et al., 1997).

Eventually realizing that the attack on the science was failing, the state agencies turned their attention to regulatory issues. Beginning in 1992 the application of PZP vaccine for deer was regulated by the Center for Veterinary Medicine at the Food and Drug Administration (FDA). Application of PZP was authorized by means of an investigational new animal drug exemption (INAD), the equivalent of INDs issued for the use of unapproved human drugs. Thus, the vaccine had official legal federal authorization. Subsequently a coalition of 16 states that disliked the concept of fertility control lobbied their respective Congressional delegations with the message to get the whole business stopped. However, FDA refused to give in to the political pressure. For states, it was "strike two."

By 2005, the regulation of wildlife contraceptives had been transferred from FDA to the Environmental Protection Agency (EPA). Shortly thereafter a second potential deer contraceptive vaccine was developed by the U. S. Department of Agriculture (USDA). This was a vaccine against gonadotropin-releasing hormone (GnRH) and was named GonaCon®. When USDA applied for registration with EPA, the states descended upon the agency. In the end they could not stop the registration, but they were successful in convincing EPA to place use restrictions on it, e.g., having to capture and tag each deer. The agencies argued that this requirement was to insure that persons harvesting deer would know if it was treated. This was despite the well-established fact that the vaccine was harmless if ingested. However, it did serve its purpose by markedly reducing the practicality of using the vaccine.

In the meantime, two smaller urban deer contraceptive field-research projects were established at the Columbus, OH, Metroparks facility and on Fripp Island, SC. In both cases the respective states approved research permits, which in itself was progress. But after several years of successful application of fertility control and decreases in population growth, both states rescinded their permits on the basis that these sites were actually "managing" deer rather than just doing research. Thus, the third phase of the states' attack on urban deer fertility control emerged, and it was spectacularly successful. It appeared that the new approach would be to establish state regulations and policies that would prevent fertility control from ever gaining traction. The approach quickly became implemented. State after state established these policies and regulations. Nebraska went so far as to amend its constitution to discourage the use of fertility control.

When GonaCon® was approved by EPA, Pennsylvania was asked to develop a state policy for urban deer fertility control. Carl Roe was then the Executive Director of the Pennsylvania Game Commission and stated publicly: "GonaCon® will never be used by the Game Commission so long as I am director." In 2012 at the Seventh International Conference on Fertility Control in Wildlife, the USDA's John Eiseman provided a list of 17 state policies, of which most were hostile to the concept of fertility control for urban deer management (Eisenman, O'Hare, & Fagerstone, 2013). By 2015 the states had largely won the deer-contraception battle through state regulations/policy.

Despite this success in blocking the application of contraceptives to urban deer management, the states still had to contend with the very impressive successes on the two federal sites, FIIS and NIST. In addition continued research had led to development of a single-injection, multi-year PZP vaccine, which would reduce the access issue and make treatment more practical (Turner et al., 2008). These successes could not be pushed aside or ignored. They kept coming back in the forms of scientific publications, popular media articles and, most importantly, strident public sentiment. Something had to be done to remove this thorn, especially since many communities with deer issues continued to explore fertility control as an option, causing the conflict to fester.

State pressure turned to the National Park Service, the parent agency for FIIS. Strategically this organization had to be reined in because it had two ongoing wild horse fertility control projects and one with wapiti as well as the FIIS project. Even more important was the fact that the NPS was a focal point for many potential fertility control projects. There were additional horses (Mesa Verde NP, Theodore Roosevelt NP), wapiti (Rocky Mountain NP, Point Reyes National Seashore), feral burros (Virgin Islands NP), bison (Yellowstone NP) and mountain goats (Olympic NP) among others, where varying degrees of pressure were being applied for the introduction of fertility control. Even more concerning to the states that were heavily entrenched in opposition to deer contraception were the multitude of potential deer projects (Indiana Dunes, Valley Forge, Gettysburg, Rock Creek Park, in Washington, DC, and several dozen other sites within the NP system).

The irony to this lies in the fact that the NPS has historically been the leading edge for application of fertility control to various wildlife populations. The single largest scientific breakthrough had occurred in an NPS unit (Assateague Island National Seashore) with wild horses, and the application rapidly spread to FIIS for deer, more horses at Cape Lookout National Seashore, wapiti at Point Reyes National Seashore, etc. So, now the states were faced with getting the NPS under control.

The precise strategy, mechanisms and intrigue behind this new effort remain obscure, but the results were soon forthcoming. In 2009, at the urging of several state agencies, the NPS met and established a set of five criteria for deer contraception in NPS units. One criterion was a contraceptive that would have 5 years of efficacy with a single administration. Such a contraceptive did not exist then, and the chances of such a contraceptive being developed are small. Together with the edict that all treated deer have to be ear-tagged (which eliminates remote treatments and increases costs in a significant manner) NPS deer contraception was made virtually impossible. But state pressure on the NPS did not stop there.

The primacy of federal law provides the NPS with all the authority they need to pursue urban/park deer fertility control, yet they deferred to the states. When asked why the NPS did not pursue deer fertility control at Valley Forge where the Pennsylvania Game Commission objected, one regional scientist for the NPS stated "we want to be good neighbors". In 2010, after 17 years of very successful deer control on a five-community block on FIIS, the NPS terminated the project, because "it had to be studied more." Eight years later there is no study and no fertility control on FIIS. And finally, in 2012, at the Seventh International Conference on Fertility Control in Wildlife, the NPS issued a policy statement on wildlife fertility control in NPS units (Wild, Powers, Monello, & Leong, 2013). Two critical items were (1) fertility control methods were considered "more acceptable in non-native species, closed populations, and highly manipulated environments" and (2) "early and active engagement with neighboring state and federal management agencies and public stakeholders is crucial for program success."

Despite this policy, the NPS actively opposed deer fertility control in "highly manipulated environments" such as Rock Creek Park in Washington, DC, and with what they consider to be "non-native species" such as horses in Mesa Verde National Park as well as on other sites. Interestingly the question of whether the horses are a native or non-native species is in itself contentious (Kirkpatrick & Fazio, 2010).

Conclusion

By 2018, wildlife fertility control was actively being applied to wild horses in more than 35 U.S. sites, including units of the NPS, BLM, U.S. Forest Service, several Indian reservations, a dozen wild horse sanctuaries, the Canadian Province of Alberta and in Hungary and Romania. Nonetheless, only a few of these are actively managing horse numbers in ongoing fashion. The technology has also spread to African elephants, where 20 game parks in South Africa are successfully managing their animals with fertility control and culling is off the Table. A herd of feral sheep in England is also being managed with a contraceptive vaccine. Two different U.S. bison populations have been treated with a contraceptive vaccine, with one realizing zero population growth in a single year. Currently, 4 deer fertility control projects are ongoing, and several have been completed in various communities. More than 200 zoos worldwide are using the same contraceptive technology for the management of more than 85 species in order to reduce or eliminate "surplus" animals, since disposition is difficult and fraught with controversy.

On the other hand, during this period the NPS sanctioned the culling of deer in Valley Forge, Rock Creek Park and several national historic sites. Yellowstone Park sent between 500 and 900 bison off to slaughter in 2014–15 in order to meet population goals. Mesa Verde National Park refused to even discuss wild horse management by fertility control, while at the same time fencing the horses out from the few available water supplies. Point Reyes National Seashore wrings its hands over a growing and damaging wapiti herd in the face of earlier demonstration that fertility control was a viable option. Hundreds of communities across the U.S. spend hundreds of thousands of dollars to have commercial "sharpshooters" come into their towns and parks and shoot urban deer. In the horse realm the Bureau of Land Management continues to remove and warehouse horses at immense expense to the taxpayer and with associated detriment to quality of life for thousands of horses. Furthermore, the inertia of insignificant use of proven PZP-based contraception continues 2 years after publication of strong evidence that it is an effective long-term contraceptive (5–6 years of infertility across 7 years) and that it really does limit population growth (Rutberg, Grams, Turner, & Hopkin, 2017).

The science of wildlife contraception has been thoroughly vetted within the scientific community through numerous publications in peer-reviewed journals and eight international conferences on the subject. At the field level the actual application of fertility control to free-ranging wildlife is not without its difficulties. The approach is labor intensive compared to other management paradigms, and not all populations will lend themselves to effective treatment and management because of differences in population sizes and habitat. Nevertheless, wildlife fertility control has proven itself a useful management tool. A more detailed discussion of field aspects of wildlife contraception is provided by Turner and Rutberg (2013).

A key consideration for the future of wildlife fertility control is the need for greater crossover of information into the public sector and to Congress about the curative capabilities of wildlife contraception for species in the dilemma of overpopulation. However, even with that accomplishment a crucial obstacle to moving forward is human nature. The desire to defend one view and attack the opposite is hard wired. While some individuals can think their way through to compromise, others cannot or will not. When individuals of the latter case are in positions of control and have decision-making power, ego and defensiveness will rule, and education toward compromise will not readily occur. Therefore, it is important to persist. The long journey continues, sustained in part by concern for pressed species and their environments and in part by those believing that fact and logic will eventually shine through the cloud cover of political agendas, cultural inertia and egocentric bias.

Every spring another cycle of birth plays out for wild horses, deer and many other species. This insurance for species preservation is strong. Across many generations species and habitats will flourish and decline. Human impacts are now figuring heavily into these patterns as part of the cost of human accomplishments.

Perhaps we as a global community can evolve sufficiently to prevent the environmental chaos that can result from continued lack of attention to these patterns. Certainly, focused local attention and action is a realistic goal. However, to accomplish this we must remove the slavery of personal bias and self-serving that derive from cultural and political indoctrinations infused across our own (human) generations. We need to think cleanly and seek the long view. Can we actually accomplish that? Yes, because knowledge and education are great vehicles of science. A positive information/education program focused on compromise and means of resolution can pave the way. Remember, humanity once believed that the world is flat. Some still do.

References

Asa, C. A., & Porton, I. (Eds.). (2005). *Wildlife contraception: Issues, methods and application*. Baltimore: Johns Hopkins University Press.

Bartholow, J. M. (2008). Economic benefit of fertility control in wild horse populations. *Journal of Wildlife Management, 71*, 2811–2819.

De Seve, C. W., & Boyles-Griffin, S. (2013). An economic model demonstrating the long-term cost benefits of incorporating fertility control into wild horse (*Equus caballus*) management programs on public lands in the United States. *Journal of Zoo and Wildlife Medicine, 44*, 34–37.

Duncan, C. L., King, J. L., & Kirkpatrick, J. F. (2013). Romance without responsibilities: The use of the immunocontraceptive vaccine porcine zona pellucida to manage free-ranging bison on Catalina Island, California, USA. *Journal of Zoo and Wildlife Medicine, 44*, 123–131.

Eisenman, J. D., O'Hare, J. R., & Fagerstone, K. A. (2013). State level approaches to managing the use of contraceptives in wildlife in the United States. *Journal of Zoo and Wildlife Medicine, 44*, 47–51.

Fayrer-Hosken, R. A., Grobler, D., Van Altena, J. J., Kirkpatrick, J. F., & Bertschinger, H. J. (2000). Immunocontraception of free-roaming African elephants. *Nature, 407*(6801), 149.

Garrott, R. A., & Oli, M. K. (2013). A critical crossroad for BLM's wild horse program. *Science, 341*, 847–848.

Kirkpatrick, J. F. (2008). Achieving population goals in long-lived wildlife (Equus caballus) with contraception. *Wildlife Research, 35*, 513–519.

Kirkpatrick, J. F. & Fazio, P. M. (2010). *Wild horses as Native American wildlife*. The Science and Conservation Cntr, Zoo Montana, Billings.

Kirkpatrick, J. F., Liu, I. K. M., & Turner Jr., J. W. (1990). Remotely delivered immunocontraception in feral horses. *Wildlife Society Bulletin, 18*, 326–330.

Kirkpatrick, J. F., & Turner Jr., J. W. (1985). Chemical fertility control and wildlife management. *Bioscience, 35*(8), 485–491.

Kirkpatrick, J. F., & Turner Jr., J. W. (1991). Reversible fertility control in non-domestic animals. *Journal of Zoo and Wildlife Medicine, 22*, 392–408.

Kirkpatrick, J. F., & Turner Jr., J. W. (1995). Urban deer fertility control: Scientific, social and political issues. *Northeast Wildlife, 52*, 103–116.

Kirkpatrick, J. F., & Turner Jr., J. W. (1997). Urban deer contraception: The seven stages of grief. *Wildlife Society Bulletin, 25*, 515–519.

Kirkpatrick, J. F., Zimmermannn, W., Kolter, L., Liu, I. K. M., & Turner Jr., J. W. (1995). Immunocontraception of captive exotic species. I. Przewalskis horse (*Equus przewalskii*) and banteng (*Bos javanicus*). *Zoo Biology, 14*, 403–413.

McShea, W. J., Monfort, S. L., Hakim, S., Kirkpatrick, J. F., Liu, I. K. M., Turner Jr., J. W., et al. (1997). Immunocontraceptive efficacy and the impact of contraception on the reproductive behaviors of white-tailed deer. *Journal of Wildlife Management, 61*, 560–569.

National Academy of Sciences. (1980). *Wild and free-roaming horses and burros: Current knowledge and recommended research*. Washington, D.C.: National Research Council.

Naugle, R.E., Rutberg, A.T., Underwood, H.B., Turner, J.W. Jr., Liu, I.K.M. (2002). Field testing of immunocontraception on white-tailed deer (*Odocoileus virginianus*) on Fire Island National Seashore, New York, USA. *Reproduction*, (Suppl.60):143–153.

Rutberg, A. T. (2013). Managing wildlife with contraception: Why is it taking so long? *Journal of Zoo and Wildlife Medicine, 44*, 538–543.

Rutberg, A. T., Grams, K., Turner Jr., J. W., & Hopkin, H. (2017). Contraceptive efficacy of primary and booster doses of controlled-release PZP in wild horses. *Wildlife Research, 44*, 174–181.

Rutberg, A. T., & Naugle, R. E. (2008). Population-level effects of immunocontraception in white-tailed deer (*Odocoileus virginianus*). *Wildlife Research, 35*, 494–501.

Rutberg, A. T., Naugle, R. E., Thiele, L. A., & Liu, I. K. M. (2004). Effects of immunocontraception on a suburban population of white-tailed deer (*Odocoileus virginianus*). *Biological Conservation, 116*, 243–250.

Rutberg, A. T., Naugle, R. E., Turner Jr., J. W., Fraker, M. A., & Flanagan, D. R. (2013). Field testing of single-administration porcine zona pellucida contraceptive vaccines in white-tailed deer (*Odocoileus virginianus*). *Wildlife Research, 40*, 281–288.

Rutberg, A. T., Naugle, R. E., & Verret, F. (2013). Single treatment porcine zona pellucida immunocontraception associated with reduction of a population of white-tailed deer (*Odocoileus virginianus*). *Journal of Zoo and Wildlife Medicine, 44*, 75–84.

Rutberg, A. T., et al. (1997). Lessons from the urban deer battlefront: Plea for tolerance. *Wildlife Society Bulletin, 25*, 520–523.

Turner Jr., J. W. (1997). Immunocontraception in white-tailed deer. In T. J. Kreeger (Ed.), *Contraception in wildlife management* (pp 147–159). Technical Bulletin 1853. Washington, D.C.: US Dept. Agriculture.

Turner Jr., J. W., Liu, I. K. M., Flanagan, D. R., Bynum, K. S., & Rutberg, A. T. (2002). Porcine zona pellucida (PZP) immunocontraception of wild horses (Equuscaballus) in Nevada: A 10 year study. *Reproduction Supplement, 60*, 177–186.

Turner Jr., J. W., Liu, I. K. M., & Kirkpatrick, J. F. (1992). Remotely delivered immunocontraception in captive white-tailed deer. *Journal of Wildlife Management, 56*(1), 154–157.

Turner Jr., J. W., Liu, I. K. M., & Kirkpatrick, J. F. (1996). Remotely delivered immunocontraception in free-roaming feral burros (*Equus asinus*). *Journal of Reproduction and Fertility, 107*, 31–35.

Turner Jr., J. W., & Rutberg, A. T. (2013). From the pens to the field: Real-world wildlife contraception. *Journal of Zoo and Wildlife Medicine, 44*(4S), S102–S110.

Turner Jr., J. W., Rutberg, A. T., Naugle, R. E., Kaur, M. A., Flanagan, D. R., Bertschinger, H. J., et al. (2008). Controlled-release components of PZP contraceptive vaccine extend duration of infertility. *Wildlife Research, 35*, 555–562.

Wild, M. A., Powers, J. G., Monello, R. J., & Leong, K. (2013). Ungulate fertility control in units of the National Park Service: Future directions. *Journal of Zoo and Wildlife Medicine, 44*, 149 (abstract).

Chapter 20
The Influence of Groupthink During the Invention of Stanley Milgram's Obedience Studies

Nestar Russell

In 1933, the same year the Nazi regime ascended to power, Stanley Milgram was born into a working class Jewish family in the Bronx in New York City. During his formative years, Milgram was perturbed by the Holocaust. Later he became a social psychologist and obtained a tenure track position at Yale University. During the many Nazi war crime trials, "ordinary" Germans in the docks—like Adolf Eichmann in Israel—typically explained that in participating in the Holocaust they were just following higher orders. This led Milgram to wonder what would happen if he ran a social psychology experiment where ordinary (American) people were ordered to inflict harm on another person. Would they also do as they were told? He designed a basic procedure that tested this question and soon afterwards had his students run the first pilot.

The result from the first trial stunned Milgram—most subjects indeed obeyed orders to inflict what appeared to be intense shocks on an innocent person. Milgram immediately sensed he had captured essential elements of the Holocaust in the laboratory setting. Thereafter he applied for funding to run an official research program so that he could better understand so-called obedience to authority. Milgram's intentions were not entirely honorable—running such an innovative research program could greatly boost his then precarious career prospects and financial security. Pre-tenure, Milgram told Jerome Bruner, a professor from Milgram's graduate program at Harvard University, "My hope is that the obedience experiments will take their place along with . . ." contributions by the biggest names in social psychology: "Sherif, Lewin and Asch" (as cited in Perry, 2012, p. 57). Whatever drove Milgram on, he anticipated enormous benefits for both scientific knowledge and himself. So what exactly did he find? What follows is a basic overview of his two baseline procedures and the counterintuitive results they produced.

N. Russell (✉)
University of Calgary, Calgary, AB, Canada

D. M. Allen, J. W. Howell (eds.), *Groupthink in Science*,
https://doi.org/10.1007/978-3-030-36822-7_20

Milgram's Baseline Experiments

The first official baseline experiment involved an actor posing as a potential subject. He entered a laboratory and encountered an apparent scientist (another actor, hereafter called the experimenter). The ostensible subject was then introduced to a waiting naïve, and actual, subject. The experimenter then told both the actual and supposed subject that the experiment they volunteered to participate in was designed to investigate the effects of punishment on learning. One person was required to be the teacher and the other the learner. A rigged selection ensured that the actor/subject was always the learner, and the actual subject the teacher. The actual subject (now teacher) watched as the experimenter secured the learner to a chair and attached an electrode to his arm. The learner was informed that the subject, using a microphone from another room, would ask them questions regarding a word-pair exercise. The learner was able to electronically transmit his answers to the subject's questions.

The subject was then taken into an adjacent room and placed before the shock generator. This device had 30 switches aligned in 15-volt increments ranging from 15 to 450 volts. The experimenter instructed the subject to give the learner a shock for each incorrect answer proffered; and each incorrect answer warranted for the learner a shock one level higher than its predecessor. No shocks were actually administered.

Upon starting, the learner regularly provided incorrect answers and, as a result, acquiescent subjects quickly advanced up the switchboard. The experimenter responded to any signs of hesitancy by the subject with one or more of the following prods:

Prod 1: Please continue, or, Please go on.
Prod 2: The experiment requires that you continue.
Prod 3: It is absolutely essential that you continue.
Prod 4: You have no other choice, you must go on (Milgram, 1974, p. 21).

If the subject attempted to clarify the lines of responsibility, the experimenter asserted: "I'm responsible for anything that happens to him. Continue please" (p. 74). At the 300 and 315-volt shock switches, the learner banged on the wall and thereafter fell silent. This silence implied that the learner had at least been rendered unconscious. The experimenter then instructed the subject to treat all subsequent unanswered questions as incorrect and inflict a shock at the next level. The experiment was deemed complete upon the subject administering three successive 450-volt shocks. Sixty-five percent of subjects (26 out of 40) inflicted every shock.

After running this experiment, Milgram and his research team ran 23 variations. For example, for the fifth experiment, Milgram decided to run a second more radical "New" Baseline, where up until the 345-volt shock switch the subject could clearly hear the content of the learner's increasingly distressed reactions (eventual panicked screams) to being "shocked." The New Baseline condition also obtained a 65% completion rate, and thereafter became the model procedure that all subsequent slight variations were based on. During the final 24th "Relationship condition," subjects were encouraged to inflict increasingly intense shocks on an eventually screaming learner who was at least an acquaintance, often a friend, and occasionally a family member (see Russell, 2014b). To clarify, prior to the experiment's start learners were covertly informed of the study's actual purpose (Will your friend follow orders to hurt you?) and then instructed on how vociferously to respond to their friend's infliction of increasingly intense "shocks." This particularly unethical variation saw the completion rate plummet to 15 percent.

Data collection took 10 months and involved a total of 780 subjects (Perry, 2012, p. 1). The amount of data collected was enormous. Despite this, to date, nobody has managed to develop a "conclusive" theory capable of accounting for Milgram's findings (Miller, 2004, p. 233).

Why Did Most Subjects Complete the New Baseline?

Despite the theoretic drought, it seems many factors, some of which I will describe below, are (perhaps cumulatively) likely to have contributed to most subjects' decision to complete the New Baseline experiment. The first such factor is termed "moral inversion" (Adams & Balfour, 1998, p. 20), which is where "something evil" (inflicting intense shocks on an innocent person) was converted by the experimenter into something "good" (advancing scientific knowledge on the effects of punishment on learning). The experimenter's higher "scientific" goals meant (apparently) the data *had* to be collected. As Milgram (1974, p.187) put it, the infliction of harm comes ". . . to be seen as noble in the light of some high ideological goal" where, by inflicting shocks, "science is served."

Another factor was the foot-in-the-door phenomenon, which is where persons are more likely to agree to a significant request if it is preceded by a comparatively insignificant request (Freedman & Fraser, 1966). For example, nearly every subject in the New Baseline inflicted the first six relatively light shocks (15–90 volts). However, in line with the foot-in-the-door phenomenon, doing so saw them comply with a small request which, unbeknownst to them, was about to be followed by some far more significant ones. The foot-in-door phenomenon is likely to have had two important consequences on subjects:

> (a) it engages subjects in committing precedent-setting acts . . . before they realize the "momentum" which the situation is capable of creating, and the "ugly direction" in which that momentum is driving them; and (b) it erects and reinforces the impression that quitting at any particular level of shock is unjustified (since consecutive shock levels differ only slightly and quantitatively). (Gilbert, 1981, p. 692)

Across many small 15-volt steps, most subjects inflicted increasingly intense and eventually dangerous "shocks."

Another likely influential factor over many subjects' decision to continue inflicting shocks was the undeniably coercive—even bullying—force of the experimenter's prods. The efficacious force of these prods was probably increased by the fact that the experimenter—a scientist—was closely associated with Yale University—a highly credible and authoritative institution of knowledge.

The final influencing factor I will discuss here was the experimenter's offer to accept all responsibility for the subject's infliction of further shocks. This offer enabled a subject to displace responsibility for their shock-inflicting actions onto the experimenter and provided the subject with an important self-interested benefit: if the subject was (apparently) not responsible for their actions, then they were under no obligation to stop the experiment. Consequently, the subject could, at the learner's expense, avoid having to engage in the predictably awkward confrontation with the experimenter otherwise necessary to stop the experiment. That is, by accepting the experimenter's offer, the subject could continue flicking the switches and—(apparently) absolved of all moral and legal culpability—simply blame the experimenter for their actions (see Russell & Gregory, 2011).

The most many obedient subjects were willing to do to help the learner avoid the intensifying "shocks" was to covertly sabotage the experiment by verbally emphasizing to the learner the correct answers to the questions. Thus, these subjects were willing to sacrifice the (apparently) all-important scientific pursuit of knowledge in favor of their self-interested desire to avoid a confrontation with the experimenter.

It seems the cumulative effect of these forces—moral inversion, foot-in-the-door phenomenon, displacement of responsibility, and appealing to the subject's self-interested desires to avoid a confrontation—probably caused most subjects to fall in line with the experimenter's groupthink desires: inflicting further shocks was (apparently) essential. And once subjects totally committed to doing as they were told, their passing of this moral Rubicon saw some engage in some rather unusual behaviors. For example, on reaching the high end of the switchboard, some subjects started anticipating the learner's screams and then attempted to talk over them, thus actively trying to avoid having to hear (neutrialize) their pained appeals. These subjects—more concerned about alleviating their stress-related pain—did not want to know what they knew: that they had committed to hurting an innocent person but preferred to remain, as termed by Heffernan in a previous chapter, *willfully blind* to this reality.

At the earliest opportunity, Milgram attempted to and eventually succeeded in publishing the first official baseline experiment (1963). This publication, which mentioned the Holocaust in its first paragraph, garnered immediate media attention and with time became Milgram's "best-known result" (Miller, 1986, p. 9). Because he thought he had captured key elements of the Holocaust in the controlled laboratory setting, Milgram likely thought the wider academic community would heap praise on his research. But the first scholarly response, by Diana Baumrind (1964) in the prestigious *American Psychologist*, was a scathing ethical critique that also questioned the external validity of the untenured Milgram's experiment. Baumrind, for example, pointed out that unlike German perpetrators during the Holocaust, Milgram's typically concerned subjects clearly did not want to hurt their victim. Thus, she remained unconvinced by Milgram's generalizations towards the Holocaust. If Baumrind was right and no parallel to the Holocaust existed, then, as she also notes, Milgram had no justification for having exposed his subjects to, as stated in his 1963 article, the following torturous experience:

> I observed a mature and initially poised businessman enter the laboratory smiling and confident. Within 20 minutes he was reduced to a twitching, stuttering wreck, who was rapidly approaching a point of nervous collapse. (Milgram, 1963, p. 377, as cited in Baumrind, 1964, p. 422)

If Baumrind was correct and harm was inflicted on innocent people for no reason at all, then the running of the Obedience studies were perhaps an example of groupthink captured in the laboratory setting. That is, through conformity and/or a desire for group harmony, somehow Milgram's many helpers—actors, research assistants, and technicians—all agreed to treat innocent people in an injurious and ultimately unethical manner. Other critics of Milgram, like Harré (1979, p. 106) for example, have alluded to this potentially groupthink connection:

> Milgram's assistants were quite prepared to subject the participants in the experiment to mental anguish, and in some cases considerable suffering, in obedience to Milgram. The most morally obnoxious feature of this outrageous experiment was, I believe, the failure of any of Milgram's assistants to protest against the treatment that they were meting out to the subjects.[1]

Milgram's research notes dated March 1962 showed he was aware of the ironic parallel between the subjects' *seemingly* harmful actions and his research team's *actually* harmful actions:

> Consider, for example, the fact --and it is a fact indeed, that while observing the experiment I ---and many others-- know that the naive subject is deeply distressed, and that...[it] is almost nerve shattering in some instances. Yet, we do not stop the experiment because of this [...] *If we fail to intervene, although we know a man is being made upset; why separate these actions of ours from those of the subject, who feels he is causing discomfort to another. And can we not use our own motives and reactions as a clue to what is behind the actions of the subject. The question to ask then is: why do we feel justified in carrying through the experiment, and why is this any different from the justifications that the obedient subject's feel?* (Stanley Milgram Papers, Box 46, Folder 163.) [Italics added]

With his unrelenting ambition to develop a psychological (individual) theory capable of explaining why most subjects behaved in "a shockingly immoral way" (Milgram, 1964, p. 849), Milgram never further pursued this more sociological (group) and no doubt disconcerting observation.

To unravel why Milgram's research team agreed to inflict harm on innocent people, I would argue it is important to analyze the start-to-finish journey that led to Milgram's destination: his perplexing Baseline/New Baseline completion rates. This "behind the scenes" approach when viewing the actual running of the experimental program is, I believe, capable of revealing some of the more important sociological forces that encouraged Milgram and his research team's groupthink

[1] Unbeknown to Harré, one of Milgram's actors, Robert J. Tracy, refused to continue performing his acting duties. According to his son, Tracy "couldn't go through with it" and walked out (see Perry, 2012, p. 226).

decision to collect a full set of ethically questionable data. It is no coincidence, as we shall see, that these group forces coincide with those that likely affected the compliant subjects' decisions to participate.

Group Forces Influencing the Research Team's Agreement to Inflict Intense Stress on Innocent People

When, after the first pilot study, Milgram decided to pursue the official Obedience research program, an obstacle likely to inhibit the realization of such ambitions became increasingly apparent. That is, because subjects during the first pilot experienced, as stated in his research proposal, "extreme tension" (as cited in Russell, 2014a, p. 412), there was a risk some of the specialists whose help he needed to collect the official data might deem the research program unethical and refuse to fulfill their essential roles.

Milgram's initial strategy to ensure that his research assistants, technicians, and actors all agreed to perform their roles was to encourage them to, as Fermaglich (2006, p. 89) put it, "view" the subjects' obedience "as an analogue of Nazi evil." Thus, much like he did with his subjects, Milgram morally converted "something evil" (imposing stress on the innocent subjects) into something "good" (generating scientific knowledge into better understanding perpetrator behavior during the Holocaust). The actor who most frequently played the role of the stress-inflicting experimenter, John Williams, for example, understood that despite his making "a man…upset," data collection was of "tremendous value," and thus the experiments "must be done" (as cited in Russell, 2014a, p. 416). Another example of moral inversion occurred when Milgram reassured his main research assistant, graduate student Alan Elms, that he did not need to worry about his "E[i]chman[n]-like" role of delivering a constant flow of subjects to the laboratory because they were all given "…a chance to resist the commands of a malevolent authority and assert their alliance with morality" (as cited in Blass, 2004, p. 99).

Although all helpers were encouraged to believe that they would be contributing to an important study, Milgram sensed that this in itself was not enough to secure everybody's long-term services. Thus, when necessary, he bolstered his moral inversion of bad into good by anticipating and then appealing to all his helpers' sometimes different self-interested desires. For example, Milgram offered actors Williams and James McDonough (the main "Learner") a generous hourly rate (which Milgram increased three times within eight months), along with the offer of a cash bonus to be paid out once all the data had been collected (Russell, 2014a, p. 416). Milgram also paid Elms an hourly rate for his services but also strengthened the attractiveness of role fulfillment by supporting the graduate students' emerging interest in the Obedience studies by publishing a journal article with him (see Elms & Milgram, 1966).

So, to promote involvement among all his helpers, Milgram basically applied what he suspected would prove to be the most successful individually tailored motivational formula—quid pro quo arrangements where benefits are provided in exchange for services rendered (Russell, 2014a, 416–417). Armed with typically similar justifications, it appears Milgram's helpers resolved the moral dilemma over whether or not to become involved in a potentially harmful study by becoming sufficiently convinced and/or opportunistically tempted into making their essential specialist contributions to data collection.

One might suspect that Milgram's helpers would have felt anxious about potentially harming innocent people, especially after weighing this risk up against the mere "scientific" and self-interested gains they hoped to obtain. This is especially so considering that during the official collection of data, at least two subjects were placed under such intense stress that they later complained that they thought they were going to have—or perhaps had—a heart attack (see Russell, 2009, pp. 104–105). However, alleviating such concerns was that as Milgram drew all his specialist helpers into role fulfillment, the issue of individual responsibility for harm infliction underwent a subtle yet powerful transformation. That is, after agreeing to perform their roles, all helpers unwittingly became links in an inherently stress-resolving and goal-directed assembly line-like bureaucratic process.

To clarify, before the official research program could proceed, Milgram had to design and then construct an inherently bureaucratic organizational process which would enable his research team to systematically and efficiently extracted data from 780 subjects. More specifically, "processing" involved training subjects, running the experiment, collecting data, and debriefing. For each subject, Milgram's research team had to complete all of these tasks within a pre-determined one-hour block so that the stage, so to speak, could be reset before the next subject's arrival at the top of the hour.

Intrinsic to all such bureaucratic processes is the division of labor (DOL)—where an organizational goal (in this case, collecting data) is subdivided into numerous tasks and then each of those tasks is allocated to a particular specialist functionary (Weber, 1976). For functionaries, however, this compartmentalization of tasks can cause a disjuncture between cause (for example, making partial contributions to Milgram's goal of collecting a full data set) and any negative effects generated by goal achievement (the infliction of intense stress on subjects). Among all functionary helpers—so-called cogs in the organizational machine—this disjuncture between cause and effect can stimulate what Russell and Gregory term "responsibility ambiguity" (2015, p. 136). Responsibility ambiguity is a metaphorical haziness, which renders debatable which functionary helper is most responsible for any harm inflicted by the wider organizational process. Importantly, responsibility ambiguity makes it difficult for arbiters to later determine who should be held to account for such harmful outcomes. This haziness can render some functionary helpers genuinely unaware of their personal responsibility. However, this haziness can also enable others to opportunistically escape shouldering responsibility because they suspect that their harmful contributions will be rewarded in the short-term and, due to the availability of plausible deniability ("I didn't know!"), never punished in the long-term. Therefore, it could be argued that the bureaucratic process structurally provided all of Milgram's helpers with the "fog" of responsibility ambiguity (Russell & Gregory, 2015).

Perhaps the most common source of responsibility ambiguity among functionary helpers working across an organizational chain is the option to displace or "pass the buck" of responsibility for their harmful contributions elsewhere (Russell & Gregory, 2015). For example, had a subject been seriously injured during data collection, Williams the stress-inflicting experimenter could, if he so chose, blame Milgram for his actions: Williams was only following his employer's instructions. Milgram, the principal investigator, was only undertaking the kind of groundbreaking research that prestigious universities like Yale pressured non-tenured faculty into pursing: he too was only doing his job. Perhaps the funders of the research—the National Science Foundation (NSF)—or the chair of Yale's Department of Psychology, Claude E. Buxton (Milgram's boss), were most responsible: they ultimately allowed, desired, and legitimized Milgram's research. The NSF and Buxton, however, did not directly hurt anyone and they certainly never condoned Milgram's pursuit of the particularly unethical Relationship condition. Perhaps, in the end the reified ideological pursuit of "scientific knowledge" was mostly to blame. The point is, as soon as a bureaucratic process forms, it suddenly becomes possible for all functionary helpers to blame someone or something else for their contributions to a harmful outcome. And because "others" were involved, it seems all sensed they could probably make their individual contributions with probable impunity. And on all realizing this, every helper thereafter only needed to concern themselves with reaping the personal benefits on offer for making their specialist contributions. This may help explain why Milgram's helpers risked partaking in such a potentially dangerous experiment.

Another subtle yet powerful effect the DOL can have on functionary helpers is termed bureaucratic momentum (Russell & Gregory, 2015). Bureaucratic momentum has usually taken hold when functionaries experience pressure to perform their specialist roles by preceding and sometimes succeeding functionary links across an organizational chain. This coercive force appears to be generated by the cumulative momentum of the many simultaneously moving functionary "cogs" bearing down and exerting pressure on one another. Functionary links often experience this coercive force to fulfill their roles in the form of peer pressure: "to get along" one must "go along." For example, in fear of causing a bottleneck or delay in organizational goal achievement, employees on a factory assembly line typically feel pressure to quickly fulfill their specialist roles. A single uncooperative functionary can—say because of moral reservations—resist such pressure; although doing so is rare because they must sacrifice whatever self-interested benefits they might otherwise have received for performing their specialist role. Also, this kind of resistance deprives other (potentially angry) functionaries from obtaining whatever benefits they anticipated receiving for organizational goal achievement. It is less stressful on everybody involved if all give in to the momentum of role fulfillment and just do their bit for goal achievement.

Bureaucratic momentum is likely to have had an influential effect during the Obedience studies. For example, to please his funders at the NSF, Milgram likely felt pressure to collect—despite any emerging ethical reservations—a full set of data. Doing so, however, required the long-term retention of the experimenter's acting services. In return for being retained over a long period of time, the experimenter—despite any emerging ethical reservations—likely felt contractually obliged to continue placing subjects under enormous stress. And, of course, it could be argued that the experimenter's seemingly unrelenting prods, like it having been "absolutely essential" the subject "continue" inflicting more shocks, saw—despite any emerging ethical reservations—the transfer of bureaucratic momentum to the last functionary link in the Obedience study's data collecting organizational chain.

The final group force I'll mention here likely to have influenced Milgram's research team was (again) the foot-in-the-door phenomenon. For example, it could be argued that after Milgram's research team agreed to undertake the first official and, relatively speaking, benign (first) Baseline condition (where the learner banged a few times on the wall), the more amenable (or perhaps desensitized) the team became to undertaking the fifth more radical New Baseline experiment (where an increasingly hysterical learner suddenly went silent). With the entire research team having agreed to undertake the more radical New Baseline, the more amenable they became to undertaking the most radical 24th and final Relationship condition where, as mentioned, subjects were pushed to inflict severe "shocks" on someone who was at least an acquaintance, often a friend, and sometimes a family member. The point being, it is unlikely Milgram's helpers would have had the nerve to run the Relationship condition at the start of the data collection process. The slippery slope of the foot-in-the-door phenomenon—small and barely perceivable steps in an increasingly radicalized direction—likely had a powerful influence on those working within the Obedience study's data-collecting bureaucracy.

In summary, much like with the obedient subjects, the forces of moral inversion, receiving self-interested benefits, displacement of responsibility, bureaucratic momentum, and the foot-in-the-door phenomenon all (perhaps cumulatively) likely exerted an influence on the research team's groupthink decision to collect a full set of ethically questionable data.

Prioritization of Milgram's Self-Interests over the Scientific Pursuit of Knowledge

It seems the reason Milgram decided to run the experimental program was because he believed the benefits—greater knowledge into mankind's destructive tendency to obey—outweighed all the costs. As he said in the draft notes of his 1974 book:

> Under what conditions does one ask about destructive obedience? Perhaps under the same conditions that a medical researcher asks about cancer or polio; because it is a threat to human welfare and has shown itself a scourage [sic] to humanity. (As cited in Russell, 2009, p. 104).

But, when Milgram decided to pursue his research program, it seemed the only people faced with paying any "costs" would be his obedient subjects (whom, as far as he was concerned, only got what they deserved for, as mentioned, failing to "assert their alliance with morality"). Again, he, on the other hand, could only envision personally benefiting from running the official experiments. But after the publication of Baumrind's (1964) critique, this all suddenly changed.

Baumrind's critique rather suddenly threatened to label his research unethically abusive and perhaps even held the potential to destroy his fledgling academic career. With *his* personal self-interests suddenly on the line, Milgram realized *he* might have to pay a high price for his earlier decision to proceed with the study. With his back against the wall—and much like those subjects who attempted to sabotage his experiments—Milgram *also* started prioritizing his self-interests over and above the so-called importance of generating scientific knowledge. That is, post-Baumrind, Milgram set about protecting his personal interests by compromising the accuracy of the knowledge he had collected—what he did and found during data collection—by massaging the truth, omitting certain facts, and even telling complete lies. Thus, like many examples of groupthink, the emergence of certain negative outcomes was followed by a carefully calculated cover up.

For example, despite encountering subjects complaining about their hearts, in his response to Baumrind (and repeatedly thereafter) a perhaps *willfully blind* Milgram (1964, p. 849) described his subjects' stress as mere "momentary excitement," a sudden change in tone that Patten (1977, p. 356) observed to be "a most astonishing about-face." In his book, Milgram noted that before each trial subjects had to sign "a general release form, which stated: 'In participating in this experimental research of my own free will, I release Yale University and its employees from any legal claims arising from my participation'" (1974, p. 64). But what he failed to disclose was, as stated in his personal notes, "The release, of course, was not used for experimental purposes, but to protect us against legal claims" (as cited in Russell, 2014a, p. 418). If Milgram honestly believed his experiments only caused "momentary excitement," why did he need legal protection?

Another omission was that although before Baumrind's critique Milgram promised to publish the Relationship condition's results, after her critique he mysteriously never mentioned the variation again (Russell, 2014b). Of course, if Baumrind's critique of the relatively benign first Baseline could, as Milgram clearly sensed, threaten the reputation of his research, one can only imagine the ethical firestorm she would have unleashed on him had he published a variation where some subjects were pushed into inflicting harmful "shocks" on a relative. And in terms of outright lies, Milgram counter-critiqued Baumrind for confusing "the unanticipated outcome of an experiment with its basic procedure," then elaborating that "the extreme tension induced in some subjects was unexpected" (Milgram, 1964, p. 848). Milgram said this despite him having earlier undertaken numerous pilot studies where, as mentioned, some subjects experienced what he termed in his research proposal "extreme tension".

It can therefore be argued that Milgram's self-interests—protecting his name, career, and the ethical reputation of his world-famous experiments—ended up being prioritized over (and thus ultimately corrupted) his espoused purest beliefs surrounding the so-called scientific pursuit of knowledge. Cementing this chapter's focus on the overlap between individual and group behavior during the Obedience experiments, at some level Milgram self-reflexively sensed a connection between his obedient subjects' self-centered decisions to prioritize their personal interests over the well-being of the learner and him prioritizing his self-interests over the subjects' well-being:

> Moreover, considered as a personal motive of the author --the possible benefits that might redound to humanity --withered to insignificance along side [*sic*] the strident demands of intellectual curiosity. When an investigator keeps his eyes open throughout a [scientific] study, he learns things about himself as well as about his subjects, and the observations do not always flatter. (As cited in Russell, 2009, p. 186)

Conclusion

Milgram naturally viewed himself as a detached, objective, and scientific observer of destructive social behavior. That is, he set up an experiment but perceived himself to be independent of the results it produced. He, however, failed to sense his own highly involved non-scientific role in the social engineering of those results. Two particular factors he remained oblivious of were, first, the subtle power inherent within the data-extracting bureaucratic process he constructed (and the necessary role it played in helping generate his surprising results— a key structural force that likely explains much of the ironic overlap in group and individual behavior). The largely invisible role of bureaucratic organization no doubt plays a key role in helping socially engineer many other "real life" examples of groupthink behavior—particularly because of its ability to promote, among all functionary links across the chain of command, feelings of responsibility ambiguity. Second, Milgram was largely unaware of the important role that his and his research team's self-interests played in both helping generate the surprising results and corrupting their scientific pursuit for new knowledge. This last point may have implications that extend beyond Milgram's laboratory walls. For example, what role did the pushes and pulls of bureaucratic organization and personal self-interest play in stifling dissent among some of the scientists working on the Manhattan Project? Finally, I am confident that Milgram's dissectible research—somewhat uniquely captured in the (semi)controlled social science laboratory—is likely to provide scholars with great insights into the inner workings of other more contemporary examples of highly destructive and seemingly unstoppable groupthink behavior, like for example, climate catastrophe.

References

Adams, G. B., & Balfour, D. L. (1998). *Unmasking bureaucratic evil*. Thousand Oaks, CA: Sage Publications.

Baumrind, D. (1964). Some thoughts on ethics of research: After reading Milgram's 'behavioral study of obedience'. *American Psychologist, 19*(6), 421–423.

Blass, T. (2004). *The man who shocked the world: The life and legacy of Stanley Milgram*. New York, NY: Basic Books.

Elms, A. C., & Milgram, S. (1966). Personality characteristics associated with obedience and defiance towards authoritative command. *Journal of Experimental Research in Personality, 1*(4), 282–289.

Fermaglich, K. (2006). *American dreams and Nazi nightmares: Early Holocaust consciousness and liberal America, 1957–1965*. Waltham, MA: BrandeisUniversity Press.

Freedman, J. L., & Fraser, C. C. (1966). Compliance without pressure: The foot-in-the door technique. *Journal of Personality and Social Psychology, 4*(2), 195–202.

Gilbert, S. J. (1981). Another look at the Milgram obedience studies: The role of the gradated series of shocks. *Personality and Social Psychology Bulletin, 7*(4), 690–695.

Harré, R. (1979). *Social being: A theory for social psychology*. Oxford, UK: Basil Blackwell.

Milgram, S. (1963). Behavioral study of obedience. *Journal of Abnormal and Social Psychology, 67*(4), 371–378.

Milgram, S. (1964). Issues in the study of obedience: A reply to Baumrind. *American Psychologist, 19*(11), 848–852.

Milgram, S. (1974). *Obedience to authority: An experimental view*. New York, NY: Harper and Row.

Miller, A. G. (1986). *The obedience experiments: A case study of controversy in social science*. New York, NY: Praeger.

Miller, A. G. (2004). What can the Milgram obedience experiments tell us about the Holocaust? Generalizing from the social psychology laboratory. In A. G. Miller (Ed.), *The social psychology of good and evil* (pp. 193–237). New York, NY: Guilford Press.

Patten, S. C. (1977). The case that Milgram makes. *The Philosophical Review, 86*(3), 350–364.

Perry, G. (2012). *Beyond the shock machine: The untold story of the Milgram obedience experiments*. Melbourne: Scribe.

Russell, N. (2014a). The emergence of Milgram's bureaucratic machine. *Journal of Social Issues, 70*(3), 409–423.

Russell, N. (2014b). Stanley Milgram's obedience to authority "relationship" condition: Some methodological and theoretical implications. *Social Sciences, 3*(2), 194–214.

Russell, N., & Gregory, R. (2011). Spinning an organizational "web of obligation"? Moral choice in Stanley Milgram's "obedience" experiments. *The American Review of Public Administration, 41*(5), 495–518.

Russell, N., & Gregory, R. (2015). The Milgram-holocaust linkage: Challenging the present consensus. *State Crime Journal, 4*(2), 128–153.

Russell, N. J. C. (2009). Stanley Milgram's obedience to authority experiments: Towards an understanding of their relevance in explaining aspects of the Nazi Holocaust. PhD thesis: Victoria University of Wellington.

Weber, M. (1976). *The Protestant ethic and the Spirit of capitalism*. Translated by T. Parsons with an introduction by A. Giddens. London: Allen & Unwin.

Chapter 21
The Physician's Dilemma: Healthcare and Bureaucracy in the Modern World

J. Kim Penberthy and David R. Penberthy

Introduction

Physicians are educated in the science of medicine and healing of patients and have traditionally been less oriented toward the business aspects of healthcare. Perfectionism, hard work, and sacrifices by physicians have helped to advance healthcare in the United States and around the globe over the past several decades. Along with the exponential scientific growth, expanded healthcare options, and growing complexities that arise, modern medicine has become increasingly regulated. This has resulted in expansion of mandatory requirements and an explosion in the growth of administrators and bureaucrats who, by the very nature of their training, focus on the "bottom line" of outcomes and costs of healthcare.

Competing incentives between physicians' way of approaching medicine and the bureaucrats' approach to healthcare has created tension for both. Physicians are feeling increasingly disenfranchised within the practice of medicine due to a myriad of factors. It is no wonder then, that physician burnout has risen over time. This burnout has been associated with distressed and disruptive physician behaviors and negative impacts on the healthcare environment and patient care.

We propose that "burnout" and related distressed behaviors of physicians are best conceptualized as a symptom of the overall dysfunction within the healthcare system. These inter- and intrapersonal mechanisms have resulted in a form of physician groupthink characterized by indignant frustration, helplessness, and inaction. We propose that the key to addressing physician burnout is larger than merely teaching physicians mindfulness strategies or improved coping skills. The goal

J. K. Penberthy (✉)
University of Virginia School of Medicine, Charlottesville, VA, USA
e-mail: Jkp2n@virginia.edu

D. R. Penberthy
Virginia Radiation Oncology Associates, Richmond, VA, USA

D. M. Allen, J. W. Howell (eds.), *Groupthink in Science*,
https://doi.org/10.1007/978-3-030-36822-7_21

cannot be to simply train physicians how to endure an increasingly burdensome and nonsensical healthcare system. We propose that physicians must instead reshape their role in healthcare, become more proactive, engage in leadership, and advocate for their profession, including pursuing common-sense approaches to treatment and increased autonomy over patient care. These behavioral and advocacy changes may renew physicians' energy and decrease burnout within the field of medicine and may even lead to reduced administrative burdens and costs, thus effecting lasting positive change in healthcare.

The Complex Character of Physicians

People who choose careers in medicine have traditionally demonstrated personality traits and aptitudes that include high intelligence, compassion, inquisitiveness, and sensitivity to others. They are also typically competitive, driven, independent, and perfectionistic (Lemaire & Wallace, 2014). The impact of such a well-intended group of high-achieving and hardworking individuals in the field of medicine has been a blessing for patients and the field of healthcare and potentially one cause of the development of a "groupthink" in physicians which has contributed to their current increased rates of dissatisfaction and burnout.

Individuals attracted to a career in medicine are motivated to help others in practical and significant ways. Most physicians understand that a career in medicine means a lifetime of service to their community and they enter this societal contract willingly. To become a physician, one must have the intellectual curiosity, capacity, endurance, and perseverance to get into and successfully complete medical school and residency programs. Simultaneously, due to the nature and intensity of the work, physicians are often more socially isolated and emotionally disconnected than individuals in other professional fields (Lipsenthal, 2005). Pre-medical collegiates are studious and independent, perhaps spending more time in the library than socializing with others. They are individuals who are achievement oriented, self-motivated, deeply engaged in academics, and invested in individual academic success (Eley, Leun, Hong, Cloninger, & Cloninger, 2016). Medical school and residency continue the indoctrination of this self-selected group.

The humanistic component of clinical competence, such as empathy and other interpersonal skills, can be eroded in medical students who are vulnerable to the rigors of medical school (Hojat, Spandorfer, & Mangione, 2013). These institutions exacerbate the natural tendencies of the individuals by making 80-hour work weeks normative and underscoring individual responsibility and achievement throughout the group. While their non-physician peers are enjoying active social lives, more pay, less demanding jobs, or starting families, young physicians in training are working in isolation and under extreme stress, collecting increasingly large debt, and making little income, with less autonomy and free time.

Most training programs are also intensely hierarchical with attending physicians setting the pace and expectations for more junior physicians in training. In our experiences, challenging senior physicians in medicine is not typically considered an option and is certainly not encouraged. If young doctors-to-be are afraid to discuss their daily challenges, learning challenges or mistakes, and fears, the isolation only becomes more extreme.

Conventional medical training, although making incremental improvements, is still highly dysfunctional. The training process exaggerates the individual's already described traits, often at the expense of innovation and social connection. It seems a basic tenet of medical training that if trainees are overloaded with responsibility and information, they will rise to the occasion, and most do. Physicians in training work long hours, get paid barely enough to survive (especially given their financial debts), and still must see ever more patients and meet other research and service demands. Too often, this leads to increased isolation or emotional distance. This tendency for emotional dissociation may be further developed in the anatomy lab, emergency room, and other places and situations where emotions are not so helpful. Physicians may learn to shut off emotions, keeping the "scientist" mindset.

These are all useful mechanisms, allowing physicians to do difficult but necessary tasks. However, such strategies often lead to additional isolation and a feeling of being "in it alone." Many physicians exhibit compulsive traits, especially what has been called the "compulsive triad" of self-doubt, guilt, and an exaggerated sense of self-importance (Spickard, Gabbe, & Christensen, 2002). Self-doubt often results from having excessively high personal standards, common in many physicians, that are often so high that the standards are difficult, or impossible, to achieve. Given these high self-expectations, such physicians often impose equally high standards on others and react strongly if colleagues or staff fail to meet them. There is some evidence that physician training and work is indeed so stressful that many physicians may meet criteria for a type of chronic stress disorder (West, Shanafelt, & Kolars, 2011). The key symptoms are intrusive thoughts, avoidance behaviors, and hyperarousal. Learned helplessness has also been hypothesized to be a factor in distressed physicians, who despite their best efforts, cannot seem to stay ahead of the workload.

Despite these stressors and pressures, the majority of physicians successfully finish their training and enter into their careers with a focus on patient care and service. They understand the commitment that medicine takes and willingly enter into this world. However, they may be forever changed by their experiences in training, and certainly many of them have learned behaviors to help them survive – including a skewed expectation of an intense workload, emotional dissociation, and little to no expectation of improvement in their situation. Many of them are chronically stressed, financially strapped, and may feel helpless (Thomas-Dyrbye & Shanafelt, 2006).

Healthcare has benefited from the hard work and dedication of such physicians. Quality medical care and prevention has blossomed, with increased access and improved treatments across the globe (Berwick, Calkins, McCannon, & Hackbarth, 2006).

Physicians work long and hard to practice a challenging profession that is also incredibly satisfying and rewarding to most of them. However, with increased success and expansion of healthcare have come increased legislation and bureaucracy, with increased administrative and management work, and the need for individuals to navigate these complexities. Thus, enter the healthcare administrator, manager, and other bureaucrats.

Increasing Role of Bureaucracy in Medicine

According the Centers for Medicare and Medicaid Services (CMS; National Healthcare Expenditures Fact Sheet, 2018), the U.S. National Health Expenditures grew to $3.3 trillion in 2016, or $10,348 per person, and accounted for 17.9% of U.S. gross domestic product (GDP). CMS projects an annual growth of 5.5%, meaning about one-fifth of U.S. GDP will be spent on healthcare by 2025 with overall GDP projection of a total economy of $25 trillion, which means about $5 trillion will be spent on the healthcare system that year. Our government along with health insurance companies, hospital systems, and other agencies has created bureaucracies to manage and direct all of this money for healthcare.

Growing numbers of healthcare regulations lead to an increased need for management to ensure compliance with these well-intentioned rules. Such work necessitates time and attention most physicians do not have due to their patient care obligations and work hours. Additionally, many physicians may not have the business knowledge and management skills to be competitive or successful in the field of healthcare administration. Thus, the healthcare system in the United States has witnessed a staggering rise in the number of non-physician administrators and managers over the past decades. The numbers from 1975 to 2010 are dramatic, to say the least, with a 3200% increase in the number of administrators compared to 150% increase in the number of physicians over that time period (Cantlupe, 2017). For perspective, the increase in physician numbers roughly kept up with population growth over this 35-year period.

Supporters say the growing number of administrators is needed to keep pace with the drastic changes in healthcare delivery over the past decades, particularly change driven by technology and by ever-more-complex regulations. To cite just a few industry-disrupting regulations, consider the Prospective Payment System of 1983, the Health Insurance Portability & Accountability Act of 1996, the Health Information Technology for Economic and Clinical Act of 2009, and The Patient Protection and Affordable Care Act of 2010. Critics say the army of administrators does little to relieve the documentation burden on physicians, while creating layers of high-salaried bureaucratic bloat in healthcare organizations.

Physicians now spend roughly two-thirds of their professional time on paperwork – mostly filling out the never-ending fields that are part of Electronic Medical Records requirements – rather than attending to patients (Sinsky et al., 2016). Remember also, that physicians do not get reimbursed for completing paperwork.

This means patients are essentially spending three times more than they should have to for their doctors' time. Simply halving doctors' paperwork could halve physicians' costs because they would have more time for productive, patient-centered work. Hospital costs are highest in the countries that have the highest administration costs (Bouchard, 2014). Research supports the fact that increased numbers of administrators is associated with increased cost of healthcare but not improved outcomes (Woolhandler, Campbell, & Himmelstein, 2003).

Hospital administrators are vital to ensuring that medical facilities run efficiently and deliver quality care, which appears to be in alignment with the goals of physicians. However, despite the appearance of alignment, differing incentives – both positive and negative – have created a disconnect between physicians and administrators. Hospital management teams are well versed in metrics including market share, revenue, and costs. They are aware when the hospital is operating with a surplus or not and are motivated to increase patient numbers and overall budget surplus.

Physicians place high value on quality patient care and will work hard for their patients. However, due to a myriad of factors including a loss of autonomy regarding patient care, requirements to complete large amounts of seemingly irrelevant or unnecessary paperwork, longer work hours, decreasing financial reimbursement, increasing threats of lawsuits, and frequent understaffing or lack of qualified and experienced ancillary healthcare workers, physicians may feel increasingly disenfranchised with the healthcare system and frustrated with their profession (Lathrop, 2017). These competing incentives between physicians' way of approaching medicine and the bureaucrats' approach to healthcare has created tension for both and has only added to the crisis in healthcare (Levine & Gustave, 2013).

Physician Distress and Burnout

What happens when people with the personalities we described – perfectionistic, high-achieving, and independent – are put under additional stress, especially when they are given immense responsibility and very little authority? This describes what has happened to physicians in modern medicine today.

Physicians are confronted with fewer resources, increasing government regulations, greater patient outcome expectations, and rising student debt (Privitera, Rosenstein, Plessow, & LoCastro, 2015). There is also more pressure to practice in specific ways, such as adhering to guidelines and pathways that limit physician autonomy, and ongoing threats of lawsuits and liability. Many physicians express dissatisfaction with the decreasing amount of time allocated to each patient and consider their workload "too heavy" (Rosenstein, 2017). Satisfaction with work-life balance has significantly declined in physicians (Shanafelt et al., 2015).

In a 2014 American Medical Association national survey, 54% of practicing physicians met criteria for burnout (Shanafelt et al., 2015). It should be noted that the issue of distress affects nearly every group of physicians ranging from interns

(Dyrbye et al., 2014; Rosen, Gimotty, Shea, & Bellini, 2006; Shanafelt, Sloan, & Habermann, 2003) to department chairs (Gabbe, Melville, Mandel, & Walker, 2002). These ever-growing strains, coupled with a competitive and demanding work environment, have led to numerous negative psychological consequences including burnout and, in some cases, suicide (Schernhammer & Colditz, 2004). Overall, physician burnout has been associated with distressed and disruptive physician behaviors as well as negative impacts on the healthcare environment and patient care (Dewa, Loong, Bonato, & Trojanowski, 2017; Rosenstein, 2015).

This increased awareness of burned out and distressed physicians has not necessarily led to increased organized efforts to address the dysfunctions in the healthcare system but instead led to a cottage industry of programs and strategies to help educate or train the physician regarding tools to help them improve coping skills or teach them to be more mindful. This approach assumes or implies that the distress, dysfunction, or burnout is the fault of the physician and their lack of abilities or perhaps their nefarious motivations.

The poor behavior of the physician is often attributed solely to the physician's lack of abilities and several programs around the country have been developed to help promote increased emotional intelligence, effective coping, and mindfulness skills in physicians. While these may be helpful skills for physicians as well as any other human being, we argue that they do not address a crucial component of physician burnout, which is related to systems issues in the modern U.S. healthcare system. These issues include unnecessary bureaucratic and paperwork burdens, ever changing and uncertain health insurance regulations, and increasing lack of autonomy of physicians to perform the advanced diagnostics, procedures, and treatments for which they trained long and hard. We posit that too often these very real underlying issues are ignored or minimized in lieu of labeling the physician as distressed, disruptive, or burned-out and advocating for education of the individual instead of reformation of the system.

The situation that physicians find themselves in can be conceptualized as a form of groupthink on the behalf of the physicians who unnecessarily accept the label of "disruptive" or "distressed" physician and continue to complain about their burdens while making no overtures to address the real underlying issues. In fact, they may not even address the presenting issue of burnout – a 2012 study revealed that 78.3% of the distressed physicians surveyed had not previously thought about seeking professional help for distress or burnout (Fridner et al., 2012)!

Challenges

Why are not physicians rising to the challenge and helping to change the current dysfunctional healthcare system? What is it about their groupthink that keeps them in such a dilemma? In the current healthcare system, most healthcare is delivered in a reactive way. Patients present with medical issues, sickness, and disease, and physicians manage their condition. In the real world, with power in the healthcare system increasingly concentrated in the administrator level, physicians have less control over day-to-day clinic and hospital operations, policy, and patient care. Control over these central issues is held by administrators and managers, the vast majority of whom have no medical training (which in and of itself, may be infuriating to physicians). These administrators implement the business models in which they were trained and the hospital or clinic is run as a business enterprise with compliance to associated regulations and policies as a focus.

Today's physicians enter into this rigid business-focused system with their own entrenched groupthink of patient-focused care along with learned expectations of perfection, dedication, and perhaps a heavy dose of learned helplessness and self-doubt, as previously described. We propose that this combination is a part of the overall problem in modern healthcare. Additional challenges for physicians include staggering student loan debts that must be paid off and thus, their focus is on maintaining employment to stay financially viable. Many are also trying to start or keep families after years of isolating training.

Some physicians may forgo the bureaucracy of insurance and provide concierge medicine, only to face their own ethical dilemma of violating their own values by "abandoning" underprivileged populations. The personality traits and learned habits of physicians may render them more likely to honor the perceived hierarchy of authority in the hospital (as they were taught to do in training) and to try and solve issues on their own or outside of the system. This may help explain why an increasing number of physicians report feeling disenfranchised with the day-to-day work of their medical practice, yet seem to do little to directly or effectively improve the situation (Dewa et al., 2017). Passivity of physicians seems to have only lead to more bureaucracy, and those physicians who do speak up may be labeled "disruptive" or "burned out" by their administration (Reynolds, 2012). Even when well-intentioned, a physician who expresses dissatisfaction with the current state of affairs could be labeled a disruptive physician, with potential significant consequences (e.g., peer review processes, costly training programs, loss of clinical privileges), which can affect their ability to work. There is an increased sense of learned helplessness regarding the physician's ability to change "the system." However, that is exactly what today's physicians must do.

Solutions

We propose that physicians' current way of thinking is not productive and is potentially harming physicians and the healthcare system. Effective solutions must include physicians working collectively to overcome the collective thought that they are powerless in the current system and asserting more control in the healthcare arena. We realize that the current healthcare system is extremely complex and ever evolving and that there is no one "magic bullet" that will solve the problem.

We propose that solving the challenges facing American healthcare will require a distinctly different type of relationship between physicians and administrators than currently exists in most health systems. This may involve helping physicians learn new skills to enhance the communication and emotional intelligence skills that they already possess. Many of these programs are currently available for physicians but are often only offered when the physician is already in trouble or having problems. We propose that offering leadership courses proactively or in medical school could help arm physicians with skills to better overcome negative groupthink tendencies and enhance wellbeing. Well-being should be considered more than simply the absence of distress.

Programs teaching mindfulness, effective communication skills, and stress reduction techniques may be key in helping to establish a resilience and effective group of physicians. Physician engagement in mindful communication programs has been associated with both short- and long-term physician well-being and positive attitudes associated with patient-centered care (Krasner et al., 2009). Mindfulness-based programs for physicians have demonstrated reduced burnout levels that may ultimately lead to a reduction in groupthink characteristics of overachievement, guilt, and avoidance (Goodman & Schorling, 2012). Increasingly, medical schools are including mindfulness education and beginning to explore the impact on physicians (Dobin & Hutchinson, 2013). Findings indicate that more research is needed and that targeted interventions may be needed to impact specific maladaptive groupthink characteristics of physicians (Daya & Hearn, 2018). These strategies alone, however, are not enough to help physicians speak up, participate, and make the dramatic and lasting changes needed in today's healthcare system. In fact, a singular focus on improving physicians' coping and interpersonal skills risks laying the sole blame and responsibility on physicians, which is not the case in such a complex system.

Positive and lasting improvements in healthcare will also entail proactive participation in administration by physicians, including physician leadership at all levels. This will necessarily entail a shift in the groupthink of physicians currently in the workforce, and thus involvement of students and early career physicians is important. One immediate strategy that may be employed is to formalize processes and structures to tap the ingenuity, innovation, and knowledge of practicing physicians. As health systems focus increasingly on maximizing value, physicians are dramatically underutilized assets. Health systems and hospitals build broad-based committees and coalitions, but there are often no physicians on them or those that are included are part-time administrators with little current clinical experience. Practicing physicians may have access to real-time knowledge and insight into problems and solutions in healthcare delivery that administrators lack. In order to implement this, there will need to be time allotted for physicians to participate in committees, and physicians will need to commit to attendance and participation. Research has demonstrated that physician involvement in strategic decision making and investments in operational capabilities are associated with improved hospital performance (Goldstein & Ward, 2004). This type of empowerment of physicians can lead to genuine insights that enable improved care and cost savings.

Another strategy is to educate physicians about the financing of healthcare in order to allow them more knowledge, power, and insight into this area of medicine. Most physicians complete their training with little or no knowledge about the financing or organization of healthcare. Nowhere in their premedical education, medical school, residency, or fellowship do they get a comprehensive education on healthcare policy, administration, finance, or organizational behavior (Mou, Sharma, Sethi, & Merryman, 2011). This can lead to mistrust and suspicion on the part of physicians especially if they have bought in to the groupthink of competitiveness, helplessness, and doubt. Spanning this gulf of knowledge can go a long way to help rebuild understanding and trust.

Physicians are increasingly interested in understanding the finance and business of medicine but only if they are actively involved in decision making and feel that their voices are heard and honored (Jain & Miller, 2012). There has been a substantial growth in physicians obtaining their Masters of Business Administration (MBA) over the past decades (Gorenstein, 2017). However, research demonstrates that after completing their education, a majority of physician-MBAs divert their primary professional focus away from clinical activity (Ljuboja et al., 2016). Progressive health administrators must invest in preparing physicians to understand how healthcare is paid for and how payment informs the structure of care delivery. Absent this understanding, there will always be a layer of mistrust and confusion that gets in the way of true constructive dialogue and engagement about how to solve problems of healthcare delivery.

The complementary idea to providing business and healthcare administration education to physicians is to teach administrators about clinical medicine. This does not necessitate that administrators obtain an M.D. or D.O., but that they are schooled enough in clinical medicine so that they can better understand the complexities of clinical care and better speak to the issues in a common language as their physician counterparts. At a minimum, administrators could better understand how care is organized and delivered on the front lines through intensive clinical shadowing that can help create mutual understanding and perhaps engender respect. Just such a thing was initiated at Mission Health in Asheville, North Carolina, where they created an "immersion day" for their board members, journalists, legislators, and regulators to experience a day at the hospital and clinics in scrubs, behind the scenes, immersed in the nuances of care delivery (Bock & Paulus, 2016). The organizers of the Mission Health project included in their article a statement from a non-physician board member who stated: "I learned more about hospitals and health care from my 10 immersion hours than 6 years sitting on our board" (Bock & Paulus, 2016, p. 1202).

What if those involved in the financing and administration of healthcare delivery came to physicians from a place of increased knowledge and respect? This would potentially go a long way to help physicians overcome their groupthink tendencies and more effectively engage to create real and lasting change. We suspect that solutions that administrators and physicians design together would then be more patient-centered and more likely to deliver value than those either side would develop alone.

Obviously, there are scores of other components of the healthcare system that could be addressed to help reduce physician and patient burden, streamline the system, and improve patient delivery and care. These include a laundry list of things to change: reduce administrative burdens of physicians, make electronic medical records more useful with less unnecessary documentation, allow increased time for adequate patient care, streamline health insurance, address liability and legal issues, increase price transparency, and reduce unnecessary regulations, to name a few.

We propose that addressing the foundational issues of physician groupthink in order to help facilitate physician wellness and improve communication between physicians and administrators are the first necessary steps to help pave the way to solving these other issues. Physicians must take back the leadership roles in medicine and healthcare and do to so, they must lay aside the groupthink characteristics that have landed them in their current dilemma. Physicians alone cannot solve healthcare's biggest problems without collaborating with talented, dedicated, and multidisciplinary administrators. Nor can these administrators solve the same problems without the robust and thoughtful engagement of physicians. Some of what we are proposing is already happening, and one big effort in particular is worth noting. Industrial heavyweights Jeff Bezos, Warren Buffett, and Jamie Dimon, with over one million employees within organizations they lead, in January 2018 announced the formation of a healthcare initiative. On June 20, 2018, they announced Atul Gawande, M.D., as the CEO of this as-yet unnamed healthcare initiative. This intentional collaboration between businessmen and practicing physicians is exactly what we believe is necessary to improve today's healthcare system.

References

Berwick, D. M., Calkins, D. R., McCannon, C. J., & Hackbarth, A. D. (2006). The 100000 lives campaign: Setting a goal and a deadline for improving health care quality. *Journal of the American Medical Association, 295*(3), 324–327.

Bock, R. W., & Paulus, R. A. (2016). Immersion day – Transforming governance and policy by putting on scrubs. *New England Journal of Medicine, 374*, 1201–1203.

Bouchard, S. (2014). Hospital budgets consumed by bureaucracy. *Healthcare Finance News.* www.healthcarefinancenews.com/new/hospital-budgets-consumed-bureaucracy

Cantlupe, J. (2017). The rise (and rise) of the healthcare administrator. *Athena Insight.* www.athenahelht.com/insight/expert-forum-rise-and-rise-healthcare-administrators

Center for Medicare and Medicaid Services. (2018). *National Healthcare Expenditures Fact Sheet.* https://www.cms.gov/Research-Statistics-Data-and-Systems/Statistics-Trends-and-Reports/NationalHealthExpendData/NHE-Fact-Sheet.html

Daya, Z., & Hearn, J. H. (2018). Mindfulness interventions in medical education: A systematic review of their impact on medical student stress, depression, fatigue and burnout. *Medical Teacher, 40*(2), 146–153.

Dewa, C. S., Loong, D., Bonato, S., & Trojanowski, L. (2017). The relationship between physician burnout and quality of healthcare in terms of safety and acceptability: A systematic review. *British Medical Journal Open, 7*, e015141. https://doi.org/10.1136/bmjopen-2016-015141

Dobin, P. L., & Hutchinson, T. A. (2013). Teaching mindfulness in medical school: Where are we now and where are we going? *Medical Education, 47*(8), 768–779.

Dyrbye, L. N., West, C. P., Satele, D., Boone, S., Tan, L., Sloan, J., et al. (2014). Burnout among U.S. medical students, residents, and early career physicians relative to the general U.S. population. *Academic Medicine, 89*(3), 443–451.

Eley, D. S., Leun, J., Hong, B. A., Cloninger, K. M., & Cloninger, C. R. (2016). Identifying the dominant personality profiles in medical students: Implications for their Well-being and resilience. *PLoS One, 11*(8), e0160028.

Fridner, A., Fridner, A., Belkić, K., Marini, M., GustafssonSendén, M., & Schenck-Gustafsson, K. (2012). Why don't academic physicians seek needed professional help for psychological distress? *Swiss Medical Weekly, 142*, w13626. https://doi.org/10.4414/smw.2012.13626

Gabbe, S. G., Melville, J., Mandel, L., & Walker, E. (2002). Burnout in chairs of obstetrics and gynecology: Diagnosis, treatment, and prevention. *American Journal of Obstetrics and Gynecology, 186*(4), 601–612.

Goldstein, S. M., & Ward, P. T. (2004). Performance effects of physicians' involvement in hospital strategic decisions. *Journal of Service Research, 6*(4), 361–372.

Goodman, M. J., & Schorling, J. B. (2012). A mindfulness course decreases burnout and improves well-being among healthcare providers. *International Journal of Psychiatry in Medicine, 43*, 119.

Gorenstein, D. (2017). *Doctors are arming themselves with MBAs to navigate a tricky health care landscape*. Marketplace, Health. https://www.marketplace.org/2017/02/15/health-care/why-doctors-are-arming-themselves-mbas-navigate-tricky-health-care-landscape

Hojat, M. A. D., Spandorfer, J., & Mangione, S. (2013). Enhancing and sustaining empathy in medical students. *Medical Teacher, 35*, 996–1001.

Jain, S., & Miller, E. (2012). Why coursework in health policy and systems should be a premedical admission requirement. *Academic Medicine, 87*(5), 550–551.

Krasner, M. S., Epstein, R. M., Beckman, H., Suchman, A. L., Chapman, B., Mooney, C. J., et al. (2009). Association of an educational program in mindful communication with burnout, empathy, and attitudes among primary care physicians. *Journal of the American Medical Association, 302*(12), 1284–1293. https://doi.org/10.1001/jama.2009.1384

Lathrop, D. (2017). Disenfranchised grief and physician burnout. *Annals of Family Medicine, 15*(4), 375–378.

Lemaire, J. B., & Wallace, J. E. (2014). How physicians identify with predetermined personalities and link to perceived performance and wellness outcomes: A cross-sectional study. *BMC Health Services Research, 14*, 616.

Levine, L. S., & Gustave, L. (2013). Aligning incentives in health care: Physician practice and health system partnership. *Clinical Orthopaedics and Related Research, 47*(6), 1824–1831.

Lipsenthal, L. (2005). The physician personality: Confronting our perfectionism and social isolation. *Holistic Primary Care, 6*(3), 19.

Ljuboja, D., Powers, B. W., Robbins, B., Huckman, R., Yeshwant, K., & Jain, S. H. (2016). When doctors go to business school: Career choices of physician-MBAs. *The American Journal of Managed Care, 22*(6), e196–e198.

Mou, D., Sharma, A., Sethi, R., & Merryman, R. (2011). The state of health policy education in U.S. Medical Schools. *New England Journal of Medicine, 364*, e19. https://doi.org/10.1056/NEJMp1101603

Privitera, M. R., Rosenstein, A. H., Plessow, F., & LoCastro, T. M. (2015). Physician burnout and occupational stress: An inconvenient truth with unintended consequences. *Journal of Hospital Administration, 4*(1), 1–8.

Reynolds, N. T. (2012). Disruptive physician behavior: Use and misuse of the label. *Journal of Medical Regulation, 98*(1), 8–19.

Rosen, I. M., Gimotty, P. A., Shea, J. A., & Bellini, L. M. (2006). Evolution of sleep quantity, sleep deprivation, mood disturbances, empathy, and burnout among interns. *Academic Medicine, 81*(1), 82–85.

Rosenstein, A. H. (2015). Physician disruptive behaviors: Five year progress report. *World Journal of Clinical Cases, 3*(11), 930–934.

Rosenstein, A. H. (2017). Physician dissatisfaction, stress, and burnout, and their impact on patient care. In P. Papadakos & S. Bertman (Eds.), *Distracted Doctoring*. New York: Springer.

Schernhammer, E. S., & Colditz, G. A. (2004). Suicide rates among physicians: A quantitative and gender assessment (meta-analysis). *American Journal of Psychiatry, 161*(12), 2295–2302.

Shanafelt, T. D., Hasan, O., Dyrbye, L. N., Sinsky, C., Satele, D., Sloan, J., et al. (2015). Changes in burnout and satisfaction with work-life balance in physicians and the general US working population between 2011 and 2014. *Mayo Clinic Proceedings, 90*(12), 1600–1613.

Shanafelt, T. D., Sloan, J. A., & Habermann, T. M. (2003). The well-being of physicians. *American Journal of Medicine, 114*(6), 513–519.

Sinsky, C., Colligan, L., Li, L., Prgomet, M., Reynolds, S., Goeders, L., et al. (2016). Allocation of physician time in ambulatory practice: A time and motion study in 4 specialties. *Annals of Internal Medicine, 165*, 753–760.

Spickard Jr., A., Gabbe, S. G., & Christensen, J. F. (2002). Mid-career burnout in generalist and specialist physicians. *American Medical Association, 288*(12), 1447–1450.

Thomas-Dyrbye, L., & Shanafelt, T. D. (2006). Systematic review of depression, anxiety and other indicators of psychological distress among US and Canadian medical students. *Academic Medicine, 81*(4), 354–373.

West, C. P., Shanafelt, T. D., & Kolars, J. C. (2011). Quality of life, burnout, educational debt, and medical knowledge among internal medicine residents. *Journal of the American Medical Association, 306*, 952–960.

Woolhandler, S., Campbell, T., & Himmelstein, D. U. (2003). Costs of health care administration in the United States and Canada. *New England Journal of Medicine, 336*(11), 769–774.

Chapter 22
Bias, Disguise, and Co-opted Science: Altruism as "Scientized" Ideology Across the English Professions—The Peculiar Case of "Ebonics"

Bradley Harris

It is widely recognized that Southern American Englishes, taken collectively, are the most widely studied dialect group across the English language. The dialects of Black Americans have generally been considered either variants of Southern English or historically rooted in Southern English, in consequence of the northern migrations of Black Americans during several periods since the Civil War and their continuing contact with relatives in the South since. The speech of Southern and urban blacks, often loosely considered a "sub-dialect" (or sub-dialects) of Southern English, has gone by a variety of names: Black English, American Black English, and, more recently, African American Vernacular English (AAVE). At times, such dialects have borne labels which hover between being descriptive for linguists and judgmental for those outside the linguistic community. The descriptor "Non-Standard Negro English," (Rickford, 2019) seen in the 1960s, comes to mind as an example of a term which vibrates somewhere near a midpoint between those poles.

To the modern professional linguist, the term *non-standard* simply means a grammatical, lexical, or pronunciative form which, as a matter of fact, is outside the generally accepted standard or preferred form for the language. Nearly everyone's speech is non-standard in some way or other. To those outside the linguist's arena, however, the term *non-standard* can—quite understandably—carry a decidedly negative judgmental flavor. In the popular imagination, *non-standard* quickly becomes *sub-standard*. And so long as the "standard," in any realm, is the pinnacle, the ideal, that which is non-standard is indeed literally sub-standard: everything which is not at the North Pole is south of it.

This chapter examines ways in which science's principles, tools, and specific findings have been co-opted by various fields within the English professions, especially linguistics and the teaching of language. Appeals to scientific authority have often underlain efforts to claim altruistic or noble purpose. Especially when linguistics is translated for popular audiences or applied purposes, some such appeals have

B. Harris (✉)
Rhodes College, Memphis, TN, USA

D. M. Allen, J. W. Howell (eds.), *Groupthink in Science*,
https://doi.org/10.1007/978-3-030-36822-7_22

involved science oversimplified, misrepresented, truncated, or distorted. Nowhere is this more evident than in claims surrounding the concept of linguistic relativism, around which an entire culture of teaching has been built. The very concept of a *language* also derives from a long-standing "scientized" tradition in historical linguistics, but now is experiencing a deconstruction as that tradition is questioned. Imported into one or more fields within the English profession, such snatches of science or the literally and figuratively capitalized *Scientific Method* become supports for theories and programs which reach beyond the journals and into the practical world, flying the flag of "scientific" legitimacy but betraying underlying ideology. The term *ebonics*, and some of the values surrounding it, give us a fine focus for examination.

The ebonics controversy was recently described in a popular work from Oxford University Press thus:

> [D]ebates were sparked when the board of a school in Oakland, California, voted to change its policy regarding the education of African American children in Standard English. Given their consistently low level of achievement in the standard language, the board resolved to extend greater recognition to the vernacular spoken by the children themselves—a variety known to scholars as African American English (AAE), and more widely as Ebonics (Horobin, 2016, p. 78).

It is less than clear that the name *ebonics* had become "widely" known at the time. The term had been coined by social psychologist Professor Robert L. Williams of Washington University in St. Louis in the 1970s (Williams, 1975) as a contraction of *ebony* and *phonics*. Williams emphasized the international aspect of the dialect and its historical origins in the slave trade and the circumstances of slaves' living conditions, not only in the United States but in the Caribbean and other Western slave-holding nations. Williams's original definition focuses importantly—as the contraction *ebonics* itself implies, to quote Williams himself—on the "science of black speech sounds and language" (Quoted in Baugh, Baugh, 2019). Attention was thus drawn to such historical factors as the inferior educational opportunities afforded to slaves, and to African Americans generally, during and since the time of slavery. African Americans simply have not largely had the same opportunities to learn standard forms of American English as have people of European ancestry. The speech of many African Americans is, no doubt, *different* from other dialects, and different from what almost anyone would call "standard American English."

Are we to consider *ebonics*, then—if we are to consider the term an appropriate one and are to use it at all—a dialect or a language? Gloria Toliver-Weddington (1979) would have it that *ebonics* is a fair term and that ebonics is a dialect of English. More specifically, she claims ebonics is what had by the late 1970s long been called Black English (and now would be by most linguists termed African American Vernacular English or AAVE) (Toliver-Weddington, 1979). Two concerns with Toliver-Weddington's account are (1) that her concern is with education, "applied linguistics," if you will, and not linguistics in the scientific sense, and (2) that she does not consider at any great length the meaning(s) of the term *dialect*. Even before we get to these, however, there is the more basic question of *what*, precisely, Toliver-Weddington would say the term *ebonics* encompasses. Does it embrace the broad and international set of speech forms to which Williams applies the term? Or does her use of *ebonics* encompass more narrowly American forms of speech? The answer is less than clear from her work. Developments since, in the theory of language and dialect, have not made the question any easier to deal with.

John Baugh rightly acknowledges the painful history of English as spoken by many African Americans. Both before and after the repeal of slavery, and ever since, he observes:

> A recurrent combination of racial segregation and inferior educational opportunities prevented many African Americans from adopting speech patterns associated with Americans of European ancestry...[G]enerations of white citizens maligned or mocked speakers of AAVE, casting doubt on their intelligence and making their distinctive speaking patterns the object of racist ridicule (Baugh, 2019).

To intrude a personal observation, I have noted, in teaching literature, writing, linguistics, and public speaking at colleges and universities in the Memphis area, such derision is sometimes so pervasive that even African American students will voluntarily apply labels such as *ignorant* or *stupid* even to specific speech patterns they themselves use, such as/aks/for *ask*,/errbody/for *everybody*, and *or either...* in place of standard *either...or*. Equally, I have, in a quarter century of living in Memphis and teaching English here, I have become quite accustomed to the ready willingness of many white Southerners to see in our shared skin color a presumed will to share in such ridicule. It has been observed by others that "the most stinging scorn for African-American mass culture is often expressed by middle-class African-Americans" (Hitchings, 2011, p. 257).

The linguistic effect of this racial clash was further problematized in 1996, in Oakland, California, when a resolution of the Oakland School Board created what Henry Hitchings called the "greatest American linguistic controversy of the last century" (Hitchings, 2011, p. 257). The resolution directed that African American students be instructed in "their primary language"—namely, for the Board, ebonics. What was important, however, was the perceived elevation of those students' brand of speech to the rank of language. Not just a narrow or local style of colloquiality. Not a mere dialect. No, this time, it was a language. Its origin, said the resolution, lay in "West African and Niger-Congo African language."

A professional linguist would have begun reply, perhaps, by insisting upon saying *languages*, plural, and pointing out that many tens, even hundreds, of languages of several families likely were involved in the linguistic origins of ebonics, including many beyond the West African and Niger-Congo regions and language groups. That linguist would likely also have pointed out that several competing theories vied for position in describing the roles of and relations between English and the slaves' languages of origin, as well as languages and dialects they encountered along the way from Africa to final destinations in America. These historical linguistic issues were not, however, the concern of the Oakland Board.

The Board sought legitimation. It wanted something for its students to stand on. Those students could not stand, it was clear, on a platform of "bad English"—a platform of indignity. The Board could not say, simply: *Our students speak non-standard English. We are going to teach them standard English.* As the Board reasoned, they might as well have said "*Our students are broken, and wrong. We are going to fix them.*" The Board, by granting to their African American students' speech the legitimacy of the brand *language*, sought to place them on an equal footing with those—largely white—students who had been able to claim the legitimacy of claiming to speak something nearer to a standard American English.

The nation was not happy. As Henry Hitchings observes, "[p]lenty of loud and poorly informed commentators" thrashed about in the popular press and semi-popular magazines, objecting strenuously to the Oakland Board's decision. At the core of their outcries was the objection that ebonics—whatever range of speech forms that term may have referred to, exactly—should not be legitimated as a dialect, let alone a language, "but simply as a corrupt and base type of English" (Hitchings, 2011, p. 257). Hitchings cites as especially vitriolic a *New York Times* piece faulting "theorists, lushly paid consultants, and textbook writers all poised to spread the gospel…that 'time that should be spent on reading and algebra [get] spent giving high fives and chattering away in street language'" (Hitchings, 2011, p. 258). To many in a population largely educated in the grammarian tradition of "proper English," the Board's legitimizing non-standard African American speech seemed a horror. Then as now, the error seemed to these objectors nothing less than a *moral* mistake. Hitchings' analysis helps explain why. He couches his account in terms of the growing English-only movement, which was already under full steam at the time of the Oakland incident.

The United States has no legislation specifying a single official language at the federal level. However, at least 31 of its states have legislation specifying English as an official language. Of these, Hawaii and Alaska have also specified one or more other languages as official. All the five inhabited U.S. territories have specified English as an official language.

Four of these have specified other official languages as well.[1] Except for Puerto Rico's Spanish, all the non-English specified official languages of U.S. states and territories are languages native to those areas. In total, then 36 U.S. jurisdictions have English as their official language and, of these, 30 have *only* English as an official language. The intent to make English official is clearly well underway. It is less than clear, however, that the English language is under threat of disappearance in America.

To speak speculatively, what may be the case is that the language is, in the minds of "standard American English" speakers, under threat of losing whatever degree of purity or correctness it may have. It is a commonplace observation, and has been for many decades, that English is "in decline." Thus, *any* departure from the bygone rules of revered and reimagined high school English teachers is to be lamented.

One does not have to be racist per se to oppose the legitimation of dialects such as those of black youth, whether termed ebonics or African American Vernacular

[1] "English Only Movement." Wikipedia. https://en.wikipedia.org/wiki/English-only_movement. Retrieved 01 July 2019.

English. One simply must be rigid. To oppose all departure from grammatical tradition—"splitting the infinitive was wrong when I was in school, and it's wrong now"—involves no necessary racial or xenophobic component. Such insistence involves only resistance to linguistic change from outside *linguistic* forces.

That said, it is clear that the "English only" movement, as framed and advanced by such figures as Theodore Roosevelt and S.I. Hayakawa, is very much directed at the consolidation of single national language as part of a unified national culture" (Hitchings, 2011). Roosevelt's century-old one flag, one language vision of America is very much alive. It is the meat and potatoes of English-only activists today. It is common fare, also, among the rank and file of citizens. Listen to any morning's or afternoon's worth of talk radio, and you are bound to hear some recitation of the notion, "*If they want to come here, they'd better learn English fast...*".

What is more, it had better be some brand of English the rest of us—white people—can readily understand. This latter demand we may take as a call for something like Standard English, or Standard American English, or as some prefer, American.

But what is that? Quirk and Greenbaum's definitive *Comprehensive Grammar* notes that, in affirming

> Students' right to their own varieties of language, many American educationalists have declared that Standard American English is a myth, some asserting the independent status of (for example) Black English. At the same time, they have acknowledged the existence of a written standard dialect, sometimes termed 'Edited American English' (Quirk, Greenbaum, Leech, & Svartvik, 2010, p. 20).

Wisely, Quirk, Greenbaum et al. have acknowledged that it is less than clear what Standard American English is. The 1800-odd pages of their grammar recognize again and again in one important sense the supremacy of dialect over language. Over and over, they note that one feature or form is acknowledged correct by speakers of one dialect but not by those of another. (One simple example: the tendency of Americans to call the alphabet's last letter *zee*, while Canadians often call it *zed*.)

We can certainly see African American Vernacular English as a dialect. Linguist William Labov prefers to see it as "a subsystem of English" with its own phonological and syntactic rules...now aligned...with rules of other dialects." He sees AAVE as both incorporating features of Southern English and as having affected Southern English. Labov is a creolist, seeing AAVE as having grown from an earlier creole similar to those of the Caribbean. Finally, AAVE has a highly developed verb-aspect system showing continuing growth of its semantic structure (Mufwene, 2001). As Seth Lerer Lerer (2007) points out, to find the full measure of distinction and substance in AAVE, we would have to look beyond the mechanics of phonology, morphology, lexicon, syntax, semantics, and the like. We must further acknowledge that AAVE is not spoken by all African Americans, that not all of the dialect's speakers are African American, and that AAVE may not be a unified dialect. History, rhetoric, theatre, and other disciplines must inform what we are to discover, as observed by Henry Louis Gates (1988).

Altruism, in its strict or literal sense, may be hard enough to find anywhere. However, it is not difficult, given a modicum of sympathy, to find a solid measure good will, good intentions at least, within the Oakland Board of Education and the educators who gave rise to their 1996 resolution, however misguided, however ill-founded it may have been scientifically and linguistically. Similarly, let us suggest also that opposing positions, however unexamined some of them may be, are not without their elements of goodwill.

What we see throughout the political side of the discussion, however—the portion occurring outside the community of professional, scientifically oriented linguists—is repeated misconstrual of concepts. Notions such as *language* and *dialect* are misconceived and misapplied. Existing definitions are ignored along with already acknowledged difficulties in definition. Also ignored were the likely natures of opposing arguments.

The linguistic community itself has experienced a long period of unsettlement on issues relevant to this discussion, and only comparatively recently has come to any degree of consensus amid discussions of the complex nature of African American Vernacular English. AAVE may not be a single dialect—hence Labov's term *subsystem of English*—and *dialect* may not be the best term for this set of speech forms. Whatever else be true, it does seem that *ebonics*—with or without the capital E Williams originally employed with the term—is not a felicitous term. Nor did it, nor will it likely ever lead to desirable results.

References

Baugh, J. *Comprehending Ebonics*. www.pbs.org/speak/seatosea/americanvarieties/AAVE/ebonics/. Retrieved 01 July 2019.

Gates, H. L. (1988). *The signifying monkey* (pp. 72–75). New York: Oxford University Press.

Hitchings, H. (2011). *The language wars: A history of proper English*. New York: Farrar, Strauss & Giroux.

Horobin, S. (2016). *How English became English* (p. 78). Oxford, UK: OUP.

Lerer, S. (2007). *Inventing English: A portable history of the language* (pp. 220–234). New York: Columbia University Press.

Mufwene, S. S. (2001). African-American English. In J. Algeo (Ed.), *The Cambridge History of the English Language* (*English in North America*) (Vol. 6, pp. 291–324). Cambridge, MA: CUP.

Quirk, R., Greenbaum, S., Leech, G., & Svartvik, J. (2010). *A comprehensive grammar of the English language*. New Delhi, India: Pearson, š1.24, p.20.

Rickford, J. R. (2019). What is Ebonics (African American English)? *Linguistic Society of America*. www.linguisticsociety.org/content/what-ebonics-african-american-english. Retrieved 02 January 2019.

Toliver-Weddington, G. (1979). Ebonics (Black English): Implications for education. *Journal of Black Studies, 9* (No. 4) [special issue].

Williams, R. (1975). *Ebonics, the true language of black folks*. St. Louis, MO: Robert Williams and Associates.

Index

D. M. Allen, J. W. Howell (eds.), *Groupthink in Science*,
https://doi.org/10.1007/978-3-030-36822-7

T

CPSIA information can be obtained
at www.ICGtesting.com
Printed in the USA
LVHW061619270420
654503LV00001B/1